Geriatric Home-Based Medical Care

Jessica L. Colburn • Bruce Leff
Mariah L. Robertson • Mattan Schuchman
Editors

Geriatric Home-Based Medical Care

Principles and Practice

Second Edition

Springer

Editors
Jessica L. Colburn
Division of Geriatric Medicine
and Gerontology
Johns Hopkins University School
of Medicine
Baltimore, MD, USA

Bruce Leff
Center for Transformative Geriatric
Research
Johns Hopkins University School
of Medicine
Baltimore, MD, USA

Mariah L. Robertson
Division of Geriatric Medicine
and Gerontology
Johns Hopkins University School
of Medicine
Baltimore, MD, USA

Mattan Schuchman
Division of Geriatric Medicine
and Gerontology
Johns Hopkins University School
of Medicine
Baltimore, MD, USA

ISBN 978-3-031-68785-3 ISBN 978-3-031-68786-0 (eBook)
https://doi.org/10.1007/978-3-031-68786-0

This Springer imprint is published by the registered company Springer Nature Switzerland AG
The registered company address is: Gewerbestrasse 11, 6330 Cham, Switzerland

Foreword

This much-anticipated second edition arrives at a time of excitement within the rapidly expanding and changing field of home-based medicine. Expertly edited by Drs. Colburn, Leff, Robertson, and Schuchman, the textbook reflects recent advances in the field and provides a roadmap for the delivery of high-value care. The invited authors, leaders in their respective areas, prepare the reader to meet the practical aspects of interdisciplinary care delivery while updating advances in care delivery, quality, outcomes, and policy. The book also serves as a foundation for the ongoing innovations in this unique and critically important field.

Dr. John Burton, a renowned leader in geriatrics, penned the forward for the groundbreaking first edition published in 2016. After briefly reviewing the history of house calls in the US, he outlined six generic trends fueling the resurgence in home-based medical care, all of which remain true to this day: (1) aging demographics, with greatly increased numbers of home-limited older adults living in the community with complex chronic conditions and disability; (2) escalating costs and financial incentives, with interest by health plans and health system leaders to shift to value-based care (e.g., fill gaps in care, reduce avoidable, recurrent hospitalizations, and deliver high-quality, cost-effective health care); (3) efforts to deliver person-centered, highly satisfying care that regains the public trust; (4) emphasis on team-based, collaborative interdisciplinary care models that are responsive to social determinants of health needs; (5) educational value of home visits for students and postgraduate trainees; and (6) advances in portable and home-based technology, including remote patient monitoring and telemedicine available in the home.

The progress is palpable, and the momentum is truly energizing. We have seen a dramatic expansion of evidence-based models of care built upon decades of field work, data analytics, and clinical performance. The changing payment landscape and the infusion of private venture capital investment have introduced a wide spectrum of home and community-based medical and social services, primary care, acute hospital-level care, and post-acute care in the home. In response to the vision of high-quality, evidence-based medical care for home-limited persons, the National Home-Based Primary Care Learning Network (improvehousecalls.org) was established. This learning community provides a quality framework and measures for the field through a combination of quality improvement and applied research.

The pandemic taught us the dangers of linking health care to brick and mortar settings and facilitated a dramatic expansion of telehealth, remote patient monitoring, and hospital-level care at home, providing yet more first-hand evidence to support these models as core elements of a high-value care ecosystem. The Hospital at Home Users Group (hahusersgroup.org) is an outstanding example of how programs can work together, share resources and best practices, develop policy standards to inform regulatory and reimbursement policies, and assure value.

Despite this enormous progress, over 25 years of waiting for "overnight" success has tested the fortitude of many in our field. When can the celebrations begin? In hiking, there is a phenomenon called the false summit, wherein the hiker reaches a peak that appears to be the end of the journey only to discover that the true summit is still looming in the distance. These false peaks can be discouraging, but the excitement of believing one is near the end propels the hiker forward. False summits can be good teachers, inviting a pause, enabling course corrections along the way, enriching the evidence base, and solidifying the best path forward.

We are almost there, a result of the enormous commitment by so many people over the years. Let us see the gap to the summit as a motivation to continually improve the care and respond to challenges met along the way.

Key questions face us:

How do we maintain fidelity to the evidence base that launched this long-awaited success and create a home and community-based healthcare delivery ecosystem that spans medical and social services?

How do we continually drive toward a vision of equity and access, including underserved populations and rural communities?

How do we evaluate the value of innovative models of care and share outcomes and best practices while navigating the intellectual property concerns of private funders?

How do we place guardrails against fraud and abuse?

How do we anticipate, prevent, and respond to unintended consequences that occur due to interests of health systems, private insurance, health plans, and private investors while supporting opportunities for home-based medicine to thrive in value-based environments?

How do we ensure that the significant savings achieved by delivering high-quality, evidence-based care get responsibly reinvested into the health and wellness of the population?

Regardless of the milepost we are currently passing in the journey, it is important to celebrate the joys of the work and the many accomplishments achieved as we work toward the goal.

The commitment displayed by those in the field is truly awe-inspiring, as are the remarkable colleagues with whom we share our work, and the patients and families who invite us into their homes and entrust us with their care.

Home-based medical care is not a quaint service or an expensive luxury—it is essential, high-value care to meet the needs of the rapidly growing population of older, seriously ill, and disabled people, and their families. Along with critically important home and community-based services, home-based medical care gives patients and families choices of where they can live and be cared for—and then supports them in their choices. Home care medicine makes sense, and it is what we want for our loved ones, and what we want for ourselves: the comforting knock on our door when we are in need. This second edition is an essential and valuable guide, further propelling home-based medicine's journey forward to fundamentally change how we deliver high-value health care.

Division of General Internal Medicine
Geriatrics and Palliative Medicine, University
of Arizona College of Medicine
Tucson, AZ, USA

Mindy Fain, MD

Preface

In the preface to the first edition of this book, circa 2016, we noted that "the health care system in the United States is changing" and then generally bemoaned the fact that home-based medical care was essentially ignored by mainstream medicine despite how much it can offer patients in an often dysfunctional and fragmented health care delivery system.

So, we repeat: the health care system in the United States *is* changing and while the pace of change may not be as fast as we would like, the arc of change is clearly bending toward health care delivery in the community and in patients' homes. Home-based medical care is ascendant.

Before the COVID-19 pandemic, there was growing interest in home-based medical care. New models of home-based care started to gain traction. A growing imperative around health care equity and addressing social determinants of health aligns with care delivery in the home setting. Multiple commercial entities hoping to disrupt health care delivery have begun to focus on delivering care in the home.

The COVID-19 pandemic added fuel to this fire. Facility-based care in hospitals, ambulatory clinics, skilled nursing facilities, and nursing homes, once viewed as the standard settings of care, were suddenly viewed with suspicion and settings for viral spread. Telemedicine, a model of care that had been stuck in the mud and underutilized for years, was adopted by clinicians and health systems around the country in a matter of weeks. The Centers for Medicare and Medicaid Services (CMS) issued dramatic regulatory flexibilities and payment relief to facilitate telehealth and new modes of home-based care, such as hospital at home. Equally important to payment modifications was the beginning of a shift in the culture of health care delivery with recognition that the home is a viable care setting for nearly all medical care except for the most intensive and high-technology care which still requires the hospital setting.

The opportunity to continue to evolve that culture and associated policy puts a full-fledged home-based medical care ecosystem within reach. Creating and training the future workforce to serve that vision is still a pressing need. This book is intended to help in that mission and is intended for clinicians who recognize the need for specialized knowledge, skills, and attitudes in providing care in the home setting, whether they are considering making their first medical house call or are already regularly caring for patients within an established home-based medical care program.

As with the first edition of this book, experts in home-based medical care from highly respected programs and institutions across the country have collaborated to create this practical reference based on decades of shared experience and solid scientific evidence. The entire text has been updated, and several new chapters and topic areas have been added.

We anticipate that the evidence base will continue to grow as this system of care expands and succeeds, along with meaningful quality assessments and outcome measures. We hope that this book serves both as a useful compendium of hands-on clinical advice and as a foundation for future development of the field of home-based medical care.

Baltimore, MD, USA — Jessica L. Colburn
Baltimore, MD, USA — Bruce Leff
Baltimore, MD, USA — Mariah L. Robertson
Baltimore, MD, USA — Mattan Schuchman

Contents

Contributors

Halima Amjad Division of Geriatric Medicine and Gerontology, Department of Medicine, Johns Hopkins School of Medicine, Baltimore, MD, USA

Peter A. Boling Division of Geriatric Medicine, Virginia Commonwealth University School of Medicine, Richmond, VA, USA

Kathryn A. Brennan Virginia Commonwealth University School of Medicine, Veterans Health Administration, Richmond, VA, USA

Melissa J. Christie Department of Neurology, UT Health Houston, McGovern Medical School, Houston, TX, USA

Jessica L. Colburn Division of Geriatric Medicine and Gerontology, Johns Hopkins University School of Medicine, Baltimore, MD, USA

Ericka L. Crouse Department of Pharmacotherapy and Outcomes Science, Virginia Commonwealth University School of Pharmacy, Richmond, VA, USA

Thomas K. M. Cudjoe Division of Geriatric Medicine and Gerontology, Center on Aging and Health, Johns Hopkins University School of Medicine, Baltimore, MD, USA

K. Eric DeJonge MedStar Washington Hospital Center, Washington, DC, USA

Jennifer Rocio Delgado Felipa Division of Geriatric Medicine, Department of Medicine, Northwestern University Feinberg School of Medicine, Chicago, IL, USA

Thomas E. Finucane Johns Hopkins Bayview Medical Center, Baltimore, MD, USA

Deborah G. Freeland Division of Geriatric Medicine, Department of Internal Medicine, UT Southwestern, Dallas, TX, USA

Lyons T. Hardy Virginia Commonwealth University School of Nursing, Richmond, VA, USA

Helen Kao Lumina Hospice and Palliative Care, Corvallis, OR, USA

Amy Kilen Johns Hopkins Community Physicians, Baltimore, MD, USA

Fred C. Ko Departments of Geriatrics and Palliative Medicine and Medicine, Icahn School of Medicine at Mount Sinai, New York, NY, USA

Won Lee Section of Geriatrics, Department of Medicine, Boston University Chobanian & Avedisian School of Medicine, Boston, MA, USA

Bruce Leff Center for Transformative Geriatric Research, Johns Hopkins University School of Medicine, Baltimore, MD, USA

Division of Geriatric Medicine and Gerontology, Johns Hopkins University School of Medicine, Baltimore, MD, USA

June M. McKoy Division of Geriatric Medicine, Department of Medicine, Northwestern University Feinberg School of Medicine, Chicago, IL, USA

Yasmin S. Meah Departments of Medicine, Medical Education, Geriatrics and Palliative Medicine, Icahn School of Medicine at Mount Sinai, New York, NY, USA

Rachel K. Miller Division of Geriatrics, University of Pennsylvania Perelman School of Medicine, Philadelphia, PA, USA

Linda Paniszyn Section of Geriatrics, Department of Medicine, Boston University Chobanian & Avedisian School of Medicine, Boston, MA, USA

Kathryn M. Rackson Division of Geriatric Medicine, Virginia Commonwealth University School of Medicine, Richmond, VA, USA

Christine S. Ritchie Division of Palliative Care and Geriatric Medicine, Department of Medicine, Harvard Medical School, Massachusetts General Hospital, Boston, MA, USA

Mariah L. Robertson Division of Geriatric Medicine and Gerontology, Johns Hopkins University School of Medicine, Baltimore, MD, USA

Mattan Schuchman Division of Geriatric Medicine and Gerontology, Johns Hopkins University School of Medicine, Baltimore, MD, USA

Anjail Z. Sharrief Department of Neurology, UT Health Houston, McGovern Medical School, Houston, TX, USA

David Skovran Department of Medicine and Medical Education, Icahn School of Medicine at Mount Sinai, New York, NY, USA

Eva P. Szymanski Division of Geriatrics, University of Pennsylvania Perelman School of Medicine, Philadelphia, PA, USA

George A. Taler MedStar Washington Hospital Center, Washington, DC, USA

Martha L. Twaddle Palliative Medicine, Northwestern University Feinberg School of Medicine, Chicago, IL, USA

Robert M. Zimbroff Division of Geriatric Medicine, University of California, San Francisco, San Francisco, CA, USA

Chapter 1
Introducing Home-Based Medical Care

Bruce Leff

Key Points

1. Home-based medical care is important in the care of frail, functionally impaired older adults.
2. Home-based medical care is highly relevant to the evolving health service delivery system in the USA and has potential to develop into a full-fledged home-based care ecosystem.
3. Formal education in home-based medical care is limited.
4. This book is intended to be a practical clinical reference for healthcare providers who practice medicine in the home, with an emphasis on home-based primary care.
5. Terminology in this field can be confusing. We adopt the term "homebased medical care" to emphasize the relevance of this practice model as part of the contemporary healthcare delivery system.

1.1 Home-Based Medical Care

Home-based medical care is coming of age and is being increasingly mainstreamed into the US healthcare delivery system. Several meta-trends have abetted this evolution. These forces include the ongoing shift in healthcare delivery from volume-based to value-based care and the recognition that typical traditional office and other facility-based care is insufficient to meet the needs of "high-need, high-cost"

B. Leff (✉)
Center for Transformative Geriatric Research, Johns Hopkins University School of Medicine, Baltimore, MD, USA

Division of Geriatric Medicine and Gerontology, Johns Hopkins University School of Medicine, Baltimore, MD, USA
e-mail: bleff@jhmi.edu

J. L. Colburn et al. (eds.), *Geriatric Home-Based Medical Care*,
https://doi.org/10.1007/978-3-031-68786-0_1

patients. The COVID-19 pandemic changed the long-standing perceptions among patients and the public at large that facility-based care is inherently "safe" and rapidly accelerated the adoption of telemedicine and virtual care modalities. Increased attention to issues related to access to healthcare, healthcare equity for minoritized populations, and the recognition that home-based medical care can ameliorate inequities has also played a role [1]. Recent advances in portable technology and remote patient monitoring facilitate higher acuity care in the home. Major health systems, commercial entities, and investors are pouring billions of dollars into home-based care. All to say that the culture of healthcare is moving toward the home.

The move to home-based medical care is based on solid health services research. Over the past several decades, a variety of home-based medical care models have been developed and tested. Figure 1.1 depicts home-based care models along a continuum on the *X*-axis from models that provide chronic/longitudinal care to those that provide acute/episodic care and on the *Y*-axis from models that are nonmedical to those that are more medical, with substantial physician and nurse practitioner involvement. Longitudinal care models include home-based primary care, home-based primary care co-management, home-based integrated medical and social care, and home-based palliative care. Episodic medical care models include hospital at home, rehabilitation/skilled nursing home care at home, emergency department care at home, and mobile integrated health—community paramedicine. Such models have been tested individually but never woven together and evaluated as part of integrated system and implemented at scale. There exists now, in the wake of the COVID-19 pandemic, an opportunity to reimagine a decentralized and distributed care ecosystem—centered in the home and community that is highly coordinated and patient-centered and less focused on traditional facility-based care [2].

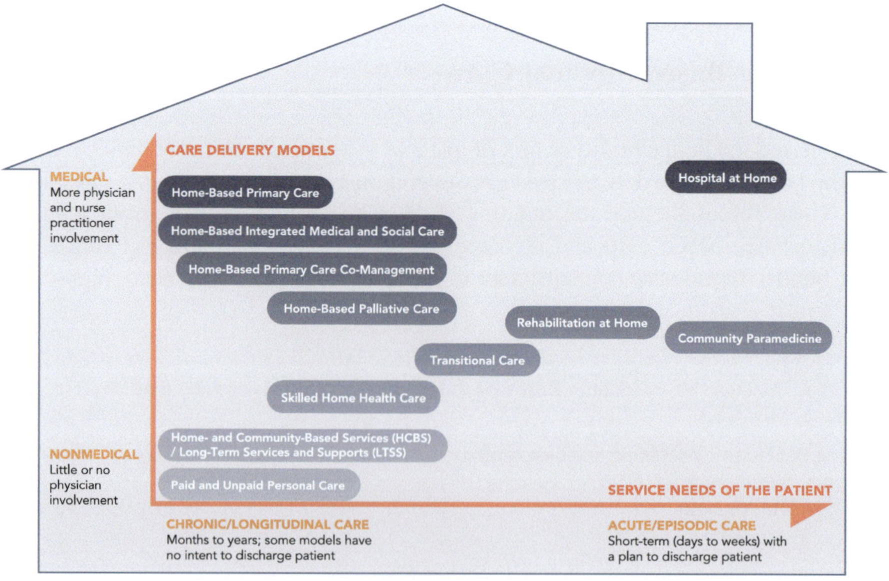

Fig. 1.1 The continuum of home-based care models

1.2 Gaps in Care Delivery Remain

While the culture of healthcare is moving toward the home and the hoped-for vision of a home-based care ecosystem evolves, significant gaps remain. There are two million older Americans who are homebound and never or rarely leave their homes; only 12% of these people receive home-based primary care. Another 5.5 million cannot leave their homes without difficulty or assistance from another person. Homebound individuals are more likely to be members of minoritized and marginalized populations, have lower educational attainment, be unmarried or without a partner, have low levels of income and self-reported health, and have depression or dementia, low functional status, and high health service utilization [3]. During the COVID-19 pandemic, the prevalence of homebound doubled to approximately 13% of adults over the age of 70 [4]. Becoming homebound is associated with nearly 70% 6-year mortality owing to many factors including higher rates of frailty and serious illness [5].

1.3 Home-Based Primary Care

As a home-based care ecosystem evolves, home-based primary care serves as a key healthcare delivery modality for homebound and seriously ill persons who cannot access or have difficulty accessing traditional office-based primary care. At its best, home-based primary care provides physician and/or nurse practitioner-led interdisciplinary team-based care. Key programmatic elements of care include patient identification, comprehensive assessment, patient risk stratification, the ability to provide key ancillary services, and urgent communication and care capabilities. The latter, identified as an utterly key component of this care, entails 24/7 call coverage with the patient able to communicate with clinicians who know them and can provide clinical advice and anticipatory guidance [6].

The evidence for home-based primary care is also robust. A systematic review of home-based primary care demonstrated that home-based primary care is associated with lower rates of emergency department visits, hospital admissions, hospital bed days of care, long-term care admissions, long-term care bed days of care, lower costs of care, and better satisfaction with care and family caregiver quality of life [7]. A more recent systematic review outlined the current state of the science in home-based primary care and noted that it is a field ripe for expansion and continued research and noted several gaps that the field needs to address while also noting that home-based primary care may help reduce health disparities, alleviate caregiver burden, and offer cost savings [8]. Home-based medicine is a critical strategy for population health management [9]; this has been recognized by the development of important policy initiatives such as the Independence at Home Act (Section 3024 of the Affordable Care Act) [10].

It is at the level of the patient and family that home-based medical care shines brightest. Seeing patients in their home provides important information that may not be discernible in the office. Imagine the patient who has experienced multiple recent hospitalizations for recurrent heart failure. The house call reveals a second-floor bathroom and a kitchen stocked with sodium-rich canned and frozen foods that a friend buys for her, because she cannot go to the supermarket herself. Only when the clinician asks about her ability to climb the stairs does the patient admit that she often "can't make it in time," so she only takes her diuretic when she goes upstairs for the evening. The clinician now proposes useful solutions for this complex set of medical, functional, and social problems contributing to the patient's recurrent hospitalizations.

By taking medical care directly to the place where the patient spends the most time, home-based medical care exemplifies patient-centered care. At home, the clinician easily assesses patient function in their own environment and helps address barriers to care and social determinants of health. Coming to see the patient at home is an unspoken endorsement of the patient's importance. As an invited guest in a patient's home, the power dynamic between patient and clinician is more balanced. This helps to build a level of trust and communication between clinicians, patients, and family members and caregivers that may be difficult to create in a typical office visit [11]. In this context, home-based primary care can also facilitate the discussion of goals of care that allow frail older adults to forgo burdensome and futile interventions at the end of life.

1.4 Workforce and Education

Unfortunately, relatively few physicians, nurse practitioners, and physician assistants are engaged in providing home-based medical care. Most clinicians receive little or no formal medical training in home-based medicine, so they are unaware that this type of care is possible [12]. This book is intended to be a practical clinical reference for healthcare providers who practice medicine in the home; the orientation is geared primarily toward home-based primary care, but its basic principles and approaches are highly applicable for providers engaged in other models comprising the home-based medical care ecosystem.

1.5 Terminology

We conclude this introduction with a note on terminology. The terms "house call" and "home visit" have commonly been used in the context of caring for patients in the clinical contexts described above. These terms are not incorrect, but these terms fail to convey the full scope of medical care in the home and may even trivialize it. When, for instance, a physician or nurse practitioner from a high-quality home-based primary care practice sees a patient at home, they are providing the patient with holistic interdisciplinary team-based care and community-based resources that address the medical, social, and functional needs of the patient and their families and caregivers. It is not simply an isolated encounter but a true system of care. Further, important stakeholders at the national level do not consistently understand the term "house call medicine" and commonly conflate it with services such as skilled home healthcare.

As such, we prefer the term "home-based medical care" to refer to house calls and home visits provided in the context of home-based primary care, home-based palliative care, and other home-based medical care models that are evolving in the ever-changing healthcare delivery system. Much of this text focuses on home-based primary care.

Further, we recognize that the language used to describe older adults who have difficulty leaving the home is important. For the purpose of this book, we will use the word "homebound" to describe these older adults, but we recognize the terminology is ever-evolving and may change in the coming years as we continue to work toward the most patient-centered language.

As care moves increasingly toward the home setting, home-based medical care will expand in scope. Please feel free to send us thoughts and ideas on topics to address in future editions via email at jcolbur1@jhmi.edu, bleff@jhmi.edu, mdewsna1@jhmi.edu, or mattan@jhmi.edu.

Jessica Colburn, M.D.
Bruce Leff, M.D.
Mariah Robertson, M.D.
Mattan Schuchman, M.D.

Acknowledgement Figure reprinted with permission from the California Healthcare Foundation 2022.

References

1. Marmot M, Allen JJ. Social determinants of health equity. Am J Public Health. 2014;104 Suppl 4:517.
2. Ritchie C, Leff B, Gallopyn N, Pu C, Sheehan O. Medical care at home comes of age. California: California Health Care Foundation; 2023. https://www.chcf.org/publication/medical-care-home-comes-age/#related-links-and-downloads.
3. Ornstein KA, Leff B, Covinsky KE, Ritchie CS, Federman AD, Roberts L, et al. Epidemiology of the homebound population in the United States. JAMA Intern Med. 2015;175(7):1180–6.
4. Ankuda CK, Leff B, Ritchie CS, Siu AL, Ornstein KA. Association of the COVID-19 pandemic with the prevalence of homebound older adults in the United States, 2011-2020. JAMA Intern Med. 2021;181(12):1658–60.
5. Ankuda CK, Husain M, Bollens-Lund E, Leff B, Ritchie CS, Liu SH, et al. The dynamics of being homebound over time: a prospective study of Medicare beneficiaries, 2012-2018. J Am Geriatr Soc. 2021;69(6):1609–16.

6. Ritchie CS, Leff B, Garrigues SK, Perissinotto C, Sheehan OC, Harrison KL. A quality of care framework for home-based medical care. J Am Med Dir Assoc. 2018;19(10):818–23.
7. Stall N, Nowaczynski M, Sinha SK. Systematic review of outcomes from home-based primary care programs for homebound older adults. J Am Geriatr Soc. 2014;62(12):2243–51.
8. Zimbroff RM, Ornstein KA, Sheehan OC. Home-based primary care: a systematic review of the literature, 2010-2020. J Am Geriatr Soc. 2021;69(10):2963–72.
9. Boling PA, Leff B. Comprehensive longitudinal health care in the home for high-cost beneficiaries: a critical strategy for population health management. J Am Geriatr Soc. 2014;62(10):1974–6.
10. Ornstein K, Levine DM, Leff B. The underappreciated success of home-based primary care: next steps for CMS' Independence at Home. J Am Geriatr Soc. 2021;69(11):3344–7.
11. LoFaso V. The doctor-patient relationship in the home. Clin Geriatr Med. 2000;16(1):83–94, ix.
12. Reckrey JM, Ornstein KA, Wajnberg A, Kopke MV, DeCherrie LV. Teaching home-based primary care. Home Healthc Now. 2017;35(10):561–5.

Chapter 2
Getting Started with Home-Based Medical Care

Mattan Schuchman, George A. Taler, and K. Eric DeJonge

2.1 Overview

This chapter aims to help providers who are getting started in the field of home-based medical care (HBMC). Home-based medical care focuses on meeting the needs of the patient and their caregiver in their place of residence. The spirit of HBMC is to serve people with conditions that make it difficult to leave the home to get care. HBMC is also valuable when medical care requires the depth of information that seeing a person in their home can provide. A core guiding principle of HBMC is to provide "the right care, for the right patient, by the right provider, at the right time, with the right tools." Whether you plan on joining an established HBMC program or thinking of starting one yourself, the concepts in this chapter are meant to serve as a guide.

In writing about HBMC, we are primarily thinking about home-based primary care (HBPC) for older adults with complex medical and social needs. HBMC is a broader term that includes HBPC as a core element. Therefore, we believe that the guidance provided in this chapter will help providers take a thoughtful and strategic approach for any HBMC endeavor.

The chapter is divided into different sections based on key considerations for operating a successful and effective HBMC practice (Table 2.1). We will conclude the chapter with a discussion of day-to-day operations in a HBPC practice.

M. Schuchman (✉)
Division of Geriatric Medicine and Gerontology, Johns Hopkins University School of Medicine, Baltimore, MD, USA
e-mail: mattan@jhmi.edu

G. A. Taler · K. E. DeJonge
MedStar Washington Hospital Center, Washington, DC, USA

J. L. Colburn et al. (eds.), *Geriatric Home-Based Medical Care*,
https://doi.org/10.1007/978-3-031-68786-0_2

Table 2.1 Key considerations for home-based medical care practices

What is the practice's mission?
Who is the intended population and what geographic area will be served?
What is the scope of home-based medical services provided and what professionals are part of the HBMC team?
What is the financial strategy for sustaining the practice?

2.2 What Is the Practice's Mission?

An HBMC practice's mission is its purpose and guiding vision. Consider what would be different in your community if your practice operated at top quality. In some cases, a mission may be expansive—e.g., provide primary care medical services for all home-limited people over 65 in your metropolitan area—or more limited, e.g., complete an in-home palliative care assessment for people discharged from your affiliated hospital with a new diagnosis of cancer. A clear mission will help answer the other key questions listed in Table 2.1. These considerations are interdependent. For example, if you primarily intend to serve a congregant housing population, a fee-for-service business models may be sufficient, but if you want to support an under-resourced geographic area, you may need to give deeper thought to case management services under a population health, value-based model.

When considering a mission, consider your practice's role in the community. Are you a long-standing and well-known anchor institution or a newcomer on the scene? Are you now an office-based practice with an established patient census that is entering the field of HBMC? Your existing community connections can affect how you build relationships and trust with community members, other medical practices, and potential referral sources. HBPC is woven into the fabric of the community and based upon the needs of the local population and environment. It is worth the effort to have conversations with community leaders, partner organizations, and other stakeholders to identify community needs. You may wish to begin by reaching out to neighborhood associations, area agencies on aging, healthcare providers, and your local hospital's community liaison.

While identifying an initial mission is a challenge, that mission may change over time as your practice develops. The mission should be revisited regularly to make sure it is still relevant. A mission also does not need to be undertaken all at once. Intermediate goals in service of your mission on 1-, 3-, and 5-year time horizons can help break the mission into more attainable parts. While revisiting the mission, these goals can be adjusted depending on the situations that your practice faces.

2.3 What Is the Intended Population and Geographic Area Served?

2.3.1 Patient Population

The HBPC population characteristics can include age, clinical conditions, functional status, and/or stage of illness. Initially, an HBPC practice needs to select a primary focus population, usually from one or more of these four major groups (see Table 2.2). Focusing on a specific group helps a practice develop strategies for financial sustainability and tailor its services to the needs of that group. Selecting a narrow population may limit the patient census and not sustain a standalone practice, while serving a broad population may present challenges in meeting a heterogeneous range of patient needs. Identifying a focus population can require some iteration, and that population may shift as the practice grows or responds to circumstances. Given the time and intention required for home visits, HBMC is well suited to focus on patients with significant medical complexity that causes limited functional status. People without home limitations and who have less medical complexity benefit more from the convenience of HBMC. Programs that cater to this population often charge additional fees to make up for the loss of revenue due to the smaller number of patients that can be seen in a day compared to an outpatient practice.

HBPC is often tailored toward older patients with chronic illness and functional disability, who account for the vast majority of this population and will be the focus of our examples. They are usually 65 years of age and over, have chronic disabling disease, and are at high risk of hospitalization [1–3]. For older adults who face obstacles getting to a doctor's office, home-based medical care provides access to primary care and can be more effective than office-based care. The patients and their families need a trusting long-term relationship with an interdisciplinary team that can offer prompt management of acute and chronic illness as well as compassionate end-of-life care.

Some HBPC practices extend services to younger populations with neurologic disability, developmental disabilities, congenital conditions, and/or severe mental illness. Other HBPC programs focus on micropopulations that require specialized

Table 2.2 Common HBPC populations

People 65 and over with severe chronic disease and disability
Younger disabled persons affected by neurologic or mental health disorders
Post-hospital or urgent care populations (without long-term primary care)
Older populations in congregate housing

medical knowledge, such as persons with ventilator dependence or people with end-stage heart disease on intravenous medication pumps or ventricular assist devices. These subgroups have technical needs that require specific personnel and specialty services.

A focus population can be defined by stage of illness or setting of care. For example, a practice may focus on the 30 days post-hospital to prevent readmissions. This focus may require that a practice loosen its criteria for functional disability and refer patients back to office-based practice as patients improve or when the 30-day period ends. Some health systems have shown modest benefits of home visits in short-term post-hospital interventions in heart failure patients that prevent hospital readmissions and to lower costs [4]. Other practices focus on end-of-life care. While many within this group are under hospice care, limitations to hospice care as well as limited access to hands-on care from a physician or advanced-practice practitioner make HBPC a needed addition to hospice care.

Some practices select a population based solely on location. For example, a practice may serve any resident of an assisted living facility or retirement community. Practices that serve patient populations in such communities can substantially increase the number of visits performed each day.

2.3.2 Geographic Area

Choice of a geographic catchment area is an essential consideration in defining practice parameters. Not doing so is a common cause of practice failure due to costs of long travel distances and greater amounts of unproductive "windshield" time. We advise that the travel radius be limited to a 20–25-min driving time. This limit can represent different mileage distances depending on the urban, suburban, or rural nature of the practice. A driving time limit enhances the ability to cluster visits each day in a smaller area, such as one zip code per provider per day, so individual visits can be less than 5–10 min apart. Driving time is the time that providers cannot see patients or safely use the phone and lessens efficiency (see "financial considerations" about potential private-pay trip charges).

To choose a geographic area, we suggest using a detailed local map with zip code boundaries, sites of senior communities, and major thoroughfares in and out of population centers. One can then map a program's service area by matching demographic data of the patient population within the driving radius. We suggest that a catchment area minimize crossing of natural boundaries such as rivers or large parks with restricted traffic patterns. Be mindful of daytime traffic congestion due to rush hours, schools, sports arenas, or large shopping malls. It helps to create clear boundaries such as natural landmarks, main roads, or county boundaries so your catchment area is easy to communicate on marketing material.

Once defined, avoid "boundary creep," except for exceptional circumstances. For example, stretching zip code boundaries beyond a 25-min driving radius may be worthwhile for high-density areas, such as continuing care retirement communities, assisted living facilities, or naturally occurring retirement communities. Once you make an exception for one patient, it is difficult to refrain from additional exceptions that further fragment the catchment zone.

When starting, a practice should assess the socioeconomic strata of patients within its territory. This information is available from US Census data tracts. High numbers of low-income patients can confer the benefits of traditional Medicaid or Medicaid waiver programs that offer social work and daily aide supports. Serving a high-income population can bring opportunities to offer private-pay services. Focusing on privileged communities may further inequality by further concentrating access to medical care and support services in affluent areas, where residents may already have a wider array of options. Service to all socioeconomic strata is particularly important in areas with histories of racial segregation or "red-lining."

Business planning and financial viability are important factors in geographic decisions. A practice needs to consider the availability of core service partners. For example, a program needs a close working relationship with a high-quality hospital and emergency department, to ensure continuity of care across these settings. The practice will also need a partner pharmacy that can deliver medications and supplies and social service agencies to organize daily support services.

A practice should assess the penetration of Medicare Advantage and Accountable Care Organizations in the area. Many health systems have access to this data in their managed care or insurance divisions. Payers recognize that groups of high-cost patients require clinical care beyond the capacity of office-based care. These payers can provide value-based payment options predicated on cost savings, which expand revenues beyond fee-for-service payments.

After defining a geographic area, the practice can identify sub-areas to allow clustering of visits and enhance daily provider efficiency. For example, if one team covers eight zip codes, providers can plan to focus visits each day on one or two contiguous zip codes to lessen driving time. Driving patterns for 1 day can either resemble a fishbone with nearby visits along a major residential thoroughfare or a small circle of visits along a clockwise path that brings you back to home base. There is mapping software that can help providers select routes between home visits to minimize driving time. As practices grow, they may wish to subdivide their geographic areas between providers. To improve commute times for staff, practices can consider where providers reside, when assigning areas.

2.4 What Is the Scope of Home-Based Medical Services Provided and What Professionals Are Part of the Team?

HBMC can come in many shapes and sizes. This section will discuss stand-alone HBPC, office-based extension practices, post-acute and urgent care practices, and some additional models of care. The models of HBMC care, the mission of the practice, and resources from outside your practice determine staffing needs. For example, if your practice is affiliated with a hospital system that provides a robust case management program, a HBMC team does not need its own case manager. For more discussion on staffing your HBMC program, see Sect. 2.6 below.

2.4.1 Home-Based Primary Care (HBPC)

HBPC practices provide a comprehensive and long-term approach to primary care at home. This longitudinal commitment involves coordinating medical and social services, usually for a population of older patients across settings and over time. An HBPC team assumes responsibility for a population with a high intensity of medical needs and, depending on the payment model, can be accountable for clinical and cost outcomes. These teams generally offer 24/7 phone access to clinical staff, urgent visits, and coordination of social and medical specialty services.

HBPC practices commonly serve frail and home-limited older patients. Many practices only accept patients aged 65 and up due to Medicare eligibility. Physicians or advanced practice providers typically provide geriatrics-focused medical care, urgent care, palliative, and end-of-life care. Specially trained RNs and/or social workers can meet the psychosocial need among this population, particularly for caregiver support, dementia education, prescription drug coverage, access to social benefits such as nutrition subsidies, the Medicaid waiver and personal caregiving services, moving to higher levels of care, and engagement with adult protective services. Proficiency with palliative care is important for all staff members since mortality for ill older adults is over 50% within 4 years of becoming home-limited [5].

HBPC, similar to any primary care practice, generates administrative work that can be performed by medical assistants or medical office coordinators. These responsibilities include outreach, screening new patients, billing, scheduling, and coordinating care with other providers such as specialists, skilled nursing facilities, hospitals, pharmacies, medical equipment suppliers, and home health agencies. Due to the high level of medical complexity, psychosocial, and administrative needs, a HBMC practice's staffing level may be similar to an outpatient practice that may serve five to ten times as many patients as the house call provider.

To support the high level of coordination and psychosocial services needed, many HBPC practices use a weighted system of assigning patients to a team, or to a provider's panel within the team, that accounts for the intensity of care needed to stabilize many of the new patients and the subset of patient with acute exacerbations of illness or social support disruption. Clearly, providers in HBPC practices carry a smaller patient panel and see fewer patients on a daily basis than in a standard office practice (see Sect. 2.6.1 for estimates on panel size). These expectations reflect the logistics of driving time and conducting visits in the home, as well as the complex care needs of the patients. Providers' panel size should enable them to focus their time and energy on patients who have the most pressing needs in order to prevent adverse outcomes. HBPC care recipients and their caregivers highly value the access to medical care [6]. The use of 24/7 phone or telemedicine coverage is a key tool to lessen emergency room use and hospitalization. A large portion of the care provided occurs outside of scheduled visits such as with phone calls between families, patients, and all team members.

2.4.2 *Office Extension Practices*

A modest approach to starting a home-based medical practice is to incorporate home visits into an existing office-based practice. This expansion can start with providers who make visits to established patients who have become homebound. In this case, the office-based infrastructure supports scheduling, phone triage, billing, prescription refills, and other administrative needs. Coordination with community agencies falls to the provider and office staff, and after-hours coverage relies on the on-call service of the office practice.

An office practice that extends itself to the home can improve the community reputation of the practice. Case-mix severity may decline for some providers as their complex patients are shifted to the providers who perform house calls. Practices that assign house calls to a nurse practitioner or physician may find that the volume-based productivity drops for those providers in order to manage more complex patients. A house call workload will generate a greater time commitment per patient [7]. Creating small panels of patients with increased medical needs has become an increasingly popular arrangement in value-based payment strategies.

Building a home-based primary care service from an office-based practice can be a starting point, but the team should set specific milestones to determine when to create an independent HBPC team. Challenges for an office extension approach include the following:

- Difficulty providing urgent visits when needed, as an office schedule limits flexibility.
- Increased on-call demands due to greater care needs of home-based patients.
- Administrative and psychosocial support needs of home limited patients may extend beyond what a typical office practice can provide.
- Practice of home-based medicine requires a distinct skill set for providers and administrative staff.
- Differences in productivity between office- and home-based medical practices require revised compensation strategies (i.e., providing incentive payments on value metrics beyond RVUs).

2.4.3 Episodic Care

Some HBMC programs, such as those tied in with health systems seeking to address specific outcomes, may only provide episodic or post-acute care for patients. For example, a practice focused on reducing 30- or 60-day readmissions may provide time-limited HBMC following a hospital discharge for congestive heart failure or for hip fracture patients. In these practices, an episodic HBMC practice sees the patient for a set period after the hospital discharge and then hands care back to their office-based primary care doctor or transition eligible patients to HBPC.

2.4.4 Innovative Models for HBMC

Many HBMC programs are emerging that provide only specific aspects of the models described above. Examples include home-based palliative care, home-based urgent care, and home-based psychosocial and case management support (hospital at home (HaH) is covered separately below.) Depending on the program's mission, the full suite of HBPC services may not be needed to benefit the patient population.

Home-based palliative care practices provide a service for people who may still be receiving primary or specialty care in an office-based setting. The insights into an individual's life gained through time spent in their home environment facilitate the trusting relationship necessary for palliative care, which includes personal conversations about symptom management and end-of-life care. Moreover, home-based palliative care enables a more nuanced assessment of the caregiver and living environment than are possible in a clinical setting. For individuals who are in the final 6 months of life, home hospice is a well-established care model. Hospice uses per-diem funding through Medicare to provide home-based medical care at the end of life, including practical and psychosocial needs such as counseling, chaplaincy, and personal care assistance.

Some health systems are exploring other ways to provide home-based urgent care. Advances in telemedicine services, particularly during the COVID-19 pandemic, have created new opportunities in this field. Some models are using community paramedics dispatched through a county or municipal emergency system to connect with providers in a control center to provide medical care and avoid unnecessary emergency room and hospital utilization. This community paramedicine model can work best in areas with a larger healthcare system where medical record review and communication with primary care providers are well-integrated. Other programs tailored to a tech savvy population interested in the convenience of HBMC have developed computer and phone software to provide this service.

2.4.5 Hospital-Level Care at Home

The most intensive application of HBMC is replacing care that would otherwise occur at a hospital, rehabilitation center, or inpatient hospice with an equivalent level of care in a person's residence. Care models such as hospital at home (HaH) can lower overall cost, increase satisfaction, and reduce iatrogenic complications such as nosocomial infection and delirium. Patients admitted to HaH are admitted to the program directly from the emergency department or, in some cases, transferred early from the hospital to HaH level of care. Admission to HaH initiates daily nursing and physician or advanced practitioner visits, as well as 24/7 support services, to provide care equivalent to hospital-level service. If patients require advanced imaging such as CT, or higher level of care such as IMC or ICU, they are transported back to the hospital.

2.5 What Is the Financial Strategy for Sustaining a HBPC Practice?

A practice needs to consider all options for creating a sustainable financial model. Long-term viability depends on close monitoring of costs and building diverse sources of revenue (Table 2.3).

A standard source of revenue for HBPC is fee-for-service billing from a primary insurance payer, of which Medicare is often the dominant entity. HBPC can bill Medicare CPT codes for home-based medical care, including evaluation and management (E&M), home health certification, care plan oversight (CPO), chronic care management (CCM), non-face-face services, and advance care planning (ACP) (Table 2.4). All these codes require detailed documentation and a vigilant billing and coding operation to submit and track collections. Detailed recommendations for billing Medicare are beyond the scope of this chapter. As value-based payment methods take hold submitting bills for service will become less important than documentation of patients' diagnoses in order to reflect medical complexity. Accurate ICD-10 coding data becomes critical in contractual negotiations under a value-based model.

Most HBPC practices in the USA struggle to achieve financial viability solely on fee-for-service Medicare revenues due to the time and costs of travel and the

Table 2.3 Revenue options for home-based primary care practices

Fee-for-service billing with a focus on high-density populations
Income from related services such as home health, pharmacy, and hospice
Shared savings or per-member per-month payments based on quality and cost reductions for health systems or payors
Private-pay fees
Philanthropy

Table 2.4 Medicare CPT and HCPCS codes used in HBPC

99347-99350	Established patient evaluation/management home visit (20–60 min)
99341-99345	New patient evaluation/management home visit (15–75 min)
99497, 99498	Initial 30 min of advanced care planning and subsequent 30 min
99496, 99495	Transitional care management visit within 7 days and within 14 days
99417	Visit duration prolonged 15 min above time billed in E&M
G0180, G0179	Certification and recertification of skilled home health episodes
G0181, G0182	Care plan oversight (CPO) for non-face-to-face time spent by a provider managing home health or hospice care
99487-99491	Chronic care management (CCM) for non-face-to-face time spent in care management activities by a provider or clinical staff

extensive time spent on care coordination, family communication, and counseling for very ill older persons. A small number of entrepreneurial HBMC companies have achieved positive financial margins on fee-for-service revenues, with rigorous billing/collections systems. Even with highly effective billing/coding operations, entrepreneurial practices have relied on other methods, such as high volumes in assisted living facilities, ancillary services such as mobile laboratory and radiology, or private-pay travel fees to achieve a positive margin.

In a fee-for-service environment, there are advantages to focusing a practice on senior congregate housing. Such settings provide economies of scale with higher volumes of patients at one site, reduced travel time, and improved fee-for-service productivity. The congregate housing also benefits when their residents receive their healthcare through a home-based primary care. An HBPC team can provide 24/7 access to lessen unnecessary 911 calls. The above factors may explain why national growth of HBPC has occurred in congregant settings [8].

Another path to financial viability entails offering other health services into a larger business entity or medical services organization. This type of diversification can make clinical and business sense, as patients who benefit from HBPC need many other services such as mobile radiology and laboratory, skilled home health, hospice, pharmacy, and/or durable medical equipment. A larger business entity that includes a wider array of home-based services creates streams of revenue, making up the net losses from HBPC fee-for-service billing.

The US health insurance system is moving away from fee-for-service toward paying for value (i.e., better health outcomes per dollar spent). In this environment, a HBPC team that can demonstrate high patient and family satisfaction and prevent high-cost events is in position to receive higher payments. Shared savings agreements require negotiation with payers such as Medicare Advantage programs or operating as an accountable care organization (ACO). The practice needs to achieve outcome metrics that are linked to shared savings and a per-member per-month coordination payment. With sufficient strategic planning and resource allocation, value-based payments can provide a significant revenue stream. As one example, the Independence at Home (IAH) Medicare demonstration project showed how this strategy can be successfully implemented to improve key quality metrics and generate shared savings for HBPC practices [9]. Another option is value-based purchasing, wherein a health system receives lump-sum payments for an episode of care for a high-risk population.

When entering value-based agreements, payers need to understand your target population and recognize that conventional metrics, such as the Medicare Advantage Star system, are less relevant for a very ill and disabled population. For example, conventional preventive care measures, such as cancer screenings and prescribing cardiovascular medications, may not be indicated for patients with limited prognosis. More useful outcome measures for the frail older population include observed/expected hospitalization rate, "days at home," patient and family experience, rate of death at home rather than in a facility, stability of functional status, and total costs of care.

Some HBPC providers have incorporated private-pay fees to supplement fee-for-service billing for services not covered by insurance. These include monthly membership fee for services such as travel time, 24/7 direct access to medical providers, and coordination of care. These arrangements can require a signed Advance Beneficiary Notice within Medicare. In the private-pay arena, the practice needs to carefully examine Medicare rules on what constitutes "uncovered" services and clarify the payment plan with new patients and families upon enrollment. Other examples of services that are billed in the private-pay market include social work case management, private duty nursing care, companion services, and other special service such as shopping, housekeeping, handyman, transportation, and nutritional programs.

In summary, the key principles to support financial viability for a home-based primary care practice are to build a rigorous billing and collections system, seek diverse streams of revenues from fee for service and value-based payments, and build a data analytics system that can track financial data and patient outcomes in real time.

2.6 Operations

The details of operating a HBMC practice will be specific to your chosen program model. The discussion below focuses on a HBPC model. Early steps to develop a HBPC team include the following:

- Identify the program leadership and, if you are working within the context of a larger healthcare organization, a champion for the program within the organization.

- Assemble the essential team members (physicians, advance practice providers (APPs), nurses, social workers, and office coordinators) by partnering, reassigning existing staff, or hiring using start-up funding from a sponsoring health system, philanthropy, or private investment.
- Make your practice known in the local healthcare community and neighborhoods (e.g., primary care practices, emergency rooms, home health and hospice agencies, social service agencies, and senior housing communities).
- Identify partner entities available to serve the target population (e.g., pharmacy delivery, durable medical equipment, skilled home health services, home-based personal care services, subspecialty physicians, and hospital care).
- Build administrative infrastructure for financial practice management and data analytics.

HBMC programs need certain essential service competencies in order to ensure delivery of excellent care to patients and their families. These capacities include the following:

- Skilled providers who can offer intensive management of serious chronic illness
- Continuity of care across settings (e.g., home, ED, hospital, skilled nursing facility, and hospice)
- 24/7 phone, telehealth, or in-person access for urgent clinical advice and triage
- Social work case management and caregiver support
- Mental health services
- Compassionate and skilled end-of-life care
- Mobile electronic health record (EHR)

2.6.1 *Staffing*

An HBPC practice needs a core team of physicians, advanced practitioners, nursing, social workers, office coordinators, and managerial staff. The clinical disciplines provide the daily direct care and coordinate specialty services needed by any population with severe chronic illness and disability. As patient census expands, the practice can subdivide into teams of providers and office staff that focus on a panel of 200–300 patients to enabling deeper relationships and trust based on familiarity and intimate knowledge of each patient and family. In the practice of one author, panel size for a full-time medical provider ranges from 150 to 200 patients, depending on efficiency of scheduling and level of administrative support. In typical urban settings, in a geographic service area of 8–10 zip codes, programs often reach a steady-state census of 600–800 patients. Reasons for this saturation point include a focus on a small subgroup of a highly targeted population and a high annual attrition rate, with annual mortality rate for the HPBC population that approaches 20–25% [5].

Beyond core staff, practices focus additional resources on development of skills that align with the practice mission, geography, and population. For example, if your mission is mostly end-of-life care, integration of pastoral and hospice services is a priority. If the population comprises a high number of Medicaid beneficiaries, practices involve higher levels of social services and community health workers to help individuals navigate the health system. If the population has significant mental health needs, then access to collaborative behavioral health and psychiatry services is essential.

2.6.2 Allied Resources

In addition to core medical and social service staff, an HBPC practice needs other specialty services (Table 2.5). For example, a larger diversified HBMC business may offer lab, radiology services, and hospice, while a smaller not-for-profit practice depends on community or independent partners to fill these needs.

2.6.3 Patient Enrollment and Management

The enrollment process starts with new patient intake. Ideally, this is a simple method for new patients and their families, with a single phone number and/or website for intake information. The office staff can determine if a prospective patient meets entry criteria with a set of simple questions on a phone or web-based tool. The initial screening asks about home-limited status, age, the presence of a reliable contact person, residence in the catchment area, interest in changing primary care provider, and confirmation of insurance eligibility. Setting clear initial expectations provides for effective future partnership with patient and family. This includes agreement on scheduling, on-call access, staff safety, expectations for length of

Table 2.5 Ancillary clinical services

Medical services	Social support services
• Mobile labs and radiology • Mental health • Emergency department and hospital care • Subspecialty services (e.g., podiatry, optometry, audiology, dentistry, other subspecialty physician care) • Medicare skilled home health agencies • Hospice care • Private ambulance and wheelchair van transportation • Inpatient rehab and skilled nursing facilities (SNF) • Pharmacy and durable medical equipment delivery	• Family and caregiver support and counseling • Legal counseling and guardianship • Coordination of personal care assistance services • Pest extermination • Home safety and accessibility modifications • Decluttering and cleaning services • Food and utility resources • Housing transitions and nursing home placement • Medicaid, Medicaid waiver, and social service application support • Pharmaceutical financial support

visits, types of providers on the team, and policies on behavior and termination of services. The practice also needs to document essential medical and social information prior to the initial visit.

Patient visit scheduling is based on patient needs and geographic efficiency. The initial visit includes a comprehensive medical, social, and functional assessment, using the "4 Ms" of geriatrics as a guide [10]. The 4 Ms are mentation, mobility, medications, and what matters. New patient visits can vary in time and often range from 60 to 90 min. The initial visit can be conducted by a physician or APP, who then makes referrals and brings in other team members based on clinical and social needs of the patient and family.

The provider who sees the patient determines the time interval until the next follow-up visit, based on the level of complexity and need. A major goal of HBPC is to prevent medical and social crises and avoidable ED visits, hospitalizations, or nursing home stays. This priority means we err on the side of frequent visits, especially for patients with unstable medical or social issues. The follow-up visit duration varies widely from 15 to 20 min for focused or stable chronic illness visits to 60–90 min for urgent or highly unstable situations. A standard approach is to confirm visits 1–2 days ahead of time, using 2–4-h windows of time for expected provider arrival. Confirmations can occur via various methods, from text and email notifications to phone calls for those who need that approach. In general, providers can see five or six patients per day in order to allow for increased visit length, travel time, and management non-face-to-face encounters with other patients. New patient encounters are longer and count as two slots. Some practices have providers that can see as many as 10–12 patients by either providing a driver/tech or focusing on congregate housing where travel time is minimal.

Providing access to urgent care within 24 h is a core element of successful HBPC programs, both for patient well-being and to prevent unneeded high-cost events. Urgent visits can displace routine visits to ensure that the team sees the highest-priority patients first. Reserving some provider slots for urgent and hospital follow-up visits allows practice to intervene promptly on unstable patients that need close attention.

HBPC practices vary in how they assign medical providers to a panel of patients. Some, as with the authors, provide a physician and APP team for each patient, where both providers know the patient and manage them jointly. This has the benefit of complementary skills and consulting from physician to APP. Other practices give a panel of 100–200 patients to the individual physician or APP, and they manage them independently as individual providers. For hospital care, continuity of goals and information can prevent unnecessary interventions and help with prompt discharge planning. Some HBPC practices are structured to have team members (RN, APP, or physician) assist in the hospital care. Most depend on hospital-based medical staff to provide the 24/7 acute care.

A core tenet of effective HBPC teams is to offer live 24/7 phone access to patients and families for urgent concerns. The HBPC team needs to provide phone triage in order to address issues promptly and manage urgent needs before they become crises. Such uninterrupted access is an important factor in preventing hospitalization and emergency room visits, which is a relief for patients and families and also leads to better value-based outcomes and cost savings. Practices in academic centers can ally with the geriatrics fellowship training program to enlist fellows to contribute to after-hours coverage.

For detailed information on conducting home visits and the necessary equipment and supplies please refer to Chap. 4.

2.6.4 Interdisciplinary Function

A HBPC team's success depends on building and sustaining a high-performing *transdisciplinary* team. On high-performing teams, everyone takes ownership from their perspective, expects each team member to do their part, and communicates freely. Teams mature from "multidisciplinary," where disciplines suggest recommendations but rely on others to form and implement a care plan, to "interdisciplinary," working together to develop a plan of care and feeling an allegiance to one another, to "transdisciplinary," recognizing where other disciplines ought to have contributions and seeking their input.

A core element of this process is a weekly team meeting. In this meeting, all team members are present to review the status of new patients, hospitalized patients, unstable patients, deaths, and any other special categories of high-risk patients, e.g., those on warfarin, insulin, or opiates. The meeting is also useful to discuss quality improvement issues in practice operations and team dynamics. Other attendees at the weekly team meeting include representatives from pharmacy, mental health, and the main partner for skilled home health services. The team can use clinical judgment and data to assign risk levels (e.g., high, medium, low) to the patients. See Table 2.6 for a sample template of the weekly team meeting. As reimbursement policies change to reward value-based outcome metrics, this template can expand to document outcomes and provide data for payors and health system partners. The team can also use this forum to document case management and coordination time and exit data.

A robust mobile electronic health record (EHR) and practice management database are essential tools for HBPC team. The mobile EHR needs viewable access from other local partners such as the hospital, home care agencies, specialists, and

Table 2.6 Interdisciplinary team meeting agenda

	Physician	NP	SW	Active issue
New patients				
Hospitalized				
Unstable				
Hospice/home health				
On hold (SNF facilities, infestation)				
Deaths and discharges				

regional health information exchanges (HIEs). Linkage to practice to the local HIE allows the practice to track patients across settings.

The IT practice database needs to produce data analytics for population-based questions (e.g., how many of our patients have had Covid or flu vaccine?), provider-specific clinical and financial outcomes, risk stratification, and utilization events. The practice management team needs capacity to query for outcomes on patient survival, vital status, emergency department visits and hospital admissions, patient and family experience, and financial collections. Such data creates the ability to prove clinical effectiveness and financial outcomes, which are important for value-based contracts, shared savings payments, and meeting future opportunities for accreditation as a high-performing practice.

2.7 Conclusion

In summary, a HBMC practice first needs to define its primary mission and the population they aim to serve. With the mission in mind, the practice must then determine a specific geographic reach, core services and staff, and financial strategy to meet the mission. Some key elements of success are finding and retaining dedicated and skilled team staff, 24/7 live access, geographic scheduling to minimize driving time, partnerships with senior congregate communities, connecting to essential specialty service partners, and developing diverse revenues that include value-based payments such as shared savings, adequate capitation, or per member per month revenues to cover practice costs.

The experience of providing HBMC is profoundly rewarding for providers, patients, and families. Visiting the home allows one to understand the patient's context and values and to create a care plan that promotes the dignity and well-being of that person and their family.

References

1. De Jonge KE, Jamshed N, Gilden D, Kubisiak J, Bruce SR, Taler G. Effects of home-based primary care on Medicare costs in high-risk elders. J Am Geriatr Soc. 2014;62(10):1825–31. https://doi.org/10.1111/jgs.12974. Epub 2014 Jul 18. PMID: 25039690.
2. Edes T, Kinosian B, Vuckovic NH, Nichols LO, Becker MM, Hossain M. Better access, quality, and cost for clinically complex veterans with home-based primary care. J Am Geriatr Soc. 2014;62(10):1954–61. https://doi.org/10.1111/jgs.13030. PMID: 25333529.
3. Federman AD, Brody A, Ritchie CS, Egorova N, Arora A, Lubetsky S, Goswami R, Peralta M, Reckrey JM, Boockvar K, Shah S, Ornstein KA, Leff B, DeCherrie L, Siu AL. Outcomes of home-based primary care for homebound older adults: a randomized clinical trial. J Am Geriatr Soc. 2023;71(2):443–54. https://doi.org/10.1111/jgs.17999. PMID: 36054295.
4. Naylor MD, Brooten DA, Campbell RL, Maislin G, McCauley KM, Schwartz JS. Transitional care of older adults hospitalized with heart failure: a randomized, controlled trial. J Am Geriatr

Soc. 2004;52(5):675–84. https://doi.org/10.1111/j.1532-5415.2004.52202.x. Erratum in: J Am Geriatr Soc. 2004 Jul;52(7):1228. PMID: 15086645.

5. Ankuda CK, Husain M, Bollens-Lund E, Leff B, Ritchie CS, Liu SH, Ornstein KA. The dynamics of being homebound over time: a prospective study of Medicare beneficiaries, 2012-2018. J Am Geriatr Soc. 2021;69(6):1609–16. https://doi.org/10.1111/jgs.17086. Epub 2021 Mar 8. PMID: 33683707; PMCID: PMC8192419.
6. LaFave S, Drazich B, Sheehan OC, Leff B, Szanton SL, Schuchman M. The value of home-based primary care: qualitative exploration of homebound participant perspectives. J Appl Gerontol. 2021;40(11):1611–6. https://doi.org/10.1177/0733464820967587. Epub 2020 Oct 22. PMID: 33090065.
7. Pedowitz EJ, Ornstein KA, Farber J, DeCherrie LV. Time providing care outside visits in a home-based primary care program. J Am Geriatr Soc. 2014;62(6):1122–6. https://doi.org/10.1111/jgs.12828. Epub 2014 May 6. PMID: 24802078; PMCID: PMC4784964.
8. Liu B, Ritchie CS, Ankuda CK, Perez-Benzo G, Osakwe ZT, Reckrey JM, Salinger MR, Leff B, Ornstein KA. Growth of fee-for-service medicare home-based medical care within private residences and domiciliary care settings in the U.S., 2012-2019. J Am Med Dir Assoc. 2022;23(10):1614–1620.e10. https://doi.org/10.1016/j.jamda.2022.06.014. PMID: 36202531.
9. Ornstein K, Levine DM, Leff B. The underappreciated success of home-based primary care: next steps for CMS' Independence at Home. J Am Geriatr Soc. 2021;69(11):3344–7. https://doi.org/10.1111/jgs.17426. Epub 2021 Aug 25. PMID: 34432890.
10. Mate K, Fulmer T, Pelton L, Berman A, Bonner A, Huang W, Zhang J. Evidence for the 4Ms: interactions and outcomes across the care continuum. J Aging Health. 2021;33(7–8):469–81. https://doi.org/10.1177/0898264321991658. Epub 2021 Feb 8. PMID: 33555233; PMCID: PMC8236661.

Chapter 3
Home-Based Care Services and Community-Based Resources

Eva P. Szymanski and Rachel K. Miller

3.1 Introduction

There are many home-based services and community resources available to support homebound patients and promote aging in place. Given the complexity of older homebound patients' needs, they often benefit from multiple services. However, the sheer number of these services, who qualifies for them, and how they are paid for can be confusing for clinicians, patients, and families. We will share a framework for available services and discuss relevant logistical details. The services discussed in this chapter are summarized in Table 3.1.

E. P. Szymanski (✉) · R. K. Miller
Division of Geriatrics, University of Pennsylvania Perelman School of Medicine, Philadelphia, PA, USA
e-mail: Eva.szymanski@pennmedicine.upenn.edu; rachel.miller@pennmedicine.upenn.edu

J. L. Colburn et al. (eds.), *Geriatric Home-Based Medical Care*,
https://doi.org/10.1007/978-3-031-68786-0_3

Table 3.1 Framework for home-based care and community resources

	Home-based medical care	Medicare-covered home healthcare services	Personal care	Center-based care	Community services
Services	– Home-based primary care – Home hospice and palliative care – Other medical professionals making house calls – Hospital at home – Rehab at Home – ED at home	*Primary* – Skilled nursing – Physical therapy – Speech language pathology *Secondary* – Occupational therapy – Medical social work – Home health aide *Additional* – Respiratory therapy	– Home health aide – Non-paid caregiver – Respite care (home or temporary facility)	– Senior centers – Adult day care centers – PACE centers	– Area Agency on Aging – Care management – Financial and legal assistance – Home repair and home modification – Transportation – Meal delivery – Faith-based services – Behavioral health
Payment	– Medicare part B – Value-based models of payment becoming more common	– Medicare part A and/or part B if has skilled need and meets qualifications	– Private pay – Medicare advantage (some plans) – Medicaid (usually waiver program) – State non-Medicaid programs – VA benefits – Long-term care insurance	*Senior centers* – Charitable and public funding *Adult day care centers* – Similar to home aide payments *PACE* – Medicare/ Medicaid	*Varies by service* – Charitable or public funding – Private pay – Cost-sharing

ED emergency department, *ADL* activities of daily living, *iADL* instrumental activities of daily living, *PACE* Program for All-Inclusive Care of Elderly

3.2 Home-Based Medical Care

Home-based medical care encompasses any type of medical care provided in the home, including home-based primary care, home hospice and palliative care, specialists who make house calls, hospital at home, and emerging models such as rehabilitation at home.

3.2.1 Home-Based Primary Care

Home-based primary care (HBPC) is exactly what it sounds like—primary care that is provided in the home, instead of the traditional office. For patients who are homebound, this greatly increases access to medical care for chronic disease management and preventative care. Home visits have also been shown to decrease Medicare costs while also reducing functional decline and overall mortality, with variable effect at preventing admission to long-term care institutions [1–5]. HBPC teams typically, though not exclusively, accept patients who meet the Medicare homebound definition (see below). The HBPC team typically includes clinicians (physicians, nurse practitioners, and/or physician assistants) available for both routine and acute home visits, nurses, access to the team for triaging questions and urgent issues, in-home labs and radiology studies, and social work and case management who are knowledgeable on home- and community-based resources, plus office and managerial staff. HBPC teams usually have geographic boundaries for practical reasons. Programs may be part of a large health system or may operate independently. The composition, admission criteria, and services offered will vary between each HBPC practice. More information about creating a HBPC practice is in Chap. 2.

3.2.1.1 A Model of Care: Veteran's Administration Home-Based Primary Care Program

The Veteran's Administration (VA) runs the oldest and largest HBPC program in the United States. VA HBPC programs started in the 1970s, and there are now over 300 HBPC programs across the country serving more than 59,000 veterans annually with multiple complex chronic diseases through an interdisciplinary team approach [6]. The interdisciplinary team is made up of a program director, physician medical director, nurse practitioner or physician assistant, nurse, social worker, rehabilitation therapists, dietician, pharmacist, and mental health provider [7]. The program provides considerable resources in the home while simultaneously producing significant overall cost saving by reducing VA nursing home days and hospitalizations [8].

3.2.2 Home Hospice and Palliative Care

Home-based palliative care provides medical care in the home for patients with serious illness and high symptom burden. Management can be provided by a patient's existing home-based primary care team as primary palliative care, or can be provided as a separate, specialty home-based palliative care team for patients with refractory symptoms. As patients get closer to end of life, they may qualify for the Medicare Hospice Benefit, which can provide additional services and support to patients, families, and caregivers as part of home-based hospice care. Home-based hospice and palliative care are discussed in more depth in Chap. 13.

3.2.3 Other Medical Professionals Making Home Visits

Other medical professionals make home visits, but availability may vary greatly depending on location. There are no search engines that can easily report availability on a national scale. Home health agencies, assisted living facilities, or the area agency on aging can provide more information about local resources. HBPC clinicians can also encourage other professionals to make home visits.

Other professions that are typically available for home visits include the following:

- *Podiatry*: routine care of foot and ankle; debridement of nails, corns, and calluses; ulcer care including diabetic ulcers; ingrown toenails; orthotics; and diabetic shoes
- *Audiology*: diagnostic hearing evaluations, hearing loss education and counseling, selection and fitting of hearing aids, hearing aid cleaning and repairs, and cerumen removal
- *Dentistry*: routine dental X-rays, exams and cleaning, treat cavities, fillings, tooth extraction, and dentures
- *Optometry*: refraction, tonometry, retinal exams, and dispensing, fitting, and adjustment of glasses

3.2.4 Telemedicine

Telemedicine is an emerging adjunct to home-based primary care, and it has grown exponentially since the start of the COVID-19 pandemic in 2020 [9]. For homebound patients, telemedicine can also greatly increase access to subspecialty care. HBPC teams can share information with telemedicine consultants (such as their in-person exam or medication review in the home) to maximize the experience. Despite being a powerful tool to increase access to medical care, there are still barriers to telemedicine, including sensory or cognitive impairments, lack of a device capable of video calls, poor Internet connection, or needing another person in the home to assist with making the call [10]. More research will need to be done on best practices for continued implementation of telemedicine for homebound older adults.

3.2.5 *Hospital at Home*

Hospital at home programs provide hospital-level care in a patient's home. Hospital at home is offered to a subset of patients with certain diseases (such as pneumonia, heart failure exacerbation, COPD, and cellulitis) and who meet specific medical eligibility criteria. Care includes home nursing; home visits by clinicians; in-home diagnostic studies such as labs, EKGs, and X-rays; and in-home treatments such as IV medications, IV fluids, and oxygen therapy. Hospital at home is meant to be a substitute for inpatient admission from the emergency department or to complete hospitalization at home. Adoption of this model has been growing over a number of years. Hospital at home was successfully evaluated in a Medicare demonstration project and has now been implemented at multiple sites across the country [11, 12]. In 2020, during the COVID-19 pandemic, the Centers for Medicare and Medicaid Services launched the Acute Hospital Care at Home initiative that waived certain regulations and allowed hospitals to implement hospital at home [13, 14].

3.2.6 *Trends in Home Care Medicine*

There is growing interest in moving aspects of facility-based care into the home. Recent pilots of home-based rehabilitation programs (SNF at home) provided home physical and occupational therapy, home nursing, and personal care services. These pilots showed improvements in functional independence and also generated cost savings compared to a traditional rehabilitation facility [15, 16]. Emergency department at home and community paramedicine models have showed reduced utilization of traditional acute care services such as emergency department visits and inpatient hospitalizations [17]. These services are part of a vision to create what has been called a "home-based care ecosystem." This ecosystem would focus on person-centered care in which individuals can receive continuous access to care in their homes, including seamless integration of HBPC, community paramedicine, ED at home, hospital at home, and SNF at home. The ecosystem would also feature interprofessional care, psychosocial care, enhanced care coordination, and more [18]. The models of care that would comprise a home-based care ecosystem are summarized in Table 3.2. Interest in these models and the home-based care ecosystem has been spurred by the COVID-19 pandemic and will likely continue to grow in coming years.

Table 3.2 Home care medicine

Model of care	Services	Team members[a]	Payment
Home-based primary care	– Primary care in the home – Routine/acute visits – In-home diagnostics – Linkage to relevant community resources	– MD/DO – NP and/or PA – RN case manager – RN – Pharmacist – Psychologist – Social work – Office staff	Medicare part B Emerging value-base payment models
Home hospice and palliative care	– Symptom management – End-of-life care – Psychosocial needs – 24/7 phone support – Higher level of care if needed	– MD/DO – NP and/or PA – Hospice RN – Hospice SW – CNA – Chaplain	Medicare hospice benefit Medicaid (varies by state) Private insurance
Hospital at home	– Acute hospital-level care – In-home diagnostics – In-home treatments (IV medications, etc.)	– MD/DO – RN – PT/OT	Medicare Acute Hospital Care at Home Initiative
Rehabilitation at home	– Post-acute care high-intensity rehabilitation in the home – SW, nursing, and personal care as needed	– PT/OT, SLP – RN – Personal care – SW – Clinician available if needed	Emerging model, payment not yet standardized
Emergency department at home and community paramedicine	– Low-acuity emergency services in the home	– EMS – Emergency clinicians – RN	Emerging model, payment not yet standardized

[a] Specific team members may vary by program

3.3 Skilled Home Health Services

The goal of skilled home health is to maximize the patient's health and function in the home, reduce acute episodes of care, and support the caregiver. Services include nursing care, rehabilitative therapy, personal assistance, and social work services. This section will discuss the types of skilled home health services, as well as the logistics of qualifying for and receiving these services. Home health services are summarized in Table 3.3.

Table 3.3 Medicare-covered home health services

Home health team members	Services provided
Nursing[a]	– Provides comprehensive patient assessment and education on disease processes, medications, diet, and self-management skills – Wound and ostomy care – Urinary catheter and gastrostomy tube changes and teaching of self-management – Injections – Infusions (intravenous hydration, parenteral nutrition, and antibiotics) – Venipuncture (venipuncture is not considered a skilled need under Medicare and will not alone qualify someone for home health)
Therapy	
– Physical therapy[a]	– Evaluates and treats to optimize functional function through use of therapeutic exercises, neuromuscular reeducation, gait training, range of motion, maintenance therapy – Evaluates for proper use of equipment to optimize physical functioning
– Occupational therapy	– Evaluates and treats to optimize functioning with ADLs (activities of daily living) and IADLs (instrumental activities of daily living) – Performs home safety evaluations, provides education, and recommends modifications to environment as needed
– Speech and language pathology[a]	– Evaluates and treats disorders of communication development, speech, language, voice, or swallowing – Assesses cognitive status and teaches patients and caregivers self-management skills
– Respiratory therapy	– In select patients, provides treatments that may include managing tracheostomies and home ventilators or designing and administering pulmonary toilet or pulmonary rehabilitation therapies
Personal care aide	– Provides assistance with ADL care needs, such as bathing, dressing, and personal care
Social worker	– Provides counseling, connection to, and assistance with applying for community resources

[a] Considered a skilled need per Medicare guidelines, other services are only provided if a patient has a diagnosis that qualifies them for a skilled need

3.3.1 Home Health Nursing

Home nurses provide comprehensive patient assessments and education on disease processes, medications, diet, and self-management skills. Goals may include improvement or stabilization in symptom control (e.g., pain, dyspnea), medication management and compliance, and improvement in knowledge of disease process and symptoms to report. Teaching and training activities may include self-administration of injectable medications, administration of oxygen, self-catheterization, maintenance of peripheral and central venous lines, administration of intravenous medications, bowel or bladder training, and proper body positioning to prevent pressure sores. Skilled nursing care can also include treatments and procedures such as wound and ostomy care, urinary catheter and gastrostomy tube changes, injections, infusions (intravenous hydration, parenteral nutrition, and antibiotics), and venipuncture. Venipuncture for the purpose of obtaining a blood sample cannot be the sole reason for Medicare home health services, but if the patient has a qualifying skilled need, venipuncture can be done as part of the plan of care. Many but not all agencies provide 24/7 nursing availability, either by telephone or with in-person nurse visits [19].

3.3.2 Home Health Therapy (PT, OT, SLP)

Home therapists provide rehabilitative treatment in the home. The goals of therapy are to maximize safety in the home environment, create and train the patient and family in a home therapy program, optimize assistive devices, attain maximum function, and possibly progress to the appropriate next level of care (such as outpatient therapy) [19].

The three main areas of therapy are described below:

- *Physical therapy* (*PT*): PT provides skilled evaluation/assessments of individuals with mechanical, physiological, and functional limitations and disabilities. PT evaluates and treats functional deficits through use of therapeutic exercises, neuromuscular reeducation, gait training, range of motion, and maintenance therapy. Treatments may include physical modalities such as heat, cold, ultrasound, shortwave, and microwave diathermy. Physical therapists also evaluate for proper use of medical equipment to optimize physical function.
- *Occupational therapy* (*OT*): OT provides skilled evaluation/assessments of individuals with mechanical, physiological, and functional limitations and disabilities with an emphasis on evaluation and treatment of deficits in ADLs (activities of daily living) and IADLs (instrumental activities of daily living). Treatment modalities include selecting and teaching task-oriented therapeutic activities (e.g., cooking); teaching compensatory techniques to improve the level of IADLs (e.g., teaching a person who lost the use of her arm due to a stroke on how to chop vegetables with one hand); designing, fabricating, and fitting orthotic and self-help devices; and providing vocational and prevocational training directed to restoration of function in ADLs. Occupational therapists can perform home safety evaluations, provide education, and recommend modifications to environment as needed. Occupational therapists are also trained to administer cognitive assessments.
- *Speech therapy* (*speech-language pathology* (*SLP*) *services*): SLP provides skilled evaluation/assessments for disorders of communication development, speech, language, voice, or swallowing. Treatments in older adults are most

commonly related to dysphagia and may include swallowing techniques or diet texture modifications. Speech language pathologists can also assess cognitive status and teach patients and caregivers self-management skills to compensate for decreasing cognition.

3.3.3 *Home Respiratory Therapy*

Though respiratory therapy (RT) is not included as one of the typical skilled home health needs discussed above, it is still a critical part of care plans for certain home-bound patients. Respiratory therapists provide treatments that may include managing tracheostomies and home ventilators, designing and administering pulmonary toilet or pulmonary rehabilitation therapies, and obtaining diagnostic testing such as spirometry or blood gas analyses [20]. Currently, respiratory therapy is considered part of the overall plan of care and is not a separately billable service during a home health period of care [19].

3.3.4 *Medical Social Work*

Medical social work is a skilled service that home-bound patients are eligible for if there are social or emotional concerns that may affect one's medical treatment or recovery. Social work services provided in the home may include counseling and connection to and assistance with applying for community resources [21].

3.3.5 *Qualifying for Skilled Home Health Services*

To qualify for skilled home health services, the patient must:

1. Have a skilled home health nursing, physical therapy, or speech therapy medical need on an intermittent basis
2. Meet Medicare's homebound definition (see below)
3. Be under the care of an allopathic, osteopathic, or podiatric doctor
4. Receive home health services under a plan of care established and periodically reviewed by a physician [19]

For the initial qualifying service, the patient must have a medical diagnosis that requires a skilled need from nursing care, physical therapy, or speech therapy. Occupational therapy, social work, and aide services can also be ordered if there is an initial qualifying skilled need, but by themselves do not constitute a basis for eligibility for Medicare reimbursement. However, the need for continued occupational therapy may be the basis for recertification of skilled home services even though it cannot be used for the initial certification.

3.3.6 Medicare Homebound Definition

For a patient to be eligible to receive covered home health services under both Medicare Part A and Part B, the law requires that a physician certify in all cases that the patient is confined to their home. The following criteria must be met:

Criterion one:

The patient must either, because of illness or injury, need the aid of supportive devices such as crutches, canes, wheelchairs, and walkers; the use of special transportation; or the assistance of another person in order to leave their place of residence.

or

have a condition such that leaving his or her home is medically contraindicated.

If the patient meets only one of the criterion one conditions, then the patient must *also* meet two additional requirements defined in criterion two below.

Criterion two:

There must exist a normal inability to leave home;

and

leaving home must require a considerable and taxing effort.

The Medicare regulation states the patient may leave the home and still be considered homebound if absences are infrequent, for short duration, or are attributable to the need to receive healthcare. They go on to provide specific examples of permitted absences from the home including therapeutic, psychosocial, or medical treatment in an adult day care program licensed or certified by a state, outpatient dialysis, outpatient chemotherapy or radiation therapy, attendance at religious services, occasional trip to the barber, a walk around the block or a drive, and attendance at a family reunion, funeral, graduation, or other infrequent or unique events [19].

3.3.7 Timing of Skilled Home Health Services

As mentioned, to receive skilled home health services, the patient must be under the care of an allopathic, osteopathic, or podiatric doctor and have a documented face-to-face visit 90 days before or 30 days after start of care, though many home health agencies require a visit prior to initiating care to ensure that the face-to-face visit happens and the agency will be paid. The face-to-face note must include the visit date and document how the patient's clinical condition (including primary diagnosis and clinical findings) supports the patient's homebound status and need for skilled services. In situations when a clinician orders home healthcare for the patient based on a new condition that was not evident during a visit within the 90 days prior to start of care, the certifying clinician must see the patient again within 30 days after admission. The specific home health services being ordered need to be documented. The initial face-to-face encounter does not need to be done by the certifying doctor. Examples include the face-to-face visit being done by a hospitalist or post-acute care provider upon discharge or by a resident physician under the supervision of the certifying physician. Under the CARES Act in 2020, nurse practitioners and physician assistants also were authorized to order home health care; however, some states limit the scope of practice of advance practice providers and so this capability is limited in some states.

Once a home health referral is accepted, the patient is required to be seen by the skilled service provider within 48 h of the referral or of the patient's return home, or on a physician ordered start date, according to the Medicare Conditions of Participation. A nurse or physical therapist performs an initial comprehensive assessment of the patient, the home, and the availability of caregivers. The patient assessment includes a history and physical along with the completion of the Outcome and Assessment Information Set (OASIS) which includes a number of baseline demographics and characteristics [22].

Home health certifications are for 60-day episodes of care. At the end of the initial 60 days, if the patient still has a skilled need, services can be recertified for subsequent 60-day episodes, with recertification required for each episode. Medicare does not limit the number of recertifications for beneficiaries who continue to be eligible. The recertification assessment must be done during the last 5 days of the previous episode. It must be signed and dated by the physician who reviews the plan of care and indicates a continued need for skilled services. Medicare also requires an estimate of how much additional time the skilled services will be required. Examples of appropriate recertification include patients with chronic urinary catheters requiring monthly and "as needed" catheter changes, wounds that have not healed and require continued skilled nursing services, and continued adjustment of medications for blood pressure control or heart failure management [19].

3.3.8 Physician Payments for Overseeing Home Health

Medicare pays physicians for reviewing and signing certifications and recertifications for home health as well as for care plan oversight (CPO) of home health medical personnel when 30 min or more are spent in a calendar month on such activities. CPO time includes discussing care with home health personnel, reviewing and signing the care plan and orders, reviewing the patient chart for issues related to home health, and completing durable medical equipment forms. Time spent on these activities needs to be documented in the chart. Time talking to patients, family members, or non-home health agency caregivers does not count toward CPO. Communication with agency personnel that is part of a home or office visit also does not count [23].

3.3.9 Choosing a Home Health Agency

Patients have the right to choose their home health agency and must be provided with care options. However, they often look to their home-based medical team for guidance.

To evaluate the quality of a home health agency, consider the following resources, questions, and strategies:

- Is the agency accredited? Accreditation is voluntary and signifies an agency meets national standards. Examples of certifying organizations include the Joint Commission (www.jointcommission.org) and the Community Health Accreditation Program (CHAP: www.chapinc.org).
- Does the agency employ all services or use subcontractors for direct clinical care?
- Does the agency specialize or have certain niche services? Examples can include heart failure care including telehealth, certified wound/ostomy nurse, lymphedema, post-orthopedic surgery rehabilitation, psychiatric nursing, pediatrics, infusion services, nutritionist, diabetic educator, and others.
- Does the agency provide culturally sensitive and linguistically appropriate care?
- How effectively does the agency communicate care needs and updates to the clinician? Are communications timely, effective, and efficient?
- How responsive is the agency in managing care?
- Do they provide 24/7 coverage, and what is their staffing on nights and weekends that can help prevent unnecessary emergency department visits?

Avoid working with agencies that may be engaged in fraudulent behavior. Some red flags include agencies that:

- Directly solicit Medicare patients by phone to whom they have not provided services
- Add on extra therapy visits to increase payments
- Continue to recertify patients when the skilled need no longer exists
- Offer payments for referrals

A good resource to ask about local home health agencies is an experienced hospital discharge planner. They will have made numerous home health referrals and will be aware of agencies that communicate well and see patients in a timely manner.

Home Health Compare (www.medicare.gov/homehealthcompare) is a website that lists all Medicare-certified home health agencies in a particular zip code and provides information on the agencies. Information includes services provided, results of 13 process measures and 9 outcomes of care measures from OASIS, and results from patient surveys (the Home Health Consumer Assessment of Healthcare Providers and Systems instrument).

3.4 Personal Care in the Home

Personal care assistants, sometimes called home health aides when part of a Medicare home health episode, provide nonmedical personal care in the home. This usually involves assistance with activities of daily living (ADLs, such as bathing, dressing, transferring, toileting, and hygiene) and/or some instrumental activities of daily living (IADLs, such as cleaning, meal preparation, and reminding to take medications). These services are incredibly important to help older adults remain at home.

Payment for home care aides can come from a few different sources that vary greatly based on an individual's circumstances. Home health aide services can be covered by Medicare if the patient has a skilled need as discussed above (e.g., nursing care) and needs hands-on personal care to maintain the patient's health or to facilitate treatment of the patient's illness or injury. The home health aide service is provided only as long as the skilled need exists, and the amount of support provided is limited to 24–35 h per week. A home health aide working under these circumstances may be able to provide additional care relevant to the skilled need such as non-skilled wound care and reinforcement of the home therapy program [24].

Outside of the context of a skilled need, Medicare does not pay for home health aides. However, some Medicare Advantage plans may cover personal care aides as part of their "supplemental healthcare benefits." For low-income individuals who qualify, Medicaid may cover personal care aides though the specific details vary by state. All 50 states and DC have Medicaid waiver programs through which individuals who would otherwise require nursing home level care may receive personal care assistance as well as other community services. For low-income individuals who do not qualify for Medicaid, there are other state programs to assist with paying for home care aides which may involve some amount of cost-sharing; details vary by state. The Veteran's Health Administration helps provide personal care aides for a subset of veterans who qualify for services [24].

"Consumer-directed" programs are also available to give individuals the option of hiring home care aides of their choice including family members, rather than aides through an agency. Consumer-directed programs are usually available through Medicaid waivers. Outside of Medicaid waiver-funded programs, similar resources may be available through veteran's benefits and insurance-funded programs [25].

Finally, in many situations, individuals will need to self-pay for personal care aides. If one has purchased long-term care insurance prior to needing assistance, those benefits can cover personal care aides. Private pay care usually costs approximately \$22–\$50 per hour depending on the level of care and geographic area. Aides can provide care ranging from a few hours per day for a few days per week to 24 h per day for 7 days per week. It is important for patients and families to make sure agencies are licensed and bonded. If patients or families hire caregivers directly rather than through an agency, it is recommended to have background checks done.

3.5 Caregivers in the Home

Caregivers provide crucial support in the home for both ADLs and IADLs. "Informal" caregivers are often family members of the person requiring care and are not paid for their services (unless utilizing a consumer-directed program as mentioned above). Caregiver burden has been associated with increased hospitalization and mortality in community-dwelling older care recipients. Providing support and reducing caregiver burden thus not only helps caregivers but may reduce adverse health outcomes for care recipients [26]. Services to assist with caregiver burden may include support groups, counseling (individual or family), education and skills training, and respite care. More information about caregiving and available resources for caregivers can be found in Chap. 14.

3.6 Community Resources

There are a multitude of community resources available to support older adults in their homes. This is in part due to a national emphasis to redirect federal dollars from institutional care (nursing homes) to home- and community-based services to enable patients to remain in the community. We will discuss the organizational structures that fund and administer community programs, review common community-based services that are available, and identify key resources for navigating the plethora of services.

HBPC programs may have a social worker, nurse case manager, or community health worker who can help participants find community resources. Private case managers can also be hired (see below). Although this section will provide background on common resources available, the full breadth of resources varies by location. Because of this variability, navigating these resources can be both overwhelming and confusing. Well-informed home-based clinicians can direct patients and families toward helpful resources. Home-based medical care practices can also develop collaborative partnerships with community resources to reduce duplication of efforts and to ensure that the provider has the most accurate information about local services. Partnerships with local resources can also serve as a key referral source for home-based medical care programs.

3.6.1 Organizational Structures and Funding for Community Resources

There are many organizations to help coordinate community resources from the national to local level. At the national level, the Administration for Community Living (ACL) is a division of the US Department of Health and Human Services that is tasked to support older adults living in the community by funding community-based services, investing in research and innovation, and advocating for older adults and people with disabilities. Among other roles, it helps support local, state, and national aging and disability networks, including but not limited to Area Agencies on Aging (AAA) [27].

Many services for older adults provided through the ACL umbrella are funded by the Older Americans Act (OAA). The OAA was initially established in 1965 and has been periodically reauthorized by Congress since then, with a goal to promote the well-being of older individuals by providing services and programs designed to help them live independently in their homes and communities. OAA national funding for programs is distributed to a region based primarily on the number of persons 60 years of age and over. All individuals 60 years of age and older are eligible for services under the OAA, although priority attention is given to those who are in greatest need. Patients are often unaware that many of the services provided through OAA are free of charge [28].

Funding from the OAA is then managed by local Area Agencies on Aging (AAA) that are on-the-ground organizations that evaluate the needs of seniors in their catchment and subcontract with local partners to fund services. Because services vary and individuals have unique needs, AAAs offer navigation services through Information and Referral/Assistance (I&R/A) programs. These programs employ information specialists who provide individualized assistance and linkage to available services. Information specialists are often accessible by telephone and in person at a local site. In addition to linking seniors with services, they can also provide assistance with housing, crisis intervention, advocacy for individuals, and more [29]. Local AAAs and more can be identified at Eldercare Locator (https://eldercare.acl.gov/).

Given community-level and regional variation, HBPC providers are advised to reach out and develop a relationship with a contact at their local AAA. This minor investment of time will yield valuable guidance but may also offer secondary benefits related to facilitated or improved referrals for your patients and timely guidance about changes in resources/eligibility.

3.6.2 *Behavioral Health*

In addition to services funded through the OAA, every community has a designated agency tasked with providing comprehensive healthcare services for seriously and chronically mentally ill patients. The agency may be the health department or a government-designated private nonprofit entity. This designated agency is typically credentialed with many governmental as well as select private payors to provide key services. Unlike traditional counseling agencies, these agencies provide comprehensive behavioral health services for seriously and chronically mentally ill patients including intensive outpatient services, 24-h crisis services, services for people with dual diagnosis of both mental health and substance use disorders, and often limited home-based services for homebound and/or seriously mentally ill clients. Many of these designated agencies have resources supporting free or reduced cost treatment for qualifying patients. There is a shortage of mental health workers in many areas of the country, especially those that provide home-based mental healthcare, so these services may be very difficult to access. Key resources include the Substance Abuse and Mental Health Services Administration (https://www.samhsa.gov/) and the Geriatric Mental Health Foundation (http://www.gmhfonline.org/), both of which have search functions to look for mental health providers based on location.

3.7 Center-Based Care and Services

Some community services are provided to many individuals at once at local senior centers. Medical and custodial care may also be provided in centers, such as in adult day care programs, as well as through the Program for All-inclusive Care of the Elderly (PACE).

3.7.1 *Senior Centers*

Senior centers are hubs that connect older adults to their community. They typically operate out of a physical location though many have provided remote services during the COVID-19 pandemic. Senior centers offer a variety of programs and services, which may include free or low-cost meals, recreational activities, educational and arts programs, fitness and wellness programs, and more. Individuals who participate in activities at senior centers must be relatively independent in their ADLs, since centers do not provide any medical or personal care assistance. Senior centers are usually funded by multiple sources including the OAA and other governmental funds, public and private grants, local businesses, fundraising, etc. There may be a small fee for individuals to participate in activities through a senior center to help maintain funding as well [30].

3.7.2 *Adult Day Care Centers*

Adult day care centers offer daytime supervision and services for individuals who cannot be left alone during the day due to medical or social circumstances. The types of adult day care centers available may vary slightly by state, but they generally provide a higher level of care, including assistance with ADLs (such as meals and toileting) and assistance with medical care (such as medication administration). Adult day care can be paid for in similar ways as personal care aides, such as through the Medicaid waiver program, non-Medicaid government assistance programs, VA benefits, long-term care insurance, or private pay [31].

3.7.3 *A Model of Care: Program for All-Inclusive Care of the Elderly*

Program for All-Inclusive Care of the Elderly (PACE) provides comprehensive services for adults aged 55 years or older who are nursing home-eligible to help them remain in the home. The PACE team is interdisciplinary and services include primary care, nursing, social work, physical and occupational therapy, recreational therapy, home health aides, nutrition, transportation, and often more. The interdisciplinary team meets frequently to help coordinate patient care. PACE provides center-based care and activities during the day, as well as care in the home as needed. Participants in PACE are typically dual-eligible for Medicare and Medicaid. When participants enroll in PACE, the program receives capitated payments from Medicare and Medicaid that are then used to pay for medical care, including any hospitalizations, and all other services provided [32]. Because of this capitated model, PACE is incentivized to provide value-based care focused on keeping older adults living in the community and out of hospitals and nursing homes. As of 2022, there are more than 100 PACE programs across 30 states. In some states, PACE is also known as LIFE (Living Independence for the Elderly) [33].

3.8 Additional Community Resources Commonly Available

Area Agencies on Aging manage funds from the Older Americans Act to provide many community resources for older adults. Commonly available resources are discussed in this section, though details vary by location. Local services can be identified through BenefitsCheckUp® (https://benefitscheckup.org/).

3.8.1 Care Management

Care managers work with family members and older adults to assess, arrange, and evaluate supportive efforts of seniors and their families to remain independent. If provided through an AAA, these services may be provided free of charge. Care managers can assess clients either at the request of medical providers, through patient self-identification, or caregiver referral. Care managers provide an exhaustive review of the patient's situation. A typical assessment includes patient goals and needs, physical and mental health, functional status, caregiver availability, transportation, environment, financial issues, legal issues, etc. Individuals and families can also hire private care managers who can provide more hands-on coordination of services and function as a "point person" for functional, medical, and social concerns.

3.8.2 Financial Assistance

While not available in every community, some areas offer no-cost benefit counseling programs that can be accessed through the Information and Referral/Assistance specialist at the local AAA to help older adults to manage their finances. Some AAA and subgrantee agencies offer paid or volunteer financial counselors who can work intensively with families to improve financial stability. Some agencies may also function as representative payees for seniors who need additional assistance.

3.8.3 Legal Assistance

More than 1000 legal aid services provide over one million hours of senior legal advice per year with funding from AAA. Services are available to persons aged 60 and over for certain types of legal matters including government program benefits, tenant rights, estate planning, and consumer problems. Legal services under Title III-B also protect older persons against direct challenges to their independence, choice, and financial security. These legal services are specifically targeted to "older individuals with economic or social needs" [34]. Most communities have a designated grantee agency to which all referrals for senior legal assistance can be made, and the lawyers available have special content knowledge. Homebound patients can receive assistance telephonically, and lawyers can visit patients at home as needed. In many cases, the local legal aid provider may also be the provider of AAA service. Eldercare Locator (eldercare.acl.gov) can direct patients and families to the local resources. The National Academy of Elder Law Attorneys (www.naela.org) also provides resources, education, and a search tool.

3.8.4 Elder Abuse Prevention Programs

Allegations of abuse, neglect, and exploitation of senior citizens are investigated by trained protective service specialists who are often affiliated with an AAA and/or a state Department on Aging. Intervention is provided in instances of substantiated elder abuse, neglect, or exploitation. While referrals will result in a comprehensive assessment, individuals with decisional capacity may decline assistance despite finding of neglect or other risks.

3.8.5 Home Repair and Home Modification Programs

Community partners may offer programs through vetted tradesmen or volunteers that help older people maintain the condition of their homes and provide repairs as needed. Home modification programs provide adaptations and/or renovations to the living environment intended to increase ease of use, safety, security, and independence. There are some local, state, federal, and volunteer programs that provide grants and loans to support these efforts, and programs may offer either fixed or reduced fee programs for eligible seniors.

3.8.6 Meal Delivery

Popularly known as "Meals on Wheels," this service delivers nutritious meals to the homes of seniors and persons with disabilities. Another resource is Congregate Meals, which provides the opportunity for persons aged 60 and over to enjoy a meal and socialize with other seniors in the community. Individuals desiring nutrition services are typically assessed for income, and the agency suggests a donation or fee to defray the cost of food. Although policies vary by community, Meals on Wheels providers often defray program fees for lower-income seniors with fundraising, and many participate in the food stamp program as well.

3.8.7 Transportation

Some communities provide reduced or no-cost door-to-door transportation for older adults or persons with disabilities who do not have private transportation and are unable to utilize public transportation. These services are often provided through local public transit agencies but can be via other organizations as well. Most senior ride programs have specific geographic service areas. There is typically an application process to be able to use these transportation services.

3.8.8 Faith-Based Resources

Many faith-based communities offer services to homebound congregants which may include meal delivery and visits from clergy people or congregants to offer companionship and support. Some communities may also have parish nurses, who provide both nursing and spiritual care. HBPC providers can encourage homebound patients to talk with their local congregations about what resources are available.

3.8.9 Community Resources for Younger Adults

Although many of the services detailed in this chapter offer specific benefits to seniors, most states also have similar services available to younger patients through their Department of Rehabilitative Services or Office of Rehabilitation Services. At a federal level, the Rehabilitation Services Administration (RSA) oversees grant programs supporting individuals with disabilities to obtain employment and live more independently. Supports include medical and psychological services, counseling job training, procurement of assistive technology, and rehabilitative training programs. More information about federally funded programs is available on the RSA web site at https://rsa.ed.gov/about/programs.

3.9 National Foundations and Associations

Table 3.4 details a number of associations and foundations which also offer support for seniors and for individuals living with certain medical conditions.

Table 3.4 National organizations for specific medical conditions

Agency	Description	Website
The ALS Association	Links to regional care and clinics Clinical trial information Printed educational material and newsletters Support groups Equipment loan programs Respite programs Caregiver resources	www.alsa.org
Alzheimer's Association	Local offices and 24-h helpline Caregiver center Online guide to helping individuals and families find the right care options; Community Resource Finder Library services Brain health quizzes and games	www.alz.org

(continued)

Table 3.4 (continued)

Agency	Description	Website
American Cancer Society	Support programs and services Patient lodging programs Road to recovery (transportation) Reach to recovery (breast cancer support) Hair loss and mastectomy products Look Good Feel Better program: helps with appearance-related side effects of treatment Online communities and support I Can Cope (online cancer education classes) Patient Navigator Program	www.cancer.org
American Parkinson Disease Association	Web site publications Young onset information guide Links to veteran services Tool to search for local services and support Research updates	www.apdaparkinson.org
Brain Injury Association of America	Information about and living with traumatic brain injury (TBI) Treatment and rehabilitation Family and caregiver information Support group resources Webinars TBI prevention Legal issues Local state chapters	www.biausa.org
Easter Seals	Easter Seals provides many services across the spectrum Senior services include: Mature workers Adult day programs In-home and center-based services Services for caregivers Medical rehabilitation National Center for Senior Transportation Military and veterans Employment and training Camping and recreation Brain health	www.easterseals.com
Muscular Dystrophy Association (MDA)	MDA clinics Support groups Equipment assistance Support for caregivers Educational resources Tips for success kit Emergency resources for MDA families	www.mda.org
Aging Life Care Association	"Find an Aging Life Care Expert Search" tool Description of typical services and benefits Standards of practice Position papers Education tools	www.aginglifecare.org

(continued)

Table 3.4 (continued)

Agency	Description	Website
National Multiple Sclerosis Society	Extensive educational publications for clinicians and laypersons Family services, insurance, and financial info Tool to search for local services and support Treatment information Current research (clinician and patient focused)	www.nationalmssociety.org
National Parkinson Foundation (NPF)	Helpline for patients Search engine for local resources including providers, centers of care, local chapters, and support groups Discussion groups Clinical trials Patient education library NPF white papers Practical tools including Parkinson's ID Bracelet, Medical Alert Card, and hospital action plan booklet Publications, online learning, webinars, and tools Multipronged training for professionals	www.parkinson.org

3.10 Summary and Key Resources

Taking care of people who are homebound and allowing them to age in place requires creating a network of support. This chapter provides a framework for the myriad services available both in the home and in the community. People may qualify for and benefit from medical care, skilled services, or personal care aides in the home. Medical and personal care are also available in centralized locations in the community. There are many additional community resources available to support older adults with social, financial, and legal needs and more. Despite the breadth of available services, getting connected to feasible and affordable care can be challenging because of differences in personal circumstances as well as regional variations in services and eligibility requirements. Home-based care providers play a crucial role in helping older adults access resources. Details have been discussed in this chapter, but we would like to summarize our key approaches to help older adults get connected to relevant resources:

- Search Eldercare Locator (https://eldercare.acl.gov/), which helps identify key aging-related agencies by location.
- Search BenefitsCheckUp® (https://benefitscheckup.org/), which helps identify key community resources by location.
- Connect with your local Area Agency on Aging.
- Work with your medical practice's social worker, who can link to relevant local resources.

References

1. De Jonge KE, Jamshed N, Gilden D, Kubisiak J, Bruce SR, Taler G. Effects of home-based primary care on Medicare costs in high-risk elders. J Am Geriatr Soc. 2014;62(10):1825–31.
2. Elkan R, Kendrick D, Dewey M, Hewitt M, Robinson J, Blair M, et al. Effectiveness of home based support for older people: systematic review and meta-analysis. BMJ. 2001;323(7315):719–25.
3. Huss A, Stuck AE, Rubenstein LZ, Egger M, Clough-Gorr KM. Multidimensional preventive home visit programs for community-dwelling older adults: a systematic review and meta-analysis of randomized controlled trials. J Gerontol A Biol Sci Med Sci. 2008;63(3):298–307.
4. Stuck AE, Siu AL, Wieland GD, Adams J, Rubenstein LZ. Comprehensive geriatric assessment: a meta-analysis of controlled trials. Lancet Lond Engl. 1993;342(8878):1032–6.
5. Stuck AE, Egger M, Hammer A, Minder CE, Beck JC. Home visits to prevent nursing home admission and functional decline in elderly people: systematic review and meta-regression analysis. JAMA. 2002;287(8):1022–8.
6. Schuchman M, Fain M, Cornwell T. The resurgence of home-based primary care models in the United States. Geriatrics (Basel). 2018;3(3):E41.
7. Geriatrics and extended care—home based primary care. VA benefits and healthcare. 2022 [cited 2022 Sep 27]. https://www.va.gov/GERIATRICS/pages/Home_Based_Primary_Care.asp.
8. Edes T, Kinosian B, Vuckovic NH, Nichols LO, Becker MM, Hossain M. Better access, quality, and cost for clinically complex veterans with home-based primary care. J Am Geriatr Soc. 2014;62(10):1954–61.
9. Hincapié MA, Gallego JC, Gempeler A, Piñeros JA, Nasner D, Escobar MF. Implementation and usefulness of telemedicine during the COVID-19 pandemic: a scoping review. J Prim Care Community Health. 2020;11:2150132720980612.
10. Kalicki AV, Moody KA, Franzosa E, Gliatto PM, Ornstein KA. Barriers to telehealth access among homebound older adults. J Am Geriatr Soc. 2021;69(9):2404–11.
11. About hospital at home. Hospital at home. [cited 2022 Sep 27]. https://www.hospitalathome.org/about-us/overview.php.
12. Leff B, Burton L, Mader SL, Naughton B, Burl J, Inouye SK, et al. Hospital at home: feasibility and outcomes of a program to provide hospital-level care at home for acutely ill older patients. Ann Intern Med. 2005;143(11):798–808.
13. Acute Hospital Care at Home. CMS.gov. [cited 2022 Sep 27]. https://qualitynet.cms.gov/acute-hospital-care-at-home.
14. Clarke DV, Newsam J, Olson DP, Adams D, Wolfe AJ, Fleisher LA. Acute hospital care at home: the CMS waiver experience. NEJM Catal. 2021:1–14.
15. Augustine MR, Davenport C, Ornstein KA, Cuan M, Saenger P, Lubetsky S, et al. Implementation of post-acute rehabilitation at home: a skilled nursing facility-substitutive model. J Am Geriatr Soc. 2020;68(7):1584–93.
16. Johnson JK, Hohman JA, Vakharia N, Zafirau W, Stilphen M, Pamer S, et al. High-intensity postacute care at home. NEJM Catal. 2021;2(6). https://doi.org/10.1056/CAT.21.0125.
17. Gregg A, Tutek J, Leatherwood MD, Crawford W, Friend R, Crowther M, et al. Systematic review of community paramedicine and EMS mobile integrated health care interventions in the United States. Popul Health Manag. 2019;22(3):213–22.
18. Ritchie C, Leff B. Home-based care reimagined: a full-fledged health care delivery ecosystem without walls. Health Aff (Millwood). 2022;41(5):689–95.
19. Medicare benefit policy manual. Chapter 7—Home health services. 2022 [cited 2022 Sep 27]. https://www.cms.gov/Regulations-and-Guidance/Guidance/Manuals/downloads/bp102c07.pdf.
20. Respiratory therapy (respiratory care). Medicare coverage database. 2021 [cited 2022 Sep 27]. https://www.cms.gov/medicare-coverage-database/view/lcd.aspx?LCDId=34430.

21. Medicare and home health care. Centers for Medicare and Medicaid Services. 2020 [cited 2022 Sep 27]. https://www.medicare.gov/Pubs/pdf/10969-medicare-and-home-health-care.pdf.
22. 42 CFR Part 484—home health services. 2022 [cited 2022 Sep 27]. https://www.ecfr.gov/current/title-42/chapter-IV/subchapter-G/part-484.
23. Care Plan Oversight and Certification/recertification services for patients receiving care through home health agencies or hospices. CGS. 2020 [cited 2022 Sep 27]. https://www.cgsmedicare.com/partb/pubs/news/2014/0514/cope25747.html.
24. Paying for home care: financial options, aid and assistance. Paying for senior care. 2020. https://www.payingforseniorcare.com/homecare/paying-for-home-care.
25. Cash & counseling programs: get paid as a family caregiver. Paying for senior care. 2019 [cited 2022 Sep 27]. https://www.payingforseniorcare.com/paid-caregiver/cash-and-counseling-program.
26. Kuzuya M, Enoki H, Hasegawa J, Izawa S, Hirakawa Y, Shimokata H, et al. Impact of caregiver burden on adverse health outcomes in community-dwelling dependent older care recipients. Am J Geriatr Psychiatry. 2011;19(4):382–91.
27. About community living. ACL administration for community living. 2022 [cited 2022 Sep 27]. https://acl.gov/about-community-living.
28. Colello KJ, Napili A. Older Americans Act: overview and funding. Congressional Research Service. 2022 [cited 2022 Sep 27]. https://crsreports.congress.gov/product/pdf/R/R43414.
29. Information and referral/assistance. USAging. [cited 2022 Sep 27]. https://www.usaging.org/content.asp?contentid=1281.
30. Get the facts on senior centers. NCOA National Council on Aging. 2022 [cited 2022 Sep 27]. https://www.ncoa.org/article/get-the-facts-on-senior-centers.
31. Paying for adult day care: financial assistance for seniors. Paying for senior care. 2020 [cited 2022 Sep 27]. https://www.payingforseniorcare.com/adult-day-care.
32. Programs of all-inclusive care for the elderly benefits. Medicaid.gov. [cited 2022 Sep 27]. https://www.medicaid.gov/medicaid/long-term-services-supports/pace/programs-all-inclusive-care-elderly-benefits/index.html.
33. Medicare PACE & LIFE Programs—state by state locations. Paying for senior care. 2022 [cited 2022 Sep 27]. https://www.payingforseniorcare.com/medicare/pace-medicare/provider-list.
34. Legal Services for Older Americans Program. ACL Administration for Community Living. 2021 [cited 2022 Sep 27]. https://acl.gov/programs/legal-help/legal-services-elderly-program.

Chapter 4
How to Perform a House Call

Deborah G. Freeland, Amy Kilen, and Jessica L. Colburn

Home visits, or visits to patients' homes for the purpose of providing medical care, are a critical element in the delivery of health services to frail homebound older adults. The previous chapters have outlined important considerations for structuring a home-based medical practice and identifying community resources for homebound patients in your geographic area. The next steps are to plan for a visit and to gather the tools you need to provide home-based medical care. These tools include not only medical equipment and access to ancillary services but also a comprehensive approach to assessment and screening that incorporates the social and functional information that is uniquely available to a home-based medical care clinician, as well as the prognosis and preferences of the individual patient. Of note, though this chapter addresses the older adult patient, it can apply to any patient seen at home.

D. G. Freeland (✉)
Division of Geriatric Medicine, Department of Internal Medicine, UT Southwestern, Dallas, TX, USA
e-mail: Deborah.Freeland@utsouthwestern.edu

A. Kilen
Johns Hopkins Community Physicians, Baltimore, MD, USA

J. L. Colburn
Division of Geriatric Medicine and Gerontology, Johns Hopkins University School of Medicine, Baltimore, MD, USA

J. L. Colburn et al. (eds.), *Geriatric Home-Based Medical Care*,
https://doi.org/10.1007/978-3-031-68786-0_4

4.1 Planning for a Visit

To start, think about the sequence of events that occur in a typical office visit. The patient arrives, registers with the receptionist, takes a seat, and completes a health questionnaire or other forms while waiting to be seen by a clinician. A medical assistant or nurse takes the patient to the clinical area to measure vital signs and enter the reason for the visit into the medical record. If needed, a medical interpreter can be connected by telephone, video, or in person to provide language interpretation for a patient. Then the clinician obtains a history, performs a physical exam, and discusses the findings and plan with the patient. Prescriptions, imaging, labs, or consultations may be ordered as part of the plan. A patient or family may meet with other team members during the visit, including a social worker in the clinic. At the end of the visit, the patient leaves with instructions on following up the plan of care. While the outline of these steps is similar, in home-based primary care the clinician will be the one performing most of these tasks.

Two unique aspects in the preparations for house calls are safety planning and adapting the visit to the home environment. Safety considerations involve awareness of one's surroundings in homes or neighborhoods and emergency preparedness prior to going out on home visits. Emergency preparedness includes knowing an exit route, positioning oneself in the home with access to the exit, and planning for how to exit if a situation becomes unsafe. Some programs also use GPS to share locations of providers who are out on visits. At the same time, we must also be aware of biases that we bring to environments; house calls often bring healthcare to communities that have been historically neglected, however, that does not inherently make them unsafe.

Visit preparation also involves adapting the visit to the home environment. In some situations, clinicians may want to consider limiting what to bring into the home to reduce exposure to harmful substances, bodily fluids, pets, or pests in the home. Providers may ask patients or family members to put pets into other rooms or to extinguish cigarettes if people are smoking in the home at the time of the visit. Once in the home, visit setup is important. Some patients may prefer to have the visit in a central location, such as the family room or kitchen, while other patients may be unable to get out of bed and require a visit in their bedroom. It is important to consider principles of trauma-informed care when doing visits in the home, to ensure patient safety and sensitivity.

A clinician may want to bring a stool or impermeable barrier (i.e., chux pad) to ensure there is somewhere to sit within proximity to the patient. Privacy considerations are important for history gathering if there are other family members in the home who the patient may not want involved in the discussion.

Many minor primary care procedures can be performed safely in the home, such as vaccine administration, phlebotomy, joint injection, and suture removal, which allows patients to avoid the burden of traveling to an office solely for these procedures. Table 4.1 lists useful equipment and supplies for a home-based medical visit.

Table 4.1 Equipment and supplies for home-based medical visits

Equipment	• Stethoscope
	• Blood pressure cuff
	• Pulse oximeter
	• Portable sound amplification device (i.e., pocket talker)
	• Otoscope/ophthalmoscope
	• Stool for sitting during the visit
	• Portable ECG machine
	• Portable handheld ultrasound device
General supplies	• Masks/face shield
	• Alcohol swabs
	• Nonsterile gloves
	• Suture and staple removal kits
	• Phlebotomy supplies (tourniquet, needles, vacutainer, tubes)
	• Sharps container
	• Microfilament
	• Chucks for procedures/wound care
	• Vaccines for administering (influenza, pneumonia, etc.)
Wound care supplies	• Sterile and nonsterile gauze pads
	• Medical tape
	• Scalpel for wound debridement
	• Sutures
	• Petroleum jelly
Joint injection supplies	• Sterile gloves
	• Topical anesthetic
	• Local anesthetic with syringes and needles
	• Injectable steroids for joint injections

Careful thought and planning must go into bringing the appropriate equipment to these visits, including a mobile electronic tablet or laptop to securely access the electronic medical record from a patient's home. Portable ultrasound may be useful for clinicians performing routine home-based medical care who have been trained in the use of handheld ultrasound. X-ray equipment for plain films might be cost-prohibitive for a clinician who is adding occasional house calls to an existing office practice; many communities have mobile imaging companies who provide these services which often are covered by insurance.

4.2 Comprehensive Home-Based Geriatric Assessment

Once the clinician has planned for and assembled the basic equipment needed for a house call, the next step is to take advantage of the array of information available by virtue of seeing the patient at home. The 4Ms framework created by the Institute for Healthcare Improvement is a person-centered approach that examines What *M*atters *M*ost to patients and their *M*edications, *M*entation, and *M*obility [1]. This framework is helpful in home-based primary care, often revealing information that would be difficult to obtain in an office visit. In addition to the 4Ms, house calls allow for an enhanced assessment of the social and structural determinants of health (SSDOH) affecting patients (see section below). Performing a physical exam in the home often looks different from one in the office. Taken together, the 4Ms framework, the SSDOH, and the home-based physical exam comprise a comprehensive home-based geriatric assessment that can identify key challenges and supports to providing personalized patient care in the home.

The approach to conducting a comprehensive assessment must be applied judiciously, considering individual patient preferences: for instance, if looking into medicine cabinets or cupboards seems important to the goals of the visit, the clinician must first ensure that the patient accepts this level of scrutiny and does not consider it an invasion of privacy.

4.2.1 The 4Ms

What Matters Most Home-based primary care provides an intimate look into how to best deliver person-centered care. It is essential to start by seeking an understanding of what matters most to patients so that the rest of the care plan can align with their specific preferences and health goals. The art of observation in the home allows clinicians to glean information about family or friend support, spiritual health, and hobbies. There may be pictures of loved ones or cherished items on display to spark these important conversations. Part of discussing what matters most may also include documentation of end-of-life preferences. Advance directive forms are state-specific and allow for patients to assign a medical power of attorney and document care preferences. These forms can then be shared across healthcare settings. Completion of advance directives at home can be challenging when lacking a notary or available witnesses and when there are difficulties with transportation to seek these services. Creative solutions can include connecting with mobile notary services or partnering with a social worker who can make a home visit.

Medications Medication reconciliation in the home can be enhanced from what is typically performed in the office or hospital because the clinician can review all the medication bottles in the house, not just the ones the patient remembers or chooses to bring to these other settings. Importantly, the list that many patients bring to ambulatory settings can be reviewed and updated in the home by direct comparison with the pill bottles. Dates and prescriber information on the prescription labels can provide clues to adherence. Over-the-counter medications, dietary supplements, and refrigerated medications are easier to reconcile and assess for proper use and storage. Medication organization quickly becomes apparent, and pillboxes can be filled or adjusted in real time. Asking open-ended questions about medication administration ("how do you take this medication?" instead of "do you take this medication three times a day?") can reveal problems with understanding or memory that may prompt changes in management, including discussion with the patient or caregivers for more assistance.

Mentation Cognitive impairment is a common contributor as to why older adults become homebound [2]. Identification, treatment, and management of dementia and other mimics such as depression or delirium are vital to supporting older adults in their home. Evidence of cognitive impairment may become apparent when touring the home in the form of reminders posted around the living space, safety measures such as child-proof door locks or missing stove knobs, unusual placement of everyday objects, or lack of grooming and general upkeep of the home. Several tools are available for screening for memory impairment and inattention. Evaluation of caregiver burden becomes particularly important for those caring for patients experiencing dementia. Managing psychological and behavioral symptoms of dementia requires a focus on behavioral interventions, and understanding the space in which the patient lives can help with generating solutions and support. If a patient can no longer use a telephone independently, they likely need 24-hour supervision. Most homebound older adults are no longer driving, but if they are continuing to drive and are showing signs of cognitive impairment, there should be a discussion about safety. For patients with cognitive impairment in assisted living facilities, the medical visit may occur without their medical power of attorney or family support present, and keeping family up to date about the medical plan is imperative (see Chap. 5 "Common Cognitive Issues in Home-Based Care").

Mobility Assessment of mobility in the home adds important information about understanding an older adult's day-to-day function. Activities of daily living (ADLs) include feeding, toileting, dressing, bathing, transferring, and walking. ADLs are the basic tasks required for minimally independent function. The home-based clinician can quickly identify problems with ADLs by noticing features of the patient's environment that may not be apparent in an office visit: the presence or degree of involvement of a caregiver, visible stains or odor of urine, and presence of assistive devices (e.g., cane, walker, wheelchair) or other durable medical equipment (e.g., total patient lift, hospital bed, bedside commode, shower chair). Patients with ADL deficits require hands-on personal assistance to function in the home, and the absence of a caregiver who can help with these basic needs may mean that the patient cannot safely remain in the community without additional support. Instrumental activities of daily living (IADLs), in contrast, are tasks necessary to continue living in the community but do not necessarily require direct physical contact with the patient. They include meal preparation, housekeeping, medication management, money management, telephone use, and transportation. Clinicians may notice a refrigerator that is empty, laundry that needs to be done, bills that need paying, or medications in disarray. Patients with deficits in IADLs can often remain safely at home if they have a caregiver who can prepare meals and medications a few days in advance and visit or call a few times a week to check for any additional needs. A key advantage of assessing functional status in the home is the ability to ask patients to demonstrate completion of a task, rather than having them simply report on their ability to perform certain activities. Hazards that may contribute to falls are easier to identify when examining balance and gait in the home. Presence of an emergency response system and other general household features (carpets, rugs, lighting) allow for a comprehensive safety assessment.

4.2.2 Social and Structural Determinants of Health

Social and structural determinants of health (SSDOH) are the conditions of the systems and places where people are born, live, work, play, worship, and age that affect a wide range of health, functioning, and quality-of-life outcomes and risks. SSDOH have a significant impact on morbidity, mortality, life expectancy, health care expenditures, health status, and functional ability for homebound older adults [3]. House calls can provide much more information about how these determinants are playing a role in patients' lives.

Consider the social and structural determinants listed in Table 4.2. Assess these throughout the visit, starting on the drive in, continued during the visit in the home, and especially when constructing the person-centered plan that aligns with what matters most.

4.2.3 Home-Based Physical Examination

There are a few unique considerations when performing a physical examination in the home. Without an exam table, the clinician will need to find different spaces in the home to maximize the performance of certain aspects of the exam. For example, assessment of jugular venous distension can be accomplished with the patient in a recliner or positioned in bed with a pillow; a hip examination can be completed with the patient lying on a bed or couch. For vaginal exams, consider bringing additional tools such as a fracture bedpan (placed upside down and padded with a towel to help prop up the pelvis for appropriate positioning), a disposable speculum, plenty of lubricant, and a flashlight or headlight to use for optimal visualization. Strategies should also be considered for providing a chaperone for genital exams.

For older patients, there are specific components to the physical exam that should be highlighted. A skin exam should include examination of the sacrum and the heels

Table 4.2 Social and structural determinants of health

Environment	• Neighborhood—presence/absence of green space, sidewalks, grocery stores • Home maintenance—yard upkeep, repairs • Exterior of home—presence of steps/ramp, functioning doors/windows, porch • Interior of home—crowding, housekeeping, privacy, pets, pests, memorabilia, stairs • General safety—rugs, lighting, smoke alarms, carbon monoxide detectors, layout of furniture, available medical equipment, presence/storage of firearms • Bathroom safety—grab bars, toilet height, shower accessibility, width of door frames for assistive device access • Kitchen safety—gas stove, cooking appliances, counter heights, chemicals, fire extinguisher
Economic stability	• Income, expenses, bills, debt • Medication affordability • Financial power of attorney • Eligibility for services: money management, Medicaid
Nutrition	• Availability, variety, and quality of foods—pantry, refrigerator, freezer • Nutritional status—obesity, malnutrition, medical diet restrictions, presence of alcohol • Tube feeding supplies • Kitchen appliances available for food preparation • Eligibility for services: SNAP benefits, Meals on Wheels
Education	• Health literacy, primary language, level of education • Access to technology—cell phone, Internet, electronic medical record portal
Community	• Social support system, neighbors, family, paid caregivers, community engagement • Cultural considerations • Mistreatment or neglect • Access to transportation—driving, public transportation
Healthcare system	• Health insurance—Medicare or Medicaid eligibility • Access to specialist care, home health services, interpretation services • Vision, dental, hearing coverage

for decubitus ulcers. This can be more time-consuming, as patients rarely wear a hospital gown and may need to undress during the visit. A foot exam can reveal neglected toenails that can impede use of proper footwear and alter gait. Sensory exams for vision and hearing can identify deficits that can make living at home independently a challenge. Check ears for cerumen impaction and ensure hearing aid batteries are operational. Oral health must not be neglected, and dentures should be checked for appropriate fit and proper cleaning. The gait exam (performed with assistive device if needed) provides clinicians with additional information about sensation, strength, balance, and coordination. Nutritional status can be observed, although weight cannot always be measured if a patient is bedbound or unable to stand. A comprehensive physical exam becomes even more improtant for someone with dementia, as they might not be able to describe concerning symptoms or answer review of systems questions accurately.

4.3 Implementing the Plan

When developing a plan of care for a patient during a home-based medical encounter, it is important to consider resources available in the home and whether a patient can access hospital or office-based resources for additional testing or procedures. Lab work can be performed by clinicians in the home and dropped off at a hospital or outpatient lab after the visit. Additionally, some areas have mobile lab services that can perform lab draws for patients at home and mobile imaging services to perform home X-ray and ultrasound imaging.

In addition to labs and imaging, referrals to specialists require additional consideration for patients who have difficulty leaving the home. Some specialists provide home-based medical care, and it is useful to have a list of resources available in the community for mobile specialists such as optometry, dentistry, and podiatry. Other specialists may be able to perform telemedicine visits for patients, which may need to be facilitated by the primary care clinician or team member if patients do not have video capability at home.

One important clinical service that can be particularly challenging to coordinate in a home-based medical practice is anticoagulation management for patients taking warfarin. Many patients can be converted to direct oral anticoagulants (DOAC), but that is not possible for some patients due to the indication for anticoagulation or the insurance coverage available to cover a DOAC. Medicare now covers the cost of point-of-care INR monitors for home use, which is one option if there is a consistent, reliable method of ensuring that the data is communicated to the clinician who is managing the warfarin dosage and monitoring. If a point-of-care monitor is not covered or if a patient and/or care partner is not able to safely use and communicate the information to a clinician, then routine lab draws in the home would be needed. This requires a system for tracking, monitoring, and adjusting the warfarin to ensure patient safety.

4.4 Screening and Preventive Care

Screening and preventive care are essential components of primary care. Traditionally, decisions around screening and prevention are algorithmic and predominantly based on age and risk factors associated with the disease being screened. However, age-based guidelines have little utility in a home-based population for numerous reasons. It is not uncommon for home-based medical practices to experience a 20–25% mortality per year [4, 5]; conventional screening and disease management guidelines become less relevant in such a population. The concept of preventive care for those with higher 1-year mortality should focus on maintaining health as much as possible while also preparing for functional decline and death.

The US Preventive Services Task Force (USPSTF) is a commonly cited resource for preventive screening guidelines [6]. Though these guidelines highlight the need to individualize screening decisions in older adults, they do not provide guidance for the provider regarding how to assess individual health status. Clinicians who have been trained to use standard guidelines for the general adult population may have difficulty reconciling the discrepancies between evidence-based recommendations and the real-life circumstances of potentially frail homebound patients.

Instead, the most important factors to consider when making screening recommendations to homebound older adults are the following:

1. Life expectancy and prognosis of the patient
2. Time to benefit from the screening test
3. Logistical considerations for tests that can only be obtained in a hospital setting
4. Alignment of these recommendations with what matters most

4.4.1 Life Expectancy and Prognosis

While age is a strong determinant of life expectancy, it is necessary to recognize the distinction between age and life expectancy. Because there is often a wide range of life expectancy at any given age, this distinction is especially important for clinicians when considering who to stop screening for various diseases. For example, approximately 25% of 75-year-old women will live at least 17 years, 50% will live at least 11.9 years, and 25% will live fewer than 6.8 years [7]. Though most guidelines still focus on a particular age at which to stop screening, as geriatric clinicians, it is more important to ask, "What is the prognosis of this older adult sitting in front of me?" An 85-year-old woman might have a longer life expectancy than a 70-year-old man; however, guidelines might incorrectly recommend screening the 70-year-old and to stop screening the 85-year-old. An approach that focuses on life expectancy is more appropriate. For this reason, it is important to factor in other variables that affect life expectancy [7].

If the patient's estimated life expectancy is shorter than the typical duration in which an asymptomatic patient develops the disease of interest and succumbs to it, then screening for that disease is likely not indicated. Knowing how to address the question of whether a patient will live long enough to develop and die from a screen-detectable disease requires an understanding of prognostication, disease, and screening test characteristics. There are several factors to consider when estimating an individual patient's life expectancy, such as age, sex, comorbidities, and cognitive and functional status. The National Vital Statistics System regularly maintains and updates this data, which is openly accessible. Not surprisingly, the higher the number of comorbidities, cognitive impairment, and functional impairment (e.g., frailty) are associated with a lower life expectancy [8, 9].

Keeping track of all these variables to render a prognosis is quite complicated and may not be feasible within the confines of a patient encounter. For this reason, it may be best to utilize calculators that can assist in generating an estimated mortality or life expectancy. Many such calculators exist which vary in complexity and incorporated variables. One commonly used website, Eprognosis (http://eprognosis.ucsf.edu), allows users to identify appropriate prognosis calculators based on patient location (clinic, nursing home, or hospital), comorbidities, functional status, and time frame for which prognosis is being considered (1–14 years). These calculators are based on population data.

It is also important to recognize that disease risk itself can change with age. This, in part, may be due to varying disease presentation (e.g., more indolent forms of breast cancer may be more common in older women) [10] but more likely is related to "competing risks." Older patients are more likely to die from causes other than the disease being screened. This concept is perhaps best exemplified by examining the number needed to screen to prevent one cancer death. These numbers go up dramatically as patients age, suggesting that it becomes increasingly challenging to prevent death from screen-detectable disease in the geriatric population.

4.4.2 Time to Benefit

In addition to estimating life expectancy, it is also important to consider certain characteristics of the screening test. Perhaps most important in the case of frail patients is the "lag time to benefit." This is the expected time that it takes for a patient to benefit from screening or treatment [11]. This information has historically been difficult to find and often was not included in the summary statement of screening guidelines. However, Eprognosis calculators now also include the time to benefit for common screening items and treatments. In the case of most cancers that are screened (e.g., breast and colon), the lag time is generally considered to be on the order of 10 years [11]. However, treating hypertension with intensive blood pressure control has a time to benefit of 1.5–2 years [11, 12].

4.4.3 Logistical Considerations for Tests and Treatments

In homebound patients, decisions regarding screening must also incorporate unique considerations of the burden of testing. The burden of screening may not only be related to completing the test but also to following up with diagnostic testing or treatments related to a positive finding. For example, performing a screening colonoscopy on a homebound patient might require ambulance transport to an endoscopy suite or hospitalization, which may not meet acute care criteria for medical necessity. False-positive results may occur with any preventive screening test and may lead to anxiety [13], as well as to recommendation for further testing, thus multiplying the burden to functionally impaired patients. If patients are functionally impaired (e.g., bedbound), some treatments such as chemotherapy may not even be offered.

Given the burden of screening on the homebound older adult, it is important to consider what can be tested or completed in the home. Though screening tests that are hospital-based (e.g., colonoscopy for colorectal cancer, CT scanning for lung cancer, bone density testing for osteoporosis) are largely infeasible for homebound patients, there are some tests that can rather easily be performed in the home. The widespread availability of home-based phlebotomy allows for hyperlipidemia screening, for example. Fecal occult blood testing or Cologuard can easily be done at home for colorectal carcinoma screening, and the increased availability of home-based radiologic and ultrasonographic testing allows for some testing, such as abdominal aortic aneurysm screening. In addition, common vaccinations such as influenza and pneumococcal vaccines can be easily administered to most homebound patients and are of higher utility than some other screening tests. Even vaccines for COVID-19 that require specific refrigeration can be successfully given in the home. Other vaccines, such as vaccines for shingles or tetanus, diphtheria, and pertussis, are typically not covered by insurance when given on a house call and may still need to be obtained through a pharmacy.

4.5 Use of Telemedicine in Home-Based Medicine

Although the primary focus of this chapter is on the in-person visit, telemedicine visits can be a useful adjunct to home-based medical care. In practical terms, the ability to offer an urgent in-person home visit can be challenging for many home-based clinicians, and telemedicine provides an opportunity for an urgent history and even partial exam, for patients and care partners who can connect via video. For patients who do not have video capability, telephone medicine is a specialized assessment skill that can bridge the gap between a patient's needs and the home-based medical practice's capabilities to provide urgent visits. Without telemedicine options for care, patients may suffer inconvenience, financial burden, or medical harm from potentially avoidable emergency department visits and hospitalizations. Sometimes the safest course of action will be to ask the patient or care partner to call 911, but often the question can be safely addressed with a visit within a few days, with labs or imaging, or with observation and follow-up telemedicine visits or telephone calls. Medications can be prescribed if the potential benefit outweighs the potential risk for harm; a common example is the use of antibiotics for uncomplicated cellulitis or urinary tract infection.

In summary, home-based medical care affords unique opportunities for the clinician to understand aspects of the patient's life that may not be apparent in the office visit. In addition, for older adults who cannot routinely leave their homes for office visits, home visits can be vital to preserving an older adult's independence in home as well as a crucial link to medical primary care.

References

1. Institute for Healthcare Improvement. Age-friendly health systems: guide to using the 4Ms in the care of older adults; 2020.
2. Ornstein KA, Liu SH, Husain M, et al. Prospective assessment of dementia on transitions in homeboundness using multistate Markov models. J Am Geriatr Soc. 2022;70(4):1117–26. Accessed 8 Nov 2022. https://doi.org/10.1111/jgs.17631.
3. Ornstein KA, Garrido MM, Bollens-Lund E, et al. The association between income and incident homebound status among older Medicare beneficiaries. J Am Geriatr Soc. 2020;68(11):2594–601. Accessed 8 Nov 2022. https://doi.org/10.1111/jgs.16715.
4. Soones T, Federman A, Leff B, Siu AL, Ornstein K. Two-year mortality in homebound older adults: an analysis of the national health and aging trends study. J Am Geriatr Soc. 2017;65(1):123–9. Accessed 8 Nov 2022. https://doi.org/10.1111/jgs.14467.
5. Ankuda CK, Husain M, Bollens-Lund E, et al. The dynamics of being homebound over time: a prospective study of Medicare beneficiaries, 2012-2018. J Am Geriatr Soc. 2021;69(6):1609–16. Accessed 8 Nov 2022. https://doi.org/10.1111/jgs.17086.
6. Lin JS, Perdue LA, Henrikson NB, Bean SI, Blasi PR. Screening for colorectal cancer: updated evidence report and systematic review for the US Preventive Services Task Force. JAMA. 2021;325(19):1978–98. https://jamanetwork.com/journals/jama/fullarticle/2779987. Accessed 8 Nov 2022. https://doi.org/10.1001/jama.2021.4417.
7. Yourman LC, Lee SJ, Schonberg MA, Widera EW, Smith AK. Prognostic indices for older adults: a systematic review. JAMA. 2012;307(2):182–92. Accessed 8 Nov 2022. https://doi.org/10.1001/jama.2011.1966.
8. Fried LP, Kronmal RA, Newman AB, et al. Risk factors for 5-year mortality in older adults: the cardiovascular health study. JAMA. 1998;279(8):585–92. Accessed 8 Nov 2022. https://doi.org/10.1001/jama.279.8.585.
9. Larson EB, Shadlen M, Wang L, et al. Survival after initial diagnosis of Alzheimer disease. Ann Intern Med. 2004;140(7):501–9. Accessed 8 Nov 2022. https://doi.org/10.7326/0003-4819-140-7-200404060-00008.
10. Tew WP, Muss HB, Kimmick GG, Von Gruenigen VE, Lichtman SM. Breast and ovarian cancer in the older woman. J Clin Oncol. 2014;32(24):2553–61. Accessed 8 Nov 2022. https://doi.org/10.1200/JCO.2014.55.3073.
11. Lee SJ, Boscardin WJ, Stijacic-Cenzer I, Conell-Price J, O'Brien S, Walter LC. Time lag to benefit after screening for breast and colorectal cancer: meta-analysis of survival data from the United States, Sweden, United Kingdom, and Denmark. BMJ. 2013;346:e8441. Accessed 8 Nov 2022. https://doi.org/10.1136/bmj.e8441.
12. Ho VS, Cenzer IS, Nguyen BT, Lee SJ. Time to benefit for stroke reduction after blood pressure treatment in older adults: a meta-analysis. J Am Geriatr Soc. 2022;70(5):1558–68. Accessed 8 Nov 2022. https://doi.org/10.1111/jgs.17684.
13. Tosteson ANA, Fryback DG, Hammond CS, et al. Consequences of false-positive screening mammograms. JAMA Intern Med. 2014;174(6):954–61. Accessed 8 Nov 2022. https://doi.org/10.1001/jamainternmed.2014.981.

Chapter 5
Common Cognitive Issues in Home-Based Medical Care

Mariah L. Robertson and Halima Amjad

5.1 Dementia

Dementia is an acquired progressive deterioration in global cognitive abilities that impairs the successful performance of activities of daily living (ADLs) due to an organic disease. In addition to loss of memory, other cognitive functions that may be impaired include language/communication, visuospatial recognition, executive function, and emotional regulation.

The disease can be devastating not only for the patient but also for the family. Caring for loved ones with dementia is a significant cause of care partner burden and burnout. Curative treatments do not exist. However, early recognition of dementia can help a patient and their family to prepare for the future, including getting finances in order, sorting out insurance issues, and discussing healthcare wishes, including goals of care, and choosing a healthcare proxy, while the patient is still able to participate meaningfully in the decision-making process.

M. L. Robertson (✉)
Division of Geriatric Medicine and Gerontology, Johns Hopkins University School of Medicine, Baltimore, MD, USA
e-mail: mdewsna1@jhmi.edu

H. Amjad
Division of Geriatric Medicine and Gerontology, Department of Medicine, Johns Hopkins School of Medicine, Baltimore, MD, USA
e-mail: hamjad1@jhmi.edu

J. L. Colburn et al. (eds.), *Geriatric Home-Based Medical Care*, https://doi.org/10.1007/978-3-031-68786-0_5

5.1.1 Epidemiology and Risk Factors

Approximately 10% of people over age 70 have significant memory loss. The frequency of Alzheimer's dementia (AD) increases with each decade of adult life, reaching at least 33% of the population over age 85 [1]. It is thought that by the year 2050, over 88 million people worldwide will suffer from dementia [1]. Dementia is the leading diagnosis associated with being homebound, with studies of homebound older adults showing dementia prevalence ranging from 29% to 52% [2].

AD is the most common cause of dementia, representing approximately 60% of patients with dementia. AD progresses slowly over time resulting in the loss of memory, thinking and language skills, and eventually behavioral changes [1]. Vascular dementia is the second most common dementia, usually the result of uncontrolled hypertension and cardiovascular disease. Vascular dementia usually affects reasoning, planning, judgment, memory, and other thought processes. Recurrent strokes may result in a presentation of a stepwise decrease in cognitive function.

Together, AD, vascular dementia, and the combination of AD plus vascular dementia account for over 80% of dementia diagnoses [3]. Approximately 4% of dementia diagnoses are due to Parkinson's disease (PD) [4], and the rest are made up of the following, less common, forms of dementia: frontotemporal dementia (FTD), progressive supranuclear palsy (PSP), and dementia with Lewy bodies (DLB). Frontotemporal dementia (FTD) is caused by the progressive degeneration of the temporal and frontal lobes of the brain resulting in significant changes in decision-making, behavioral control, emotion, and language [5]. PSP can result in a dementia that causes gait and balance problems, as well as visual disturbances [6, 7]. DLB is a progressive dementia that affects thinking, reasoning, and independent function and is characterized by visual hallucinations, delirium, and signs of parkinsonism, including muscle rigidity [8].

Risk factors for dementia include increasing age, family history of AD, vascular disease, alcoholism, PD, diabetes, and vitamin deficiencies [1].

5.1.2 Differential Diagnosis/Etiology

An important reason to evaluate cognitive impairment thought to be caused by dementia is to exclude modifiable or treatable causes. Medications and their side effects are frequently culprits and should be reviewed and considered first. The Beers Criteria include many potentially harmful medications for older adults [9]. Table 5.1 lists many of the key medication classes known to affect cognition. Some other common modifiable factors that can contribute to cognitive impairment are depression, hearing impairment, physical inactivity, alcohol and other substance use disorders, vitamin deficiencies, and thyroid disease [10]. Brain neoplasm is a very rare cause of dementia. Certain symptoms accompanying memory loss may serve as

Table 5.1 Medication classes that can affect cognition

Anticholinergics
Antihistamines (particularly first generation)
Overactive bladder treatments
Antispasmodics
Antidepressants (specifically paroxetine and TCAs)
Antipsychotics
Benzodiazepines
Opioids
Sedative hypnotics (e.g., zolpidem, eszopiclone)
Steroids

Table 5.2 Causes of non-Alzheimer's disease (AD)-related cognitive impairment

Type of non-AD-related cognitive impairment	Related symptoms
Normal pressure hydrocephalus	Wide-based gait, urinary incontinence Change in gait occurs well in advance of cognitive changes
Parkinson's disease	Resting tremor, stooped posture, masked facies
Dementia with Lewy bodies	Parkinsonian features with visual hallucinations, psychiatric features
Frontotemporal dementia	Changes in decision-making, increased disinhibition, poor control of emotions, problems with language
Progressive supranuclear palsy	Gait and balance problems, as well as visual disturbances
Brain neoplasms	Seizures Focal findings on neurological exam
B12 deficiency	Ataxia, fatigue, and easy bruising

clues for possible etiologies. Table 5.2 shows a list of symptoms frequently seen with non-AD-related cognitive impairment.

5.1.3 Diagnostic Approach in the Home

Evaluating a patient in the home environment presents a unique opportunity for the clinician to gather information not usually apparent during an office visit. In addition to the known clinical criteria for all-cause dementia [11] noted in Table 5.3, when evaluating a patient in the home for cognitive decline, the assessment will utilize similar evaluation tools as in an office-based setting: a thorough medical history including reviewing all medications, a physical exam with neurological exam and gait assessment for ambulatory patients, and a formal cognitive assessment.

Unique to home-based care, the effects of a person's cognitive dysfunction can be assessed by observing the condition of a person's home environment and how the

Table 5.3 Clinical criteria for all-cause dementia [11]

Cognitive or behavioral symptoms that:	
1.	Interfere with ability to complete usual activities
2.	Represent decline from previous functioning
3.	Are not explained by delirium or major psychiatric disorder
4.	Are detected through combination of history, including from knowledgeable informant, and objective clinical assessment
5.	Involve at least two of the following domains:
	– Impaired ability to acquire and remember new information
	– Impaired reasoning, handling of complex tasks, or poor judgment
	– Impaired visuospatial abilities
	– Impaired language function (speaking, reading, writing)
	– Changes in personality, behavior, or comportment

patient functions in their environment. Additionally, being able to spend time speaking with their family care partners is invaluable. In the office setting, patients are often able to present their "best side," coming in well-groomed and nicely dressed. Stepping into someone's home, you immediately begin to gather information about your patient before even laying eyes on them—clutter, disorganized medications, papers strewn about, an empty fridge, bare walls—which may all provide some insight into how someone is functioning on a day-to-day basis.

Care partners play a critical role in the care of people with dementia and it is important to assess their well-being. Please see Chap. 14.

5.2 History

A person with dementia may not be an adequate informant. It is important to include family members and care partners within and outside of the interview to obtain further history. With the patient's or proxy's consent, additional relevant history can be obtained from friends, home care workers, housekeepers, neighbors, home care nurses, previous medical providers, doormen, pharmacists, Meals on Wheels representatives, and home/community social workers.

Specific historical elements are important in the evaluation of a patient with dementia:

- Cognitive history (worsening short-term memory, word-finding difficulty, behavior changes/emotional lability)
- Functional and fall history (driving, falls, gait disturbance, changes in ADLs/IADLs)
- Head trauma (loss of consciousness)
- Stroke history (vascular disease history, remnant symptoms from prior stroke, arrhythmias, hypertension)
- Seizure history

- Movement disorder history (tremor, parkinsonism)
- Work and educational history (when stopped working and why, what they did for work, highest completed level of education)
- Recreational habits (alcohol, tobacco, cannabis, other substances)
- Eating habits (eating more sweets, dietary changes, involuntary weight loss)
- Sexual history and history of prior sexually transmitted infections (treated or untreated)
- Behavioral disturbance (onset of behavior changes, visual changes, hallucination, depression, paranoia)
- Caregiver and family support system
- Genitourinary history (any new urine/bowel incontinence)

5.3 Medication Review

Being in a patient's home affords you the opportunity to perform a thorough and accurate medication reconciliation. Seeing how your patients keep and manage their medications provides useful information about their ability to manage their medical conditions. Ask permission to look in the patient's medicine cabinets, on the kitchen counter, dining room table, bedroom tables, drawers, etc. Call the patient's pharmacy to confirm questionable medications. Check dispense dates on prescription bottles or pill packs, which provides information regarding adherence to medications. Performing a "pill count"—emptying a bottle's contents and counting the number of pills inside, looking at the fill date on the bottle, and then calculating the number of pills that should be left—can lead to valuable information regarding your patient's ability to manage their medications. Conduct a thorough review of all prescribed and over-the-counter medications, paying particular attention to medications that can alter cognition. See Table 5.1 and the Beer's Criteria [9] for a comprehensive list of medication classes that may affect cognition.

In later stages of dementia, it may be more challenging to administer medications due to behavioral issues and changes in swallow function. The benefits of many medications may not outweigh the challenges and risks of taking them. This is an important time to decide which medications may need to be continued or, when essential, to convert them to formulations that can be crushed or are in liquid form.

5.4 Physical Exam

When conducting a thorough physical examination, be sure to gather the following information, which helps with staging dementia and in some instances may also help determine if there is a modifiable cause for the memory loss [12]:

- Vital signs: orthostatic blood pressures (especially if patient has a history of syncope/dizziness)
- Skin: assess for infected decubitus ulcers or skin or soft tissue infections
- Eyes: cataracts, visual impairment, double vision, extraocular movement
- Ears: cerumen impaction, hearing loss
- Cardiac: murmurs, irregular rhythm, pacemaker/automated implantable cardioverter defibrillator (AICD)
- Neuro: carotid bruits, cranial nerves, deep tendon reflexes, tremor, rigidity, bradykinesia, myoclonic twitching, agnosia, apraxia, aphasia, gait disturbances

5.5 Cognitive and Functional Assessment Tools

If feasible, conduct cognitive and functional assessment tests without family or care partners present to avoid distractions or potential patient embarrassment. It is important to put the patient at ease. Explain the findings and recommendations to the patient. Obtain consent, when possible, to share findings with family members/care partners. Choose the appropriate cognitive assessment tool based on your clinical findings and the amount of time you have available.

Table 5.4 lists some commonly used cognitive assessment tools available and the amount of time they take to administer. These cognitive tools may be influenced by patient's age, educational level, language, attention, visuospatial ability, and reduced attention. In combination with a good history and physical examination, these tools are usually sufficient to make a diagnosis.

Table 5.4 Cognitive status assessment tools [10]

Test	Description	Scoring	Limitations	Time to administer
Mini-Cog	Consists of recall of three unrelated words and clock drawing test	If no words recalled, diagnosis is dementia If one or two out of three words recalled, look at the clock draw test. If abnormal, diagnosis is dementia If all numbers on the clock are presented in the correct sequence and the hands display the correct time, no dementia	Quick screening test, not diagnostic Requires the physical ability to write or draw	<5 min

(continued)

Table 5.4 (continued)

Test	Description	Scoring	Limitations	Time to administer
GPCog	Screening test that includes both a patient questionnaire with orientation, recall, clock drawing, and current events and an informant questionnaire to gather family/caregiver perspective. Specific to the primary care setting and not influenced by cultural or linguistic background	Patient score: 9 = no impairment, no informant testing 5–8 = more information required from informant 0–4 = cognitive impairment, work-up indicated	Requires the physical ability to write or draw	4 min for patient portion 2 min for informant portion
Mini-Mental State Examination (MMSE)	Tests a broad range of cognitive functions including orientation, recall, attention, calculation, language manipulation, and constructional praxis	Maximum score is 30; score must be adjusted based on education, language, and age; <24 implies dementia	Limited by education level, literacy, and language. The patient should have at least an eighth-grade education and be fluent in English Test is copyrighted	10 min
Montreal Cognitive Assessment (MoCA)	Tests a broad range of cognitive functions including orientation, memory recall, visuospatial relations, sustained attention, verbal fluency, and executive function. Available in 35 languages or dialects. MoCA Blind available for visually impaired patients	Maximum score is 30; <26 implies mild cognitive impairment or dementia (dementia diagnosis dependent on presence of associated functional impairment)	Limited by education level and literacy Test is copyrighted	10 min

(continued)

Table 5.4 (continued)

Test	Description	Scoring	Limitations	Time to administer
Saint Louis University Mental Status Exam (SLUMS)	Tests a broad range of cognitive functions including attention, orientation, recall, registration, digit span, visual spatial, and executive function. Available in many different languages	Maximum score is 30 27–30: normal if HS educated 21–26: mild neurocognitive disorder 0–20: indicates dementia Adjust two points lower for non-HS educated patients	Developed in the veteran population and less tested in more diverse populations	4–10 min
PHQ-2 and PHQ-9	Concise tool to screen and assess for major depression and for monitoring treatment and changes in depression	If score 1 or 2 on the PHQ-2, suggested next step is to complete the PHQ-9 0–4 normal 5–9 mild 10–14 moderate 15–19 moderate to severe 20–27 severe	Designed to be self-administered, which may be impacted by literacy and education level	2–5 min
Geriatric Depression Screening—15	It is a series of 15 yes/no questions	0–4 considered normal 5–8 indicates mild depression 9–11 indicates moderate depression 12–15 indicates severe depression	Successful in differentiating depressed from nondepressed	10 min

5.5.1 *Tests*

The home-based clinician may consider appropriate lab work to diagnose modifiable causes of cognitive changes. Table 5.5 lists laboratory tests to consider ordering and what each test evaluates.

Obtain consent to gather medical records for any previous head imaging studies, electrocardiograms, EEG, and lab results for comparison. Neuroimaging can be helpful in the exclusion of secondary causes of dementia, such as masses or normal pressure hydrocephalus, and a finding of medial temporal lobe atrophy on MRI, for example, supports a clinical diagnosis of AD [10, 13]. New imaging modalities have emerged including fMRI and amyloid PET scanning; however, these are primarily

Table 5.5 Laboratory tests for evaluating modifiable causes of cognitive changes

Laboratory test	Evaluating for
Complete blood count (CBC)	Possible infection, immune disorders, anemia, blood disorder
Comprehensive metabolic panel (CMP)	Metabolic disturbance (e.g., hyponatremia), kidney, liver disorders
Calcium level	Parathyroid, malignancy
Thyroid-stimulating hormone (TSH) level	Thyroid, endocrine disorders
Vitamin B12, folate, iron level	Nutritional, vitamin deficiency
Erythrocyte sedimentation level	Signs of inflammation
RPR	Neurosyphilis
HIV, hepatitis	Viral infections
Lyme titers	Affecting central nervous system
Urine analysis and urine toxicology screening	Blood, protein, rarely infection (though testing and treating infection should be limited to those who are symptomatic and should be supported by culture data), substances that could be affecting cognition
Drug levels: e.g., dilantin (phenytoin), digoxin	Drug toxicity affecting cognition

used in research studies and are not meant to replace a physical exam and clinical diagnosis of dementia. Normal brain imaging does not rule out dementia.

In situations where you cannot obtain past records or the patient has not had any past imaging, it is important to use your clinical judgment as to whether you think it is of value to obtain imaging. Clinical context always matters. In a patient with a history of high blood pressure and strokes, with a stepwise decline in cognition, imaging is unlikely to reveal anything other than vascular changes. NPH will present with clinical exam findings; you do not need a CT or MRI to rule it out. Did you find a focal deficit on the neurologic exam? Is there something about the patient's presentation or history that points you away from thinking their cognitive changes are due to AD or vascular dementia? Would it be incredibly challenging to get them out of the home to obtain imaging? Will the results change your management based on the goals of care? These are all questions to consider before deciding to recommend imaging. In patients with a history consistent with AD and non-focal neurological examination, our practice is to forego brain imaging if it would be difficult to obtain.

5.5.2 *Pharmacologic Treatment*

5.5.2.1 Alzheimer's Disease

Medications indicated for Alzheimer's dementia have been shown to have a minimal effect on slowing the progression of disease. As such, the mainstay of treatment is not pharmacological.

Medications should be used cautiously under close monitoring, particularly given the fact that homebound older adults are already at high risk for polypharmacy [14]. The mantra "start low, go slow" should be considered when it comes to dosing of these medications. Medications for Alzheimer's dementia have shown to minimally improve scores on cognitive function tests but still have not shown improvement in the ability of patients to perform activities of daily living (ADL) or instrumental activities of daily living (IADL), which would be more likely to translate into improvement in the quality of life of these patients.

Cholinesterase inhibitors (AChEI) and noncompetitive *N*-methyl-D-aspartate (NMDA) receptor antagonist are currently the medications approved for Alzheimer's dementia. There is no difference in the efficacies of the different cholinesterase inhibitors [15].

Medications approved for the treatment of dementia are described in Table 5.6. Often patients' family members will ask to start their loved one on a medication they have seen advertised to help people with dementia. We take this as an opportunity to educate them on the limited efficacy of these medications as a means of setting realistic expectations. If it is the family's wish to try one of the medications, we review the potential major side effects of the medications and offer a 6–12-month trial, making it clear that they can stop the medication at any time if they are concerned about side effects. After 6–12 months, we review together whether any beneficial changes have been observed, and if not, we do not write a new prescription. The pharmacologic treatment of vascular dementia focuses on management of risk factors for hypertension and hyperlipidemia to avoid further deterioration of the vascular system in the brain.

At times patients come to us on more than one memory medication at a time. In many cases, by the time someone is homebound, they are in the later stages of dementia, and we discuss deprescribing these medications in a stepwise manner as the likelihood they are benefiting the patient is lower at this stage. Though they may be used concurrently and have different mechanisms of action, there is no clear evidence that the combination of cholinesterase inhibitors and NMDA receptor agonists improves cognition in meaningful ways. However, being on multiple medications may cause untoward side effects. If a patient or family wishes to continue multiple medications, enhanced monitoring of side effects or significant progression of dementia is warranted.

Recently, new medications that target amyloid plaque protein deposits in the brain have come on the market (including aducanumab and lecanemab) for treating mild AD [16]. Unfortunately, these medications have not been as effective as hoped and have significant side effects including brain swelling and bleeding. Most homebound older adults with dementia would not qualify for these medications because of the stage of their dementia and associated risks of treatment outweighing benefits. For this reason, we have not included these medications in Table 5.6.

Table 5.6 Pharmacological treatment for dementia

Medications	Dosing	Major side effects
Cholinesterase inhibitors		
Donepezil (Aricept)	Mild to moderate dementia	Neuro: seizures, syncope, altered sleep with vivid dreams, neuroleptic malignant syndrome (NMS)
	5 mg PO QHS for 4–6 weeks, then increased to target dose of 10 mg PO QHS	Cardiac: symptomatic bradycardia
		MSK: muscle cramps
		GI: nausea, diarrhea, anorexia
Rivastigmine (Exelon, Exelon patch)	Mild to moderate AD	Neuro: seizures, syncope, depression, hallucinations
	1.5 mg PO BID, increased by 1.5 mg PO BID Q2 weeks as tolerated to target dose of 6 mg PO BID Some studies have shown improvement in side effects when given in three times daily dosing	Cardiac: bradycardia, hypotension GI: vomiting, diarrhea, peptic ulcer, GI bleeding
	Transdermal patch:	Skin irritation can occur with the transdermal patch. Rotate sites to avoid irritation when possible
	4.6 mg patch daily for 4 weeks, increased to 9.5 mg patch daily for 4 weeks, and then increased to target dose of 13.3 mg patch daily	
	Mild to moderate PDD	
	1.5 mg PO BID, increased by 1.5 mg PO BID Q4 weeks as tolerated to target dose of 6 mg PO BID	
	Transdermal patch:	
	4.6 mg patch daily for 4 weeks, increased to 9.5 mg patch daily for 4 weeks, and then increased to target dose of 13.3 mg patch daily	

(continued)

Table 5.6 (continued)

Medications	Dosing	Major side effects
Galantamine (Razadyne and Razadyne ER)	Mild to moderate AD	Neuro: syncope, dizziness
	Regular:	Cardiac: bradycardia
	Start 4 mg PO BID, increased to 4 mg PO BID Q4 weeks as tolerated to maximum of 12 mg PO BID	GI: vomiting, nausea, anorexia, weight loss. Give med with meals to improve these symptoms
		Renal: renal impairment or failure
		Liver: hepatotoxicity
	ER:	
	Start 8 mg PO QAM, increased by 8 mg PO QAM Q4 weeks to maximum of 24 mg PO QAM	
	If either form is stopped for more than 3 days, medication must be restarted at 8 mg and retitrated up	
	Medication should be renally dosed, not advised for patients with liver problems	
Noncompetititve N-methyl-D-aspartate (NMDA) receptor antagonist		
Memantine (Namenda)	Moderate to severe AD	Neuro: dizziness, headache, somnolence, anxiety
	Start 5 mg PO daily, increased to 5 mg PO BID at 1 week as tolerated, and then increased by 5 mg weekly to a maximum of 10 mg PO BID	Pulm: dyspnea
		GI: vomiting, constipation
		GU: urinary incontinence
		MSK: back pain

AD Alzheimer's dementia, *BID* twice a day, *ER* extended release, *GI* gastrointestinal, *GU* genitourinary, *MSK* musculoskeletal, *PO* by mouth, *PDD* Parkinson's disease with dementia, *QAM* every morning, *QHS* at bedtime

5.5.2.2 Behavioral and Psychological Symptoms of Dementia (BPSD)

Neuropsychiatric symptoms in dementia are very common and expected and can, in many cases, be very difficult for care partners to manage in the home [17]. Some of the prevalent behavioral and psychological symptoms among community-dwelling residents with dementia are repetitions, apathy, depression, agitation, aggression, delusions, anxiety, hallucinations, and wandering [18]. As a person living with dementia progresses in their disease process, it can be increasingly challenging for them to communicate their needs and understand the things happening around them.

5.5.3 Managing the Behavioral and Psychologic Symptoms of Dementia (BPSD) Through Non-pharmacologic Means

The mainstay of treatment for dementia behavioral symptoms is non-pharmacologic. Caring for someone afflicted with dementia involves a multipronged approach to help improve the quality of life of the patient and care partners, manage active symptoms, and plan for the future.

Non-pharmacological interventions can benefit the care partner/family by alleviating some more challenging behavioral manifestations of dementia.

Educating patients and caregivers about dementia is an important first step. Assess patient, family, and caregiver knowledge about the disease process. Ask the patient, family, and care partners to explain in their own words what their understanding of dementia is and how it is affecting them. Educating care partners family, friends, and homecare workers about the disease process will assist in improving communication for timely interventions to reduce or eliminate behaviors.

Early referral to any of the following resources can give needed support to families caring for loved ones with dementia: social workers within your own practice, in a Medicare-certified home health agency, or in the community, the Alzheimer's Association, or the Department of Aging. These resources help reinforce your teaching in the home and also may offer support groups.

Effective communication with the patient is a mainstay in managing disruptive behaviors due to cognitive impairment, especially in the early stages of the disease process. Be sure to allow adequate time for the patient to communicate their thoughts. Communication can be facilitated through visual cues, by remaining at the patient's eye level and speaking softly and slowly in a quiet place. If the patient uses glasses or hearing aids, be sure to make them available [19].

Agitation, aggression, confusion, irritability, delusions, and hallucinations are common and persistent behavioral symptoms that may have multiple etiologies. The most frequent cause of the behavioral change may be related to acute delirium, discussed later in this chapter, or to modifiable environmental factors.

Careful clinical observations often reveal environment-related causes for behaviors. Finding the trigger is essential in reducing or eliminating the behaviors.

A three-step ABC approach may be used to identify the behavior disturbance.

1. *Antecedents*: What are the triggering events to minimize or eliminate?
2. *Behavior*: Describe the behavior in detail. How often does it occur, how and where it is most likely to happen, and how long does it last?
3. *Consequences*: How does the caregiver, family member, or home care worker react to reinforce or deter the activity, and what happens when the activity ceases?

Identifying trigger events and working to navigate them in patient-centered ways can help to reduce, eliminate, or prevent the events.

Conduct a home environment assessment; dementia behaviors can be brought on by triggers from the home environment. Table 5.7 shows interventions to improve behaviors that are responses to the home environment.

Structured activities can also decrease behaviors of dementia. Write out a prescription with one personal care goal for the patient who declines bathing or personal care. Provide visual or sensory cues such as colorful calendar to indicate events, bathing, toileting, meals, exercise, or bedtime.

Sensory stimuli intervention, such as doll therapy, music, and reminiscing therapy, can be done in the home by care partners to help reduce anxiety and worry.

Table 5.7 Behaviors seen in dementia, possible environmental triggers, and suggested interventions [19]

Behavior	Trigger	Therapeutic intervention
Awake at night	Bright light during nighttime	Make living area bright, preferably with natural light, during the daytime
		Turn off TVs and radios at night
		Lower shades/curtains at night
		Use night lights
Pacing	Dark room/poor lighting	Add upward-facing light fixtures
	Sensation of confinement	Place pictures over doorways to prevent wandering
	Shadows can trigger visual hallucination	Place stop signs as visual cues
		Paint the walls with neutral colors
Refusing to shower	Fear of falling, fear of being unclothed with "strangers"	Place a colorful bathmat in tub so the patient can see there is a bottom to the tub, allow them to bathe partially clothed or in their swimsuit, great resource: bathing without a battle [20]
Overstimulation	Elevated noise level, multiple external stimuli	Reduce noise level on television, move to a less high-traffic space (e.g., small children, kitchen noises)
Restlessness	Room temperature too cold or too hot	Monitor and adjust room temperature to comfort level, remove or add layers to help with temperature regulation

Doll therapy enhances participation in activities of daily living and personal care. Dolls have been found to be useful in reducing anxiety, withdrawal behaviors, depression, and mild agitation [21]. The Alzheimer's Association has an online Alzheimer's store where therapeutic products such as dolls can be purchased. Family members, care partners, nurses, and home care workers can use the therapeutic object when behaviors emerge as a means of engaging participation.

Music therapy has demonstrated decreases in overall agitation during personal care. Ask family members to choose the music and to monitor the patient's reactions to the music being played. Classical, nature, and instrumental music may be soothing during meals, during sleep, or when agitated [22].

Reminiscence therapy is used to decrease behaviors such as agitation, anxiety, or confusion. Patients become engaged in open-ended questions about their life. Using open-ended questions allows the patient to tell their story. If available, have them look at a picture album and describe the events in the pictures. An enjoyable event in their past is not confusing to them and they often become engaged.

Supportive care for family and caregivers is invaluable [14]. Spending time in your patients' homes lets you see the depth and breadth of supportive care provided to your patients by those around them and at the same time gives you a fuller sense of which care partners may need more support than others. Acknowledge all the work they do in the home and ask how they find time for themselves, what they do to relax, and whom they turn to for support. Most care partners have unmet needs for resource referrals and caregiver education. Encourage care partners to educate themselves about the disease as well as non-pharmacologic management by providing resources and problem-solving skills.

The Alzheimer's Association is an important resource for many care partners, including their 24-h call line. Home medical providers should refer appropriate patients to home nursing agencies for home safety evaluations and care partner education. A referral to social work or case management can be used to educate care partners about community resources such as day or night programs, as well as potential options for respite care arrangements. See "Further Reading" at the end of the chapter for additional information, and please see Chap. 13 for more details on supporting care partners.

A detailed discussion of pharmacologic management of dementia and delirium behaviors will be highlighted below in the delirium section.

5.5.4 *Prognosis*

Discussing prognosis with patients and their families is important. While the decline of a patient with dementia tends to follow a known course, the timeline is often difficult to predict. Dementia is a terminal illness. The prognosis for AD is typically 7–10 years after diagnosis but can range from 1 to 25 years [23]. However, once a patient has advanced dementia and is bedbound, relying on others for all their care, the 6-month mortality rate is 25%, with a median survival of 1.3 years [23].

Table 5.8 Stages of dementia

Stage	Description
Mild/early[a]	Subtle deficits in short-term memory or other cognitive domains, decreased knowledge of current or recent events, some deficit in memory of personal history, decreased ability to perform complex tasks such as handling finances, medications, or technology
Moderate/middle[a]	Requires assistance with additional complex or instrumental activities of daily living and then basic activities of daily living (dressing, bathing, toileting); unable to survive independently; difficulty recalling major aspects of their lives; increasing disorientation to time; behavioral symptoms more common or significant
Severe/late	Diminished verbal abilities; decreased awareness of environment and situation; incontinent; requiring help with all basic activities of daily living including feeding; declining psychomotor skills with worsened mobility
End-stage	Characteristics of severe stage plus loss of ability to ambulate, sit, or hold head up without assistance; loss of ability to smile; hospice agencies will also consider additional comorbidities and experience of secondary conditions such as delirium, recurrent or intractable infections or sepsis, decubitus ulcers, recurrent fevers, weight loss or malnutrition, inability to maintain hydration, aspiration pneumonia, dysphagia, or diminished oral intake

[a] Cognitive domains most significantly affected during mild and moderate stages may vary based upon dementia type

The cause of death for either usually stems from difficulty in moving, eating, and swallowing—pressure ulcers, aspiration pneumonia, and urinary retention with associated infection. Over 50% of patients with advanced dementia who have an episode of pneumonia will die in the next 6 months [23]. Table 5.8 shows the stages of dementia and common characteristics of each stage.

Previously, it was thought that feeding tubes would prevent aspiration among people with dementia who could no longer feed themselves. This is not true. Feeding tubes do not prevent aspiration or provide any mortality benefit; they may cause pain and discomfort and deprive a patient of potential comfort and enjoyment that feeding and eating can provide. Talking with families about these findings is helpful when feeding tube consideration arises [24, 25]. Patients with vascular dementia tend to die from stroke, heart disease, or infection. Patients suffering from FTD and PSP have a shorter life expectancy given earlier age of onset and worse prognosis [26].

Regular discussions with care partners concerning likely future events in the course of dementia should be undertaken. At each visit thereafter, it is helpful to end by giving them a brief summary of where you see the patient at this point of time and what interventions may help them remain comfortable at home. End-of-life issues, including palliative care and hospice referral, are discussed in Chap. 13.

Dementia clinical practice guidelines [27] are available to facilitate comprehensive, systematic person-centered care for older adults with dementia. Table 5.9 summarizes key aspects of comprehensive dementia clinical care across existing practice guidelines.

Table 5.9 Dementia clinical care recommendations consistent across different guidelines [27]

Care domain	Description
General non-pharmacologic management	• Incorporate values, cultures, and specific needs in care plans and interventions • Encourage exercise and recreational activities • Encourage participation in cognitively stimulating activities • Be aware of abuse risk and report as required by law • Provide information at all stages on available community and medical resources • Regularly re-evaluate disease progression, including cognitive and functional decline
Management of cognitive symptoms	• Involve patient and family in pharmacotherapy decision, including discussion of medication risks, benefits, and side effects • Assess and monitor changes in medications, effects, and adherence at every visit • Educate caregiver on expected changes, communication, and support strategies
Evaluation and management of behavioral symptoms	• Assess for behavioral symptoms at regular intervals • Identify and treat delirium that may be contributing • Emphasize non-pharmacologic strategies to address behavioral symptoms • Use medications sparingly, only after non-pharmacologic approaches have failed. Low doses should be used and carefully uptitrated; taper and discontinue when possible • Advise patients and families on the risks and benefits prior to starting medications
Evaluation and management of mood and other symptoms	• Evaluate for comorbid depression • Non-pharmacologic therapy is recommended first • In severe disease or after failed non-pharmacologic therapies, use an antidepressant • Assess for pain and constipation
Evaluation of safety	• Evaluate and advise on driving ability, following state laws for reporting • Assess and address home safety, fall risk, and wandering risk • Consider other potential safety issues, such as self-managing medications and cooking
Caregiver support	• Regularly evaluate and address caregiver needs • Cognitive behavioral therapy or psychotherapy is beneficial for caregivers facing psychological morbidity • Anticipate financial impact and discuss potential benefits available
Decision-making and advanced care planning	• Discuss use of advanced directives and identify surrogates for medical and legal decision-making • Discuss advanced planning regarding cardiopulmonary resuscitation, including discussion of poor outcomes in advanced dementia. Complete medical orders for life-sustaining treatment if available within state regulations • Assess patient decision-making capacity
Palliative care	• End-of-life issues should be discussed with patients and families as appropriate • Tube feeding is discouraged

5.6 Delirium

Delirium is a clinical syndrome characterized by an acute and fluctuating change in cognition and attention. Delirium, both in its hyperactive and hypoactive forms, is distressing for family and patients and associated with increased care partner burden [28]. Hyperactive delirium is the more recognizable form of delirium, noted for mood lability, hallucinations, delusions, and agitation. Hypoactive delirium is more frequently missed or misdiagnosed, as it usually presents as lethargy; family and medical professionals often mistake it for depression or fatigue. Both forms of delirium are associated with increased morbidity and mortality. Treatment is focused on diagnosing and treating the underlying condition causing the delirium.

While the literature mainly focuses on delirium in the hospital setting, it is a common occurrence among homebound patients in response to changes in medications, environmental changes, and symptoms such as pain which can lead to confusion, anxiety, and agitation. Delirium is appropriately challenging and distressing for patients and their care partners and is important to identify and manage as an urgent concern.

5.6.1 *Risk Factors*

Risk factors for delirium include dementia, advanced age (over 65), illness, and polypharmacy and medication changes. It is estimated that 30–40% of cases of delirium are preventable [29]. Up to two-thirds of older adults with delirium have underlying dementia [30].

5.6.2 *Etiologies*

The etiologies of delirium are diverse and multifactorial, often reflecting the consequences of an acute medical illness or effects of a drug [30]. Common underlying causes of delirium include the following:

- Medication side effects, withdrawal and interactions (see Table 5.1)
- Infection
- Volume depletion/dehydration
- Pain
- Constipation
- Sleep deprivation
- Metabolic imbalances—e.g., calcium, sodium, or glucose
- Hypoxia
- Ischemia
- Sensory deprivation—e.g., are they missing their glasses or hearing aids?

- Environmental changes—e.g., a recent move, a hospitalization, and change in caregiver
- Substance withdrawal—e.g., alcohol, tobacco, or other substances [28, 30–32]

5.6.3 Investigations at Home

Delirium is a clinical diagnosis; there is no lab test or imaging study that provides greater accuracy in the diagnosis of delirium than the confusion assessment method (CAM) algorithm. The diagnosis of delirium can be made quickly (sometimes within seconds) at a patient's bedside without any lab tests or studies.

The CAM algorithm is a quick, validated screening tool, with high sensitivity and specificity [33]. The CAM algorithm assesses the patient for: (1) acute onset of confusion with a fluctuating course, (2) inattention, (3) disorganized thinking, and (4) altered level of consciousness [34].

Since its development, many different derivations of the CAM have been developed, including the 3D CAM, a 3-min assessment tool that is effective and easily applied at bedside in the home [35]. See Table 5.10 for the details fo the CAM assessment method [34–36].

Table 5.10 Confusion assessment method algorithm [34]

Criteria	Assessment method
1. Acute onset and fluctuating course	Caregivers and family members are often the best sources for this information. Did the confusion present over hours to days? Do the symptoms fluctuate during the course of a day?
2. Inattention	Observe the patient—are they easily distracted, or over-absorbed in a task, such as picking at the bed sheet?
	Two ways to test attention are as follows:
	Asking the patient to recite the months of the year backward (abnormal if unable to do so correctly)
	Digit span test: Having the patient repeat a series of random numbers presented at a rate of 1 per second. First, give a two-number sequence and if the patient repeats the sequence correctly, then give a three-number sequence. Continue adding one digit to each subsequent sequence. A digit span of less than 5 is considered to be abnormal
3a. Disorganized thinking	Ask patient an open-ended question, such as "Describe your medical condition"
	Listen for rambling, incoherent speech, or tangential thought process
3b. Altered level of consciousness	Does the patient respond to their name?
	Overall, would you rate the patient's level of consciousness as alert (normal), vigilant (hyperalert), lethargic (drowsy, easily aroused), stupor (difficult to arouse), or coma (unarousable)? Any answer other than "alert" counts

If patients have either 1 or 2 and 3a or 3b, it is considered a positive screen for delirium, warranting further work-up and intervention

5.6.3.1 History

If the cause of the delirium is due to a general medical condition, the diagnosis can often be made with a good history, thorough physical examination, and basic laboratory testing. The history should focus on the reversible risk factors listed above, including a thorough review of prescribed and over-the-counter medications in the home, looking for high-risk medications.

5.6.3.2 Physical Exam

Examination of the patient should focus on the potential causes, including an exam for signs of infection, pain, and shortness of breath. Constipation and urinary retention are especially common causes in homebound persons.

5.6.3.3 Tests

Labs and imaging should be ordered as guided by physical exam findings. Consider ordering a complete blood count (CBC), comprehensive metabolic panel (CMP), urinalysis and/or bladder scan when signs of infection or retention are present, and/or chest X-ray (CXR) if concern for pulmonary findings or possible infection. Additional labs should be based on specific symptoms. Treatment of asymptomatic bacteriuria in delirious patients is not recommended unless a urinary catheter is present [37], and a head CT is not warranted in the absence of focal findings.

5.6.4 Non-pharmacologic Management of Delirium

Successful treatment of delirium requires correction of all remediable factors. Given the multifactorial nature of delirium, especially in older adults, it may not be possible to identify a single cause.

Nondrug therapy is key and should be the initial course of action. Frequent engagement, gentle reorientation, and socialization for patients with delirium or who are at risk for delirium are key maneuvers. It is important to maintain a routine and schedule as much as possible. Take advantage of the home setting by having care partners present patients with familiar photos and objects found in the home (much like discussed above in the non-pharmacologic management of dementia). Instruct the care partner to ask the patient to name the people in pictures, and if they cannot remember, do tell them who is pictured and ask about the person or event documented. If family members and friends live near, let them know that it can be helpful to remain a presence in their loved one's life, visiting with consistency when possible.

Sensory deprivation can lead to delirium and can be improved by providing adequate sensory input. Ensure patients wear their eyeglasses and hearing aids, if appropriate. Encourage care partners to sit with the patient at various times during the day, such as at meals and when watching television. Encourage conversation about topics of interest.

Medication effects may be improved by removal of an offending agent and the observation of the patient. Non-pharmacologic treatment of pain can include massage or pressure point therapy. Hypoxia can be rectified by giving supplemental oxygen. Remind care partners to pay careful attention to nutrition and hydration status, as older patients do not feel the same sense of thirst and/or may have difficulty accessing food and drink. Assistance with meals, including possible hand feeding and offering drinks, may be necessary to reverse hunger or volume depletion. Facilitate the adoption of healthy sleep–wake cycles in patients at risk for delirium and encourage night sleeping by reducing environmental stimuli within the home, including turning off televisions and radios at night and opening window blinds and increasing home light sources during the day.

Educate the patient's family and care partners that recovery from delirium can be a slow process even after the underlying cause is addressed and reversed. Patients may remain delirious for weeks to months despite resolution of the underlying cause.

5.6.5 Pharmacologic Treatment of Dementia and Delirium

As noted above, the non-pharmacologic approach is the mainstay in symptom control in both dementia and delirium, but providers do turn to antipsychotics when they are having great difficulty managing patients' behaviors or acute delirium without medication, or when the patient or care partner is unsafe due to the patient's behaviors. While some of these medications can be, at least initially, very sedating (which may offer care partners some respite from an extremely agitated patient), they have not been shown to be effective in ameliorating the behavioral disturbances they are used to treat [17, 38, 39], and they carry a black-box warning stating that older adults with dementia-related psychosis treated with conventional or atypical antipsychotic drugs are at an increased risk of death compared to placebo [40].

Prescribing an antipsychotic to treat psychosis, aggression, or agitation in someone with dementia and overlying delirium must be done with caution and the understanding that overall, the adverse effects have been found to outweigh any benefits. Table 5.11 shows medications used by many clinicians to manage delirium as well as the behavioral symptoms in dementia. All uses of these medications to treat behavioral disturbances associated with dementia are off-label.

Initiate drug therapy cautiously to manage agitation in delirium, and be prepared to discontinue or change medications if the patient's agitation does not respond. These medications are meant for short-term use; once the patient's agitation is well controlled and the underlying cause for the delirium is addressed, begin to taper these medications slowly until they can be discontinued.

Avoid opioids, benzodiazepines, and cholinesterase inhibitors if possible in patients with delirium. Sedating agents are thought to worsen or prolong delirium. Cholinesterase inhibitors have not been shown to be effective in improving delirium [40].

Table 5.11 Pharmacologic treatment for agitation associated with delirium and dementia [36]

Medications	Dosing	Major side effects
Antidepressants		
Citalopram	Start at 10 mg daily and uptitrate, usually waiting at least 1–2 weeks but as long as 4 weeks to see maximal benefit. Can increase to 20 mg max for patients >40 years of age	Neuro: mania or hypomania in undiagnosed bipolar, serotonin syndrome
		Cardiac: QT prolongation
		Heme: bleeding (particularly in combination with antiplatelet, anticoagulating, or NSAID medications)
		Renal: hyponatremia
		GU: sexual dysfunction
		Bone: increased fragility fractures
		Ophthalmologic: acute angle closure glaucoma
Typical antipsychotic		
Haloperidol (Haldol)	Start 0.5 mg PO BID, titrate to lowest effective dose first by increasing frequency to max of q4h, then increasing dose with a maximum of 10 mg PO q4h	Neuro: TD, dystonia, EPS, NMS, seizures
		Cardiac: hypotension, hypertension, QT prolongation, torsades de pointes, arrythmias, sudden death
		Pulmonary: pneumonia
		Heme: agranulocytosis, neutropenia, leukopenia
Atypical antipsychotics		
Olanzapine (Zyprexa, Zyprexa Zydis)	Start at 2.5 mg daily, increase to BID as needed, titrating up to a maximum of 5 mg BID	Neuro: NMS, TD, EPS, stroke syncope, seizures
		Endocrine: severe hyperglycemia
		Cardiac: hypotension, hyperlipidemia
		GI: hepatotoxicity, pancreatitis
		Pulmonary: dysphagia, aspiration
		Heme: anemia, thrombocytopenia, agranulocytosis, neutropenia, leukopenia
		Renal: rhabdomyolysis
		Heme: agranulocytosis, neutropenia, leukopenia

(continued)

Table 5.11 (continued)

Medications	Dosing	Major side effects
Risperidone (Risperdal)	Start at 0.25 mg PO daily, titrate to lowest effective dose first by increasing frequency to BID, then by increasing dose by 0.25 mg per week, with a maximum of 4 mg total daily	Neuro: EPS, TD, NMS, seizure, syncope
		Cardiac: TIA, stroke, hypotension, QT prolongation
		Endocrine: severe hyperglycemia
		Psych: suicidality
Quetiapine (Seroquel, Seroquel XR)	Start at 25 mg PO BID, titrate to lowest effective dose, to a maximum of 100 mg BID	Neuro: EPS, TD, NMS, dystonia, seizures, syncope
		Endocrine: hyperglycemia
		Cardiac: TIA, stroke, hypotension
		Psych: suicidality, depression
		Heme: agranulocytosis, neutropenia, leukopenia

BID twice daily, *EPS* extrapyramidal symptoms, *NMS* neuroleptic malignant syndrome, *PO* by mouth, *TIA* transient ischemic attack, *TD* tardive dyskinesia

References

1. 2022 Alzheimer's disease facts and figures. Alzheimers Dement. 2022;18(4):700–89.
2. Yang M, Pajewski N, Espeland M, Easterling D, Williamson JD. Modifiable risk factors for homebound progression among those with and without dementia in a longitudinal survey of community-dwelling older adults. BMC Geriatr. 2021;21(1):561.
3. O'Brien JT, Thomas A. Vascular dementia. Lancet. 2015;386(10004):1698–706.
4. Aarsland D, Zaccai J, Brayne C. A systematic review of prevalence studies of dementia in Parkinson's disease. Mov Disord. 2005;20(10):1255–63.
5. Gomperts SN. Lewy body dementias: dementia with Lewy bodies and Parkinson disease dementia. Continuum (Minneap Minn). 2016;22(2 Dementia):435–63.
6. Bang J, Spina S, Miller BL. Frontotemporal dementia. Lancet. 2015;386(10004):1672–82.
7. Armstrong MJ. Progressive supranuclear palsy: an update. Curr Neurol Neurosci Rep. 2018;18(3):12.
8. Savica R, Grossardt BR, Bower JH, Boeve BF, Ahlskog JE, Rocca WA. Incidence of dementia with Lewy bodies and Parkinson disease dementia. JAMA Neurol. 2013;70(11):1396.
9. American Geriatrics Society 2019 updated AGS Beers Criteria® for potentially inappropriate medication use in older adults. J Am Geriatr Soc. 2019;67(4):674–94.
10. Ranson JM, Rittman T, Hayat S, Brayne C, Jessen F, Blennow K, et al. Modifiable risk factors for dementia and dementia risk profiling. A user manual for Brain Health Services—part 2 of 6. Alzheimers Res Ther. 2021;13(1):169.
11. McKhann GM, Knopman DS, Chertkow H, Hyman BT, Jack CR, Kawas CH, et al. The diagnosis of dementia due to Alzheimer's disease: recommendations from the National Institute on Aging-Alzheimer's Association workgroups on diagnostic guidelines for Alzheimer's disease. Alzheimers Dement. 2011;7(3):263–9.
12. Arvanitakis Z, Shah RC, Bennett DA. Diagnosis and management of dementia: review. JAMA. 2019;322(16):1589–99.
13. Bonifacio G, Zamboni G. Brain imaging in dementia. Postgrad Med J. 2016;92(1088):333–40.
14. Lyketsos CG, Colenda CC, Beck C, Blank K, Doraiswamy MP, Kalunian DA, et al. Position statement of the American Association for Geriatric Psychiatry regarding principles of care for patients with dementia resulting from Alzheimer disease. Am J Geriatr Psychiatry. 2006;14(7):561–73.

15. Birks JS. Cholinesterase inhibitors for Alzheimer's disease. Cochrane Database Syst Rev. 2006;2016(3).
16. Woloshin S, Kesselheim AS. What to know about the Alzheimer Drug Aducanumab (Aduhelm). JAMA Intern Med. 2022;182(8):892.
17. Cummings J, Ritter A, Rothenberg K. Advances in management of neuropsychiatric syndromes in neurodegenerative diseases. Curr Psychiatry Rep. 2019;21(8):79.
18. Lyketsos CG. Mental and behavioral disturbances in dementia: findings from the Cache County Study on memory in aging. Am J Psychiatry. 2000;157(5):708–14.
19. Teri L, Rabins P, Whitehouse P, Berg L, Reisberg B, Sunderland T, et al. Management of behavior disturbance in Alzheimer disease: current knowledge and future directions. Alzheimer Dis Assoc Disord. 1992;6(2):77–88.
20. Barrick AL, Rader J, Hoeffer B, Sloane P, Biddle S. Bathing without a battle. 2nd ed. Berlin: Springer; 2008.
21. Fitzsimmons S, Barba B, Stump M. Sensory and nurturing nonpharmacological interventions for behavioral and psychological symptoms of dementia. J Gerontol Nurs. 2014;40(11):9–15.
22. Cohen-Mansfield J. Nonpharmacologic interventions for inappropriate behaviors in dementia: a review, summary, and critique. Am J Geriatr Psychiatry. 2001;9(4):361–81.
23. Mitchell SL, Teno JM, Kiely DK, Shaffer ML, Jones RN, Prigerson HG, et al. The clinical course of advanced dementia. N Engl J Med. 2009;361(16):1529–38.
24. Gillick MR. Rethinking the role of tube feeding in patients with advanced dementia. N Engl J Med. 2000;342(3):206–10.
25. Finucane TE, Christmas C, Travis K. Tube feeding in patients with advanced dementia. JAMA. 1999;282(14):1365.
26. Kertesz A. Frontotemporal dementia/Pick's disease. Arch Neurol. 2004;61(6):969–71.
27. Ngo J, Holroyd-Leduc JM. Systematic review of recent dementia practice guidelines. Age Ageing. 2015;44(1):25–33.
28. Chai E, Meier D, Morris J, Goldhirsh S. Geriatric palliative care: a practical guide for clinicians. New York: Oxford University Press; 2014. p. 190–5.
29. González M, de Pablo J, Fuente E, Valdés M, Peri JM, Nomdedeu M, et al. Instrument for detection of delirium in general hospitals: adaptation of the confusion assessment method. Psychosomatics. 2004;45(5):426–31.
30. Fong TG, Tulebaev SR, Inouye SK. Delirium in elderly adults: diagnosis, prevention and treatment. Nat Rev Neurol. 2009;5(4):210–20.
31. Clegg A, Young JB. Which medications to avoid in people at risk of delirium: a systematic review. Age Ageing. 2011;40(1):23–9.
32. Young J, Murthy L, Westby M, Akunne A, O'Mahony R. Diagnosis, prevention, and management of delirium: summary of NICE guidance. BMJ. 2010;341:c3704.
33. Wei LA, Fearing MA, Sternberg EJ, Inouye SK. The confusion assessment method: a systematic review of current usage. J Am Geriatr Soc. 2008;56(5):823–30.
34. Inouye SK. Clarifying confusion: the confusion assessment method. Ann Intern Med. 1990;113(12):941.
35. Marcantonio ER, Ngo LH, O'Connor M, Jones RN, Crane PK, Metzger ED, et al. 3D-CAM: derivation and validation of a 3-minute diagnostic interview for CAM-defined delirium. Ann Intern Med. 2014;161(8):554.
36. Breitbart W, Alici Y. Agitation and delirium at the end of life. JAMA. 2008;300(24):2898.
37. McKenzie R, Stewart MT, Bellantoni MF, Finucane TE. Bacteriuria in individuals who become delirious. Am J Med. 2014;127(4):255–7.
38. Schneider LS, Tariot PN, Dagerman KS, Davis SM, Hsiao JK, Ismail MS, et al. Effectiveness of atypical antipsychotic drugs in patients with Alzheimer's disease. N Engl J Med. 2006;355(15):1525–38.

39. Rubino A, Sanon M, Ganz ML, Simpson A, Fenton MC, Verma S, et al. Association of the US Food and Drug Administration antipsychotic drug boxed warning with medication use and health outcomes in elderly patients with dementia. JAMA Netw Open. 2020;3(4):e203630.
40. Overshott R, Karim S, Burns A. Cholinesterase inhibitors for delirium. Cochrane Database Syst Rev. 2008;2008(1):CD005317.

Further Reading

Alzheimer's Association. www.alz.org.
Alzheimer's Association Store. www.alzstore.com.
American Delirium Society. www.americandeliriumsociety.org.
Hospital Elder Life Program (HELP) for prevention of delirium. www.hospitalelderlifeprogram.org.
National Academy of Elder Law Attorneys. www.naela.org.
National Association of Home Care. www.nahc.org.

Chapter 6
Common Neurologic Issues

Melissa J. Christie and Anjail Z. Sharrief

6.1 Introduction

The home-based medical practitioner will frequently encounter patients with neurological diseases and conditions that are often superimposed on chronic medical conditions. An understanding of common neurological conditions both at an anatomical and functional level and the impact of medical conditions on the symptomatology will empower a home-based practitioner with the tools to provide optimal neurologic care to this population.

6.2 Stroke

In the United States, approximately 85% of all strokes are ischemic in etiology, while intracerebral hemorrhage and subarachnoid hemorrhage are responsible for the remaining 15% [1]. Transient ischemic attack (TIA) refers to stroke signs and symptoms that resolve in <24 h without residual deficits. TIA often precedes ischemic stroke, and appropriate investigation following TIA can prevent a more devastating ischemic event [2]. Practitioners who care for patients who are homebound will need to be especially familiar with up-to-date stroke management [3]. In the home-based medical care setting, it is important to determine whether a patient has suffered a TIA or stroke, to determine when to seek care immediately for stroke, and to implement secondary prevention measures for recurrent stroke.

M. J. Christie (✉) · A. Z. Sharrief
Department of Neurology, UT Health Houston, McGovern Medical School, Houston, TX, USA
e-mail: melissa.j.christie@uth.tmc.edu; Anjail.Z.Sharrief@uth.tmc.edu

J. L. Colburn et al. (eds.), *Geriatric Home-Based Medical Care*,
https://doi.org/10.1007/978-3-031-68786-0_6

6.2.1 Advanced Directives

Management of a patient with acute neurological change thought to be related to acute stroke will depend on patient's advanced directives. If the patient is severely neurologically impaired at baseline, has a history of multiple prior strokes, and does not wish to be hospitalized for an acute event, a palliative or home stroke care support approach should be instituted.

However, if a patient's preferences do not discourage hospitalization for a treatable acute neurological event, acute hospitalization may be required for stroke management.

6.2.2 Diagnosing an Acute Stroke in Homebound Patients

Diagnosis of acute stroke should not be delayed, as acute stroke is treatable and delays in treatment can lead to avoidable disability. If a practitioner learns of acute onset stroke symptoms prior to assessment in the home, the patient or family member should be instructed to call 911 immediately in order to receive timely emergency care. For ischemic stroke, acute treatment with thrombolytic therapy within the first hour after symptom onset leads to two times higher likelihood of good function outcome compared to patients who present later, and treatment for large vessel occlusion is available within 24 h [4, 5]. Therefore, patient or families who call a practitioner with symptoms of acute onset of symptoms represented by the sudden onset of various symptoms (Table 6.1) should be instructed to call 911 immediately. If a provider is not aware of the acute onset of symptoms prior to arrival at the home, or if symptoms have been present for several days once the provider is notified, the level of acuity can be determined from clinical history combined with a rapid neurological assessment.

6.2.3 Level of Acuity

A practitioner examining a patient in the home-based setting with an expected acute neurologic change should begin with assessment of the patient's level of consciousness. The presence of stupor (physical stimulation required for patient response) or coma (no response to physical or verbal stimulation) suggests diffuse cerebral dysfunction which can be related to primary neurologic etiology (intracerebral hemorrhage, massive ischemic stroke, basilar artery stroke, status epilepticus) or from secondary etiology (toxic, metabolic, or infectious). While evaluation of cranial nerves and careful history may help to distinguish primary neurologic from toxic, metabolic, or infectious causes of stupor or coma, any primary or secondary neurologic insult resulting in stupor or coma requires emergent hospital evaluation and

Table 6.1 Localization of stroke symptoms

Brain region	Hemisphere	Functional region	Stroke symptom
Cortex	Left	Language	Speech fluency or language (aphasia)
		Vision	Visual field defects
		Sensorimotor	Right-sided sensory impairment and/or hemiparesis or hemiplegia involving the face, arm, and leg
		Cognition	Inability to read and/or write
	Right	Sensorimotor	Left-sided sensory impairment and/or hemiparesis or hemiplegia
		Vision	Visual field defects
		Higher sensory processing	Neglect of left side of body Inability to recognize body parts and depth perceptual problems
	Structures	**Stroke symptoms**	
Subcortex	Internal capsule	Pure unilateral motor weakness (face, arm, or leg weakness) Dysarthria with weakness or clumsiness	
	Basal ganglia/ thalamus	Pure unilateral motor weakness (face, arm, or leg weakness) Dysarthria with weakness or clumsiness Pure sensory loss (face, arm, leg) Mixed motor and sensory symptoms	
	Brainstem	Cranial neuropathies and unilateral or bilateral weakness (e.g., locked-in syndrome)	
		Pure motor weakness (face, arm, or leg weakness) Dysarthria with weakness or clumsiness Ataxia with hemiparesis	
Cerebellum		Vertigo	
		Nystagmus	
		Nausea/vomiting	
		Truncal or appendicular ataxia	

management unless the patient has previously indicated a wish against this. In the case of stupor or coma, a practitioner caring for a homebound patient should immediately facilitate rapid evaluation in the hospital.

For patients with intact consciousness, a concise and pertinent history followed by a rapid neurological evaluation can help to further determine the acuity of management. A set of specific questions can help to identify whether a patient may be a candidate for acute stroke treatment: When was the patient last seen in his/her usual neurologic state? Was onset of symptoms witnessed? Did the patient awaken with symptoms? Does the patient have any current deficits (by report or rapid assessment).

These question helps to determine the approximate time of symptom onset. Ischemic stroke can be treated with IV thrombolytics (tissue plasminogen activator or tenecteplase) within 4.5 h of symptom onset [6, 7]. Some patients may also be eligible for acute thrombolytic therapy if they awaken with symptoms, even if last seen normal was prior to 4.5 h of symptom onset [8].

In most places, thrombolytic therapy is only available in an emergency department; however, mobile stroke units or ambulances equipped with a CT scanner and thrombolytic treatment are increasingly present in cities across the United States. Treatment in mobile stroke units is safe and is associated with better outcomes because of the speed with which thrombolytic therapy can be administered [9]. When emergency services are activated, EMS notification about stroke symptoms may help to facilitate management in the most appropriate setting.

In addition to IV thrombolytic therapy for acute ischemic stroke, mechanical thrombectomy is another evidence-based treatment for patients with a subset of ischemic stroke presenting withing 24 h of symptom onset [5]. Endovascular treatment with mechanical thrombectomy for patients with stroke resulting from large vessel occlusion is associated with improved outcomes [5]. While patients with stroke resulting from large vessel occlusion will often present with more severe disability and/or with cortical symptoms (aphasia, neglect, impaired vision), the etiology of stroke cannot be determined solely from neurological symptoms. Therefore, any patient may be eligible for stroke treatment within 24 h of symptom onset, and rapid evaluation is essential to determine eligibility.

While headache and impaired consciousness may be hallmarks of severe intracerebral hemorrhage or subarachnoid hemorrhage, this is not always the case. It is not possible to accurately and consistently distinguish ischemic stroke from hemorrhagic stroke on the basis of symptoms alone. Depending on the cause of hemorrhagic stroke, emergent management with blood pressure medication or surgical treatment may be indicated. Any patient with acute (24 h) and focal onset of neurological symptoms, regardless of presumed etiology, requires emergent neurological assessment.

Patients with suspected stroke, but who are outside of the 24-h ischemic stroke treatment window may likely still need hospital evaluation, but the practitioner may have additional time to determine the best location and ideal mechanism for transport to the facility depending on the specific timing, severity of symptoms, and patient and family preferences.

6.2.4 Conducting a Home-Based Stroke Assessment

For patients in whom emergency assessment is not required, or after 911 has been activated for patients requiring emergency assessment, the home-based provider can proceed with additional questions and a basic neurological assessment. These queries can help to exclude stroke mimics, give clues to specific etiology, and localize the stroke (Table 6.1).

6.2.5 *Additional Questions*

- Which medications are the patient taking?
  - Important medications to query about include use of anticoagulants, antiplatelet agents, antihypertensives, opioids, antihyperglycemic drugs, and anticonvulsants.
- Has the patient been adherent to prescribed medications?
  - Acute withdrawal of antithrombotic therapy, whether intentional (holding for procedure) or unintentional, can predispose to ischemic stroke, especially in patients with high-risk medical conditions (atrial fibrillation/mechanical valve) or prior ischemic stroke.
- Has the patient had similar symptoms in the past?
  - Prior similar symptoms that have previously resolved could suggest TIA, seizure, recrudescence of stroke symptoms do to concurrent infectious or metabolic issues, or even complex migraine.

6.2.6 *Physical Exam*

1. Obtain vital signs (e.g., blood pressure, heart rate, temperature, oxygen saturation) and a bedside fingerstick glucose.
2. Perform a basic neurological exam:
   (a) Assess level of consciousness (discussed previously). Determine the level of stimulus needed to arouse the patient and maintain arousal (voice, touch, or pain).
   (b) Evaluate orientation (person, location, time).
   (c) Evaluate language—aphasia:
      - Have patient repeat a sentence: "Today is a sunny day."
      - Have the patient name three objects.
      - Have the patient follow three simple commands: Raise your right arm, stick out your tongue, and show me two fingers with your left hand.

   (d) Evaluate speech (dysarthria):
      - Have the patient repeat the following words: Mama, tiptop, thanks, and 50 to determine if speech is articulate/clear or if there is evidence of dysarthria.

   (e) Evaluate gaze:
      - Ask the patient to follow your finger in horizontal and vertical directions.

- A gaze preference to one side, while at rest, suggests the presence of a visual field defect and/or neglect from a hemispheric stroke.
- A centered gaze at rest with impaired eye movement(s) indicates a brainstem lesion.

(f) Check for facial weakness:

- Carefully observe their lower face for weakness at rest.
- Ask them to smile and observe for weakness.
- Check for eye closure weakness by gently pulling up on their upper eyelids against resistance.

(g) Check for limb weakness:

- Have patient raise each arm in front of them separately for a count of 10.
- Have them do the same for each leg separately (counting to 5).
- Drifting downward or difficulty elevating the limb confirms weakness.

(h) Test sensation and extinction:

- Test tactile sensation by using a cotton swab or pinprick comparing both sides of the face, arms, and legs.
- If the patient has intact sensation, ask them to close their eyes and simultaneously test sensation on both arms and legs to determine whether the patient is demonstrating extinction to one side.

(i) Assess for dysmetria or ataxia:

- Conduct finger–nose–finger and heel–shin tests on both sides to determine the presence of limb ataxia.
- Overshooting or past-pointing and clumsiness during these tests suggest cerebellar involvement.
- Note that these tests will not rule out truncal ataxia.

(j) If the patient complains of dizziness without other clear findings on exam, you may cautiously ask them to walk. Note, some patients may have primarily truncal ataxia, which can be very disabling, but may not be noticeable until they sit or walk.

6.2.7 *Strategies for Home-Based Management of Subacute Stroke and TIA*

As is it not possible to distinguish between ischemic and hemorrhagic stroke by symptoms alone, the approach to acute home-based management, in a situation where the patient has determined that they would not want to return to a hospital, may be limited.

If stroke symptoms have been present for several days and the patient has minimal disability, it is reasonable to obtain an outpatient MRI to determine the stroke type. A CT scan may be helpful but has limited resolution to detect small ischemic strokes and may not be able to distinguish ischemic from hemorrhagic stroke in the subacute setting. Additional studies should be used to determine stroke etiology after stroke type has been determined (Table 6.2).

The etiology or mechanism of ischemic stroke guides treatment. Ischemic stroke etiology is typically characterized according to the TOAST classification scheme as (1) small vessel disease, (2) large vessel disease, (3) cardioembolic, (4) cryptogenic (undetermined), or (5) stroke of other determined cause [10].

6.2.8 Management of Stroke Risk Factors in Patients with Subacute Stroke [11]

Secondary prevention guidelines provide recommendations about medication dosing and approaches following a TIA or stroke [11].

Blood Pressure Control

- Blood pressure may be elevated acutely in the setting of ischemic or hemorrhagic stroke. In the setting of ischemic stroke, slow BP lowering can begin after 24 h of symptoms onset, whereas for hemorrhagic stroke, BP lowering should begin

Table 6.2 Diagnostic studies for patients with acute and subacute stroke [11]

Study type	Specific studies	Use
Neuroimaging studies	1. Brain CT 2. Brain MRI	• Determine stroke type (ischemic or hemorrhagic) • Help to determine stroke etiology (infarct appearance)
Vascular imaging	1. CTA head and neck 2. MRA head and neck 3. Carotid Doppler 4. Transcranial Doppler	• Help to determine stroke etiology • Evaluate for intracranial or extracranial atherosclerosis or large vessel etiology
Cardiac imaging	1. Transthoracic echo 2. Transesophageal echo 3. Cardiac MRI 4. Cardiac CT	• Help to determine stroke etiology (cardioembolic source)
Cardiac rhythm assessment	1. EKG 2. Prolonged cardiac monitoring (external and internal)	• Help to determine stroke etiology (atrial fibrillation)
Laboratory assessment	1. Lipid panel 2. Hemoglobin A1c 3. Hypercoagulable studies (when indicated)	• Characterizes prevalence and control of risk factors • May help to determine etiology

CT computed tomography, *EKG* electrocardiogram, *MRI* magnetic resonance imaging, *MRA* magnetic resonance angiogram immediately. In the subacute setting, aggressive BP control should be held until stroke etiology is determined and vascular imaging obtained (Table 6.2), because rapid BP lowering in the setting of severe stenosis can lead to increased risk for stroke [6].

Antiplatelet and Anticoagulation Therapy

- For mild ischemic stroke and TIA, initiation of dual antiplatelet therapy with aspirin 81 mg and clopidogrel 75 mg or aspirin 81 mg and ticagrelor 90 mg BID for a short duration of (typically 21–30 days) may be indicated to reduce the risk of recurrent stroke. Long-term aspirin therapy (81 mg) is indicated as first line for patients with ischemic stroke not secondary to atrial fibrillation or other cardioembolic source. Long-term use (>90 days) of dual antiplatelet therapy is not indicated for stroke prevention and may be associated with harm [11].
- For moderate to severe ischemic stroke, initiation of aspirin or clopidogrel if aspirin allergic is indicated [11].
- If a patient requires anticoagulation for atrial fibrillation or other cardioembolic etiology (atrial or ventricular thrombus or mechanical valve), the addition of antiplatelet therapy for stroke prevention is typically not indicated [11]. The choice of anticoagulant depends on patients' specific risks and should be based on best available data for safety and stroke prevention.
- Depending on the risk of recurrent events from the cardioembolic source, and depending on the size of ischemic stroke, initiation of anticoagulation therapy may be delayed for up to 14 days to prevention hemorrhagic transformation [6].

Lipid Management

- Initiation of high-intensity statin therapy is associated with reduced risk of ischemic stroke recurrence. High-intensity statin therapy should be initiated immediately after TIA or ischemic stroke [11].

Blood Sugar Management

- Blood sugar should be checked and maintained within normal limits after acute ischemic stroke [6].

6.2.9 Supportive Management in Home Setting for Acute or Subacute Stroke

6.2.9.1 Neurological Disability

- Depending on stroke location, disability after stroke may manifest with aphasia, neglect, dysarthria, dysphagia, hemiparesis, vision loss, ataxia, or gait instability.
- Physical therapy, speech therapy, and occupational therapy aid in recovery after stroke. In the homebound setting, home therapy assessments and treatment can aid in neurologic recovery for patients with subacute ischemic or hemorrhagic stroke [12].

6.2.9.2 Dysphagia Management

Patients with acute stroke are at risk for dysphagia [13]. Dysphagia can increase the risk of aspiration events and aspiration pneumonia after stroke [13]. Bedside assessment of dysphagia can be performed with a basic bedside swallow evaluation. NG tube may need to be placed if dysphagia is suspected. A home-based swallow assessment may be indicated to determine if a modified diet is required or if a patient should remain NPO following an acute stroke.

6.2.9.3 DVT Prophylaxis

Patients with acute ischemic or hemorrhagic stroke are at risk for deep vein thrombosis and pulmonary embolism. DVT prophylaxis should be considered for homebound patients with acute or subacute ischemic stroke at high risk for DVT because of impaired mobility and hemiparesis or hemiplegia [14]. DVT prophylaxis is also indicated for hemorrhagic stroke and typically can be initiated with 48 h of hemorrhagic stroke onset [15].

6.2.10 Home-Based Management of TIA [2]

If a patient's neurological deficit is not resolving within 1 h or has not completely resolved over 24 h, it is recommended to send the patient to the emergency department for evaluation or manage their condition as an acute stroke in the home setting.

Complete resolution of the neurologic deficit necessitates determining patient's stroke risk factors. The ABCD2 score [16], which takes into account age, blood pressure, and clinical symptoms, is one of the most widely used scores to use to risk stratify TIA patients for the likelihood of having a stroke.

6.2.11 Risk Stratify Based on ABCD2 Score

- Age ≥60 (1) point
- BP >140/90 (1) point
- Clinical symptoms with focal weakness (2) points
- Speech impairment w/o weakness (1) point
- Duration ≥60 min (2) points or 10–59 min (1) point

Scores greater than 6 suggest a greater than 10% stroke risk within 1 week and closer to 20% chance in 90 days. Two limitations of this score are that (1) it does not include posterior circulation symptoms and (2) it does not factor in stroke mechanism. Nonetheless, it is a good tool to use for risk stratification, especially when combined with other tests (Table 6.2). Patients suspected of having a TIA should be evaluated for stroke etiology and screened for risk factors including hypertension, diabetes, hyperlipidemia, and atrial fibrillation. Based on a patient's goals of care and projected life expectancy, a pragmatic approach to managing the following risk factors should be employed to sustain an optimal quality of life:

1. Begin treatment with dual antiplatelet therapy if patient does not have contraindications. Dual antiplatelet therapy should continue for 21–30 days and then aspirin alone should be initiated [2].
2. Aim for BP <130/80 mmHg, which can be slowly lowered with antihypertensive agents beginning within 24 h after symptom onset [11].
3. Aim for glycemic control—AIC<7.0.
4. Aim for LDL cholesterol <70.
5. Evaluate for the presence of intracranial or extracranial atherosclerotic disease.
6. Evaluate for the presence of atrial fibrillation with EKG or long-term monitoring.
7. Evaluate for the presence of sleep apnea.

6.2.12 Management of Homebound Chronic Stroke Patients

Determine patient's level of disability and tailor therapy based on residual symptoms. Physical, occupational, and speech therapists are often required for management and retraining of limb movements, gait, cognitive, and speech/language deficits. Such therapy in an enriched interactive environment reduces overall disability and provides opportunity for stroke patients to regain a level of independence. Worsening of chronic stroke symptoms should prompt an evaluation for infectious or metabolic causes by the home-based provider.

Individuals managing chronic stroke patients should be aware of other complications that all contribute to the quality of life in patients with stroke. These include fatigue, depression, anxiety, pain, sleep apnea and other sleep disorders, bowel and bladder dysfunction, and spasticity [17–20]. Providers should be aware of these complications and evaluate and manage them as they would with any patient. Management of spasticity is covered in the section on "Spinal Cord Injury."

6.3 Parkinsonism

Parkinsonism is a general term that refers to a group of neurological disorders that cause movement disorders, including Parkinson's disease. The cardinal symptoms of parkinsonism are a constellation of bradykinesia along with muscle rigidity, tremor, and postural instability.

Bradykinesia is most important for the diagnosis and is characterized as a decrease of rapid sequential movement on examination with lack of spontaneous, automatic movements. Its clinical manifestations include small handwriting that tends to trail off (micrographia), reduced facial expression (masked facies), and/or reduction in vocal intonation (hypophonia).

Rigidity, or muscle stiffness, is related to increased muscle resistance during passive limb movement that produces a ratcheting feeling similar to a "cogwheel." Very mild rigidity usually requires coactivation maneuvers of the contralateral limb in order to elicit it.

Postural and gait changes in parkinsonism are characterized by a stooped posture, reduced stride length producing a shuffling appearance to the gait, and multipivot turning. In addition, impairment or loss of postural reflexes places many of these patients at risk of falling. A pull test, in which the examiner stands behind the patient and pulls them backward while monitoring the number of steps they need to recover without assistance, is often utilized. Greater than two steps to recover or the need of the examiner to prevent them from falling is abnormal.

Furthermore, these patients can develop gait freezing, whereby they stutter step in place or one or both feet suddenly seemed pasted to the floor when walking normally or through small spaces such as doorways, turning, and/or upon initiating walking. Failure to compensate by holding on to someone or an assistive device increases the risk of falling. This can be seen late in the disease course for Parkinson's disease (PD), but rather early on among the atypical parkinsonism syndromes.

6.3.1 *Classification and Treatment of Parkinsonism*

6.3.1.1 Parkinson's Disease

Parkinsonism results from either a degenerative disease or an acquired etiology (e.g., medications, toxins, infections, vascular). Among the degenerative causes, Parkinson's disease is the most common, and an accurate diagnosis is predicated upon a clinical assessment, which clinical-pathological studies [21] have shown to have a greater than 90% accuracy. This is based on the presence of an asymmetric bradykinesia with at least one concomitant symptom: muscle rigidity, tremor, and/or postural and gait instability. Importantly, PD typically begins with symptoms on one side of the body, with eventual progression to bilateral symptoms after a few years, although asymmetry of symptom severity is retained throughout the disease. The tremor of PD is primarily present at rest involving the fingers, usually the thumb and index, to produce the characteristic pill-rolling tremor. Tremor abates during action and tends to re-emerge after a brief delay. Further supportive features include a slow progression with sustained, robust levodopa response.

Distinguishing PD from atypical parkinsonism has both treatment and prognostic implications, as the latter conditions do not respond well to levodopa and have a more rapid and deleterious clinical course. The atypical parkinsonism syndromes include progressive supranuclear palsy (PSP), corticobasal degeneration (CBD), multisystem atrophy (MSA), and dementia with Lewy body (DLB) [22].

6.3.1.2 Treatment of Parkinson's Disease

The treatments for PD are symptomatic with levodopa being the gold standard. It is reasonable to start symptomatic treatment in the early stages of the disease when the level of severity is starting to adversely impact quality of life and daily activities [23]. See Table 6.3.

6.3.2 Motor Symptom Management

- Levodopa is considered the first-line therapy in patients older than 70 years. Providers should initiate levodopa in immediate-release formulations with a titration to at least three times per day. Nausea related to levodopa can be treated with extra carbidopa or domperidone taken with each dose of levodopa. Should patients develop levodopa-induced hallucinations or psychosis, incorporating pimavanserin or low-dose quetiapine into the regimen is often efficacious [24].
- The dopamine agonist class or monoamine oxidase (MAOB) inhibitors can be utilized early on in patients less than 70 years who are cognitively intact. Short-acting dopamine agonists are administered three times per day. Long-acting formulations exist for both pramipexole and ropinirole and can be used once a day. The rotigotine patch is utilized daily and should be changed and applied on different body regions (e.g., upper limbs, torso, back) at the same time each day to ensure continuous benefit. There are no clinical data demonstrating superiority

Table 6.3 Pharmacological treatment for Parkinson's disease [23, 24]

Medication class	Formulations	Initial doses	Clinical considerations
Levodopa	Carbidopa/levodopa, ODT	Start 25/100 mg three times per day	Nausea
			Light-headedness
			Hallucinations
Dopamine agonists	Pramipexole	Start 0.25 mg three times daily, max 4.5 mg daily	Impulse control disorders
			Hypersomnolence
			Cognitive deficits
	Pramipexole extended release	Start 0.375 daily, max 4.5 mg daily	Hallucinations
	Ropinirole	Start 0.25 mg three times daily, max 24 mg daily	
	Ropinirole extended release	Start 2 mg daily, max 24 mg daily	
	Rotigotine TD	Start 2 mg daily, max 8 mg/24 h	
MAO-B inhibitors	Selegiline	5 mg twice daily	Dizziness, headache, dyspepsia
	Rasagiline	1 mg daily	

of one agonist over another. Dopamine agonists can cause excessive sedation, sleep attacks, hallucinations, and impulse control disorders (e.g., gambling, hypersexuality, shopping). It is important to screen patients for these potential side effects, as reduction in dose or discontinuation of the medication is ameliorative [24].

Patients on long-standing levodopa therapy can develop "wearing-off" episodes also known as motor fluctuations. As the disease progresses, the hours of good motor response ("on" time) per dosing interval decrease, while precipitous "off" periods increase. This along with the emergence of dyskinesia, involuntary muscle movement flowing from one region of the body to another, reduces a patient's quality of life. A summary of medication treatment strategies is contained in Table 6.4.

Dystonia is an involuntary contraction of muscle groups that causes abnormal twisting or repetitive movements or postures. Common focal dystonias that can develop in PD include the following:

- Cervical dystonia
- Blepharospasm (involuntary eyelid closure or spasms) or eyelid opening apraxia
- Hand dystonia
- Lower limb dystonia (e.g., toe curling or foot dystonia)
- Camptocormia (abnormal anteroflexion of the trunk)
- Pisa syndrome (lateral flexion of the trunk)

Table 6.4 Management approaches for motor complications and dystonia in Parkinson's disease

Motor fluctuations/wearing "off"	Increase levodopa dose and/or dosing frequency
	Add COMT-I
	Add MAOBI
	Switch levodopa formulation to carbidopa levodopa extended-release capsules (Rytary)
	Add a dopamine agonist
	Utilize apomorphine SC injections, apomorphine sublingual, or inhaled levodopa formulations as rescue medication
Dyskinesia	Reduce dose or frequency of levodopa
	Discontinue COMTI
	Discontinue MAOBI
	Add amantadine 100 mg three to four times daily
Focal dystonia	
Cervical Blepharospasm/eye-lid opening apraxia Hand dystonia Camptocormia Lower limb Pisa syndrome	Baclofen (start 5 mg three times daily, max 80 mg daily divided)
	Low-dose benzodiazepines (clonazepam, diazepam, lorazepam) dosed two to three times daily
	Trihexyphenidyl (2 mg two to three times daily, max 12–15 mg daily divided)
	Botulinum toxin injections

COMTI catechol-*O*-methyl transferase inhibitor, MAOBI Type-B monoamine oxidase inhibitor

In order to manage motor fluctuations, dyskinesia, and other involuntary movements such as dystonia, it is important to initiate discussions with a neurologist who is willing to offer management guidance, even if the patient is unable to come in to a neurology office visit. Many neurology clinics also offer telemedicine evaluations for patients unable to leave the home environment.

There is little to no superiority data for the different classes of antidystonic agents. Uses of these therapies are based on the patient's tolerance and the existence of other underlying medical comorbidities. Botulinum toxin injections have emerged as the first-line treatment choice for many of the focal dystonias, due to its targeted clinical efficacy and minimal risk of constitutional and cognitive adverse effects.

6.3.3 Surgical Strategies

As the disease progresses, pharmacological permutations not only become more complex, but the propensity for side effects increases.

6.3.4 Deep Brain Stimulation

Deep brain stimulation (DBS) is an effective treatment for the management of the cardinal Parkinson's motor symptoms, including refractory tremor. It should be considered in patients who have idiopathic PD and not atypical variants, demonstrate robust levodopa response, lack dementia or signs of atypical parkinsonism, and have motor complications (e.g., motor fluctuations, dyskinesia) requiring higher dopaminergic dosages [23].

Compared to the best medical therapy, DBS produces longer "on" time for patients with dramatic reductions in wearing offs, dyskinesia, and medication burden. It can also benefit focal dystonia that emerges as a consequence of disease progression or levodopa complication.

6.3.5 Carbidopa/Levodopa Intestinal Gel

This specially formulated enteral gel is particularly useful for a patient with advanced PD with motor complications, who also has cognitive dysfunction and/or dysphagia that affects oral intake. It significantly increases "on" time while reducing dyskinesia by continuously infusing carbidopa/levodopa through a gastrostomy–jejunostomy tube (PEG-J) 16 h per day.

6.3.6 *Nonmotor Symptom Management (Refer to Table 6.5)*

Table 6.5 Nonmotor symptom management in Parkinsons' disease [23, 24]

	Symptom	Treatment	Adverse effects
Autonomic	Constipation	Refer to Table 6.10	
	Orthostatic hypotension	Midodrine 2.5 mg three times daily, can titrate to 10 mg three times daily	Hypertension, nausea, headache
		Fludrocortisone 0.1 mg daily, max 0.3 mg daily	Hypertension, electrolyte abnormalities
		Droxidopa 100 mg three times daily, titrate to max 600 mg three times daily	Hypertension, headache
	Urinary incontinence	Refer to "Sphincter Dysfunction in Spinal Cord Injury"	
Sleep disorders	REM behavioral disorder	Clonazepam 0.25 mg at bedtime, titrate to max 1 mg at bedtime	Sedation and confusion
	Fragmented sleep	Improve sleep hygiene	
		Melatonin 6–15 mg at bedtime	Somnolence
		Mirtazapine 7.5–15 mg at bedtime	Same as melatonin
		Trazodone 25–100 mg at bedtime	Somnolence, headache, dizziness
Sialorrhea		Botulinum toxin injections to salivary glands	Dysphagia, pain at injection site
		Glycopyrrolate 1–2 mg two to three time daily, max is 8 mg daily	Anticholinergic effects
Neurobehavioral	Depression	SSRI	Gastrointestinal symptoms, sexual dysfunction
		SNRI	Same as SSRI
		TCA	Anticholinergic effects, heart block, gastrointestinal symptoms
	Anxiety	Benzodiazepines	Daytime sleepiness, confusion
		Change dosing of levodopa if symptom correlated with timing of medication	

(continued)

Table 6.5 (continued)

	Symptom	Treatment	Adverse effects
	Hallucinations/ agitation	Quetiapine 12.5–50 mg daily or BID, high doses can lead to worsening parkinsonism	Sedation, extrapyramidal symptoms
		Pimavanserin 34 mg daily	Nausea, QTc prolongation
		Donepezil 5 mg daily, max 10 mg daily	Gastrointestinal symptoms, heart block, bradycardia
		Rivastigmine: Oral 1.5 mg twice daily, can titrate to 6 mg twice daily	Same as donepezil
		Rivastigmine: Transdermal 4.5 mg daily, can titrate to 13.3 mg daily	
	Cognitive impairment or dementia (PDD)	Donepezil 5 mg daily, max 10 mg daily	Gastrointestinal symptoms, heart block, bradycardia
		Galantamine 4 mg daily, can titrate to 12 mg daily	Same as Donepezil
		Memantine 5 mg daily, can titrate to 20 mg daily or divided	Dizziness, headache, confusion
		Rivastigmine: oral 1.5 mg twice daily, can titrate to 6 mg twice daily	Same as Donepezil
		Rivastigmine: Transdermal 4.5 mg daily, can titrate to 13.3 mg daily	

SSRI selective serotonin reuptake inhibitor, SNRI serotonin and norepinephrine reuptake inhibitor, TCA tricyclic antidepressant, PDD Parkinson's disease dementia

6.3.7 Autonomic Dysfunction

- Constipation should be managed with stool softeners and increased daily water and fiber intact. Enemas, suppositories, lubiprostone, and linaclotide may be utilized in severe cases.
- Orthostatic hypotension can emerge in advanced stages of Parkinson's disease. Midodrine, fludrocortisone, and droxidopa can be used.
- Sialorrhea—Glycopyrrolate, atropine, and botulinum toxin injections to salivary glands can be used.
- Urinary incontinence from detrusor hyperreflexia is prevalent in the PD population and must be distinguished from benign prostatic hyperplasia, which is also common in men above 65 years. Detrusor hyperactivity can be treated with medications such as oxybutynin or tolterodine (refer to "Sphincter Dysfunction in Spinal Cord Injury").

- Dysphagia—Presence or history of dysphagia should prompt the home-based clinician to recommend that patients wait to be in the medicated "on" phase before eating, change their food consistency to soft or puree, take small portions, and do a chin tuck with gentle cough after swallowing. An evaluation by speech-language therapy to investigate extent of swallowing difficulty and risk for aspiration will be important to obtain. Severe symptoms may necessitate artificial nutrition if such measures are consistent with the patient's overall condition and goals of care.

6.3.8 Sleep Disorders

- REM behavioral disorder (RBD) is a sleep disorder whereby a patient acts out their dreams during REM sleep. Vocalizations or flailing arm and/or leg movements are common symptoms of RBD. Treatment with melatonin is first line with addition of low-dose clonazepam at bedtime being efficacious in severe cases (i.e., hitting bed partner, falling out of bed).
- Fragmented sleep or incomplete non-restful sleep is common among PD patients. Conservative therapies such as relaxation methods, reduction in daily caffeine intact, and avoiding watching television or using a computer at night are recommended. Pharmacological agents to consider include melatonin, mirtazapine, or trazodone.

6.3.9 Neurobehavioral

- Serotonin reuptake inhibitor (SSRI), tricyclic, or serotonin norepinephrine reuptake inhibitor (SNRI) antidepressants may be used for treatment of depression, anxiety, and/or apathy.
- Quetiapine is an atypical neuroleptic that can be used for managing hallucinations or emotionally dysregulated behaviors (e.g., paranoid delusions) that can emerge late in the disease course. Pimavanserin is an inverse agonist/antagonist of serotonin that was specifically developed for treatment of Parkinson's disease psychosis and has less risk of worsening motor symptoms of Parkinson's disease.

6.3.10 Botulinum Toxin Injections for Parkinsonism

Botulinum toxin injections are very effective in treating a wide spectrum of symptoms in parkinsonism, such as dystonia, sialorrhea, and bladder dysfunction. These injections should be done by a trained physician. They are covered by most commercial insurances, Medicare, and Medicaid. Its effects are realized over 3–7 days after the injection(s) and benefit can last up to 12–16 weeks. In order to minimize the development of antibodies to the toxin, low doses are used initially, treatment intervals are 3 months, and booster injections are avoided.

6.3.11 Dystonia

Botulinum toxin injections are the first-line treatment for cervical dystonia, blepharospasm, eyelid opening apraxia, and focal hand dystonia and a treatment of choice for lower limb dystonia. Limb injections may require use of electromyography (EMG), ultrasound, or electric stimulation guidance to identify the muscles to be injected and, therefore, should be done in a hospital or clinic setting.

6.3.12 Sialorrhea

Botulinum toxin injection to the parotids/submandibular glands is considered the treatment of choice for sialorrhea, especially when oral anticholinergic (e.g., glycopyrrolate) medications have limited benefit and/or are not well tolerated.

6.3.13 Neurogenic Bladder

Botulinum toxin injection to the bladder's detrusor muscle has been shown to be effective in reducing detrusor overactivity and improving incontinence and bladder capacity in medication refractory neurogenic bladder. The injections oftentimes require anesthesia, but the benefits can last up to 9 months before a repeat treatment is needed. These are typically performed by a urologist or urogynecologist.

6.4 Multiple Sclerosis

Multiple sclerosis (MS) is a chronic, progressive, neurologic disease that, in its primary form, causes patient's great morbidity and functional compromise. Characterized by attacks of neuronal inflammation, demyelination, and degeneration at different times and in differing locations of the central nervous system (CNS), MS affects over 2.5 million people worldwide and about 350,000 in the United States [25]. While the patient's diagnosis of MS will likely be known and a primary reason for referral for home-based medical services, understanding the clinical type, baseline symptoms, and general prognosis/course is important for a provider to best provide anticipatory guidance and recognize symptoms that may signify acute exacerbation and/or progression of disease.

Because the lesions of MS can affect any part of the central nervous system, the clinical symptoms vary widely in type and severity, including both motor and autonomic systems (see Table 6.6). The most common clinical type of MS, relapsing/remitting MS (RRMS), affects 85% of patients and is usually characterized by recovery after an attack. However, a subset of those with RRMS may develop secondary progressive MS (SPMS) in which there is progressive deterioration in function with every attack. Together with primary progressive MS (PPMS), characterized by later age at onset and lack of discrete attacks, and progressive/relapsing MS (PRMS), which overlaps with PPMS and SPMS, these types collectively make up 15% of all diagnoses and are those most likely to experience significant disability and benefit most from medical and personal care services in the home.

While prognosis varies by clinical type, in general, patients with clinical diagnoses of MS experience progressive neurological and functional disability, and about 80% of patients have some functional limitations 15 years after onset. In some studies, 80% of patients required assistance with ambulation by 25 years after onset. Death from MS rarely occurs from the diagnosis itself but rather due to complications of the resulting debility (e.g., aspiration pneumonia or infection). Management of patients with MS as they age, whether in a traditional or home-based setting, can also be challenging as their functional disability may be compounded by other

Table 6.6 Common symptoms of multiple sclerosis

Weakness of limbs
Spasticity
Optic neuritis
Visual blurring
Diplopia
Sensory symptoms (e.g., paresthesia, hyperesthesia)
Pain
Ataxia
Bladder dysfunction
Constipation
Cognitive dysfunction
Depression
Fatigue
Sexual dysfunction
Facial weakness
Vertigo
Heat sensitivity
Lhermitte's symptom
Paroxysmal motor and/or sensory symptoms
Cranial neuropathies V, VII, IX neuralgias and/or spasms
Facial spasms or contracture

chronic conditions associated with overlapping symptoms, such as cerebrovascular disease or diabetes mellitus. Exacerbations of these chronic conditions may also cause worsening of their MS symptoms [25].

6.4.1 *Disease-Specific Management of MS*

Several agents have been shown to reduce rates of attacks, severity of disease, and new or total number of lesions on MRI (Table 6.7). Little is known, however, about long-term efficacy of these treatments. In general, patients with MS who are receiving home-based medical care and have been in the care of a neurologist either are already taking a disease-modifying agent or have stopped because of lack of response or inability to tolerate appropriate options.

The timing, selection, titration, and response monitoring of specific agents should always be made in consultation with a neurologist, as certain medications are more effective with specific clinical types of MS and many have contraindications or adverse effects that may worsen other chronic conditions. Some medications such as the INF-b treatments require monitoring of liver function tests and white blood cell count, so coordination of home-based labs and communication of results with the neurologist are ideal to reduce burden on the patient.

Table 6.7 Therapies for multiple sclerosis

Agent	Clinical considerations
Interferon-b	Subcutaneous injection
	Injection site reactions
	May cause flulike symptoms
	Monitor LFTs, CBC for hepatotoxicity, lymphopenia
Glatiramer acetate	Subcutaneous injection
	Injection site reactions
	Systemic reactions after injections (15%)
	Lipoatrophy
Ocrelizumab	IV infusion
	Infusion reactions
	Upper respiratory infections
	Herpes infections
Natalizumab	Monthly IV infusion
	Risk of PML with long-term treatment
	Hypersensitivity reactions
Fingolimod	Oral dosing
	Monitor LFTs, CBC for hepatotoxicity, lymphopenia
	First-degree heart block or bradycardia

The home-based medical provider should advise the patient regarding feasibility of treatment administration, as traveling for monthly infusions (if home-based infusion services are unavailable) may not be possible for a sufficiently debilitated patient, who will need specialized travel arrangements or alternate therapies. Additionally, a caregiver, rather than the patient, may need to be trained to administer subcutaneous injections such as interferon-b or glatiramer. As with all patients taking any immunosuppressant therapy, patients and their caregivers should be aware of their higher risk for infection, and providers should be vigilant for indicative signs and symptoms.

For patients who have progressive neurologic deterioration with the absence of relapses, experience unwanted side effects, or determine that the burden of a treatment is outweighing its benefits due to the severe stage of MS or another condition, and/or changes in prognosis or goals of care, it is reasonable to discuss discontinuation of disease-modifying therapies.

6.4.2 Management of MS Exacerbations

When an acute deterioration in function occurs, the first consideration is to ascertain whether the acute clinical worsening is due to an MS "attack" or "flare" signifying new disease activity (i.e., a new neurologic lesion) or attributed to an MS exacerbation from a metabolic, infectious, or environmental process (e.g., temperature change).

MS exacerbation typically manifest as worsening of underlying residual deficits or re-emergence of past symptoms related to a known demyelinating lesion. Resolution of the medical trigger oftentimes improves the symptoms without need for glucocorticoids.

Therefore, for a patient or caregiver who reports an acute change in baseline function, a thorough history, physical, and appropriate lab work and/or imaging should be performed looking for a non-MS etiology such as an infection, new or changed medications, a pressure ulcer or other evidence of traumatic injury, evidence of organ dysfunction, new urinary retention, fecal impaction, exacerbation of a concomitant chronic condition, or even change in recent activity or location.

If there is no other identifiable cause of the acute decline and symptoms are new and/or severe enough to cause dysfunction, then glucocorticoid treatment is the standard management, though there is little evidence of long-term benefit. If home-based intravenous (IV) services are available, methylprednisolone 1000 mg/day via IV for 3–5 days is preferred. A steroid taper is typically not required following pulse dose steroid administration. Equivalent doses of oral dexamethasone or methylprednisolone can be substituted for the IV portion of therapy but are associated with increased risk of GI complications such as gastritis or ulcers. Especially if patients have other chronic conditions, it is important to anticipate and manage common side effects of even short-term glucocorticoid therapy such as hyperglycemia, fluid retention, GI complications as already described, electrolyte disturbances (e.g., hypokalemia), and emotional lability. Acute symptoms of MS that are refractory to glucocorticoid therapy may require hospital admission for plasma exchange therapy.

6.4.3 Management of MS Symptoms

Whether or not patients with MS are receiving disease-modifying therapy, aggressively managing symptoms related to the motor, sensory, and functional effects of MS is important to maintain function, improve quality of life, and prevent complications. Management in the home setting is ideal as therapies can be delivered by multiple disciplines, tailored to be most appropriate to the patients' home setting, and reinforced by training caregivers if capable. The management rationale for each symptom is general and does not modify this incurable disease; certain symptoms are also more responsive to treatment than others. Therefore, constant symptom assessment, titration of dosing or intensity of symptom management, and patient education are important and necessary in managing expectations [25, 26]. The type of symptom and optimal management are summarized in Table 6.8.

6.4.4 Palliative Care and Hospice

In addition to assessing and managing symptoms in a patient whose MS has progressed, the home-based medical provider should effectively communicate the current status and possible course of the disease to the patient and caregivers [27, 28]. Furthermore, excluding other diagnoses, discussing treatment options, and providing resources for emotional and spiritual support are also important. As symptoms become severe and difficult to treat and/or a patient's overall clinical status is declining, it is appropriate to review a patient's prognosis and their goals of care and discuss referral to hospice and even an inpatient hospice admission to control certain symptoms more aggressively.

Table 6.8 Management of multiple sclerosis symptoms

Symptom	Management
Sensory	
Neuropathic pain	Gabapentin (900–3600 mg/day, divided doses)
	Pregabalin (50–200 mg two to three times/day)
	Duloxetine (30–120 mg daily)
	Venlafaxine extended release (37.5–225 mg daily)
	Tricyclic antidepressants (10–100 mg at bedtime)
	Acetaminophen; NSAIDs; opiates
Nystagmus	Gabapentin (300–600 mg four times/day); memantine (5–10 mg twice/day)
Temperature intolerance	Environmental modification; adequate room ventilation
Motor	
Cerebellar ataxia/tremor	Clonazepam (0.5–2 mg/day, divided doses); mysoline (25–150 mg/day); propranolol (60–320 mg/day, divided doses if not extended release); trihexyphenidyl (2–15 mg/day, divided doses); occupational therapy; deep brain stimulation
Dysphagia/dysarthria	Speech/language therapy; nutritional aids; artificial nutrition/hydration
Spasticity (see "Spasticity" in "Spinal Cord Injury" section of this chapter)	Physical therapy; botulinum toxin injections; systemic oral drugs (e.g., tizanidine (2 mg two to three times/day, max 36 mg/day), baclofen (5–10 mg three times/day, max 80 mg/day), gabapentin (100–900 mg three times/day, max 3600 mg daily), diazepam (2–5 mg one to two times/day, max 60 mg/day)); intrathecal baclofen pump
Functional	
Fatigue/weakness	Workup for associated conditions; physical therapy; dalfampridine (10 mg two times/day); amantadine (100 mg two or three times/day); methylphenidate (5–10 mg two times/day)
Bladder dysfunction (See "Sphincter Dysfunction" in "Spinal Cord Injury" section of this chapter) • Detrusor hyperreflexia • Detrusor dyssynergia/atony	Behavioral techniques; oxybutynin (2.5–5 mg, two or three times/day); tolterodine (2 mg two times/day); intravesicular botulinum toxin Terazosin (1–20 mg daily); bethanechol 190–50 mg three or four times/day, max 150–200 mg daily); intermittent urinary catheterization
Constipation	Stepwise bowel regimen
Depression	Antidepressants; talk or behavioral therapy
Cognitive dysfunction	Management of associated conditions; donepezil (5–10 mg daily), memantine 10 mg twice daily

6.5 Spinal Cord Injury/Traumatic Brain Injury

6.5.1 *Management of Spasticity*

Spasticity is a velocity-dependent increase in muscle tone resulting from an upper motor neuron (UMN) lesion due to spinal cord and/or traumatic brain injury (SCI/TBI), stroke, multiple sclerosis, and other chronic neurological conditions causing motor dysfunction. The clinical manifestations can range from a subtle increase in resting tone on examination to hyperexcitability of antigravity muscles causing impaired dexterity and restricted joint mobility.

Clinically, the pattern of increased muscle tone of spasticity presents in the upper extremity with excessive flexion of fingers and adduction of thumb, resulting in a "thumb in palm" clenched fist deformity, often with flexion and pronation of the larger muscles of the arm. In the lower extremity, adduction of the hips, knee and plantar flexion, inversion of ankles, and hyperextension of the big toe are the most common findings. Clonus, exaggerated tendon reflexes, muscle weakness, and spasms as a result of spastic co-contraction (inappropriate activation of antagonistic muscles during voluntary activity) are also seen. Sudden worsening of a known diagnosis of spasticity can be due to many factors including noxious somatic or visceral stimuli (see Table 6.9), primary disease progression, or a new neurological process. Therefore, the home-based clinician should do a thorough evaluation to treat and/or refer for further diagnostic workup.

Chronic spasticity can lead to contractures, which tend to restrict movement of joint, ultimately fixing it in a deformed painful position. Timely diagnosis and management of spasticity are important to prevent such complications and optimize function. Furthermore, complications result both from unaddressed spasticity and from associated debility such as falls, pain, pressure ulcers, infections, and contractures. There is little robust evidence to base clinical guidelines for spasticity management; current recommendations are based on expert recommendations for a multidisciplinary approach that combines both pharmacologic and nonpharmacologic agents.

Table 6.9 Potential triggers of worsening spasticity

Visceral: constipation/impaction, UTI, dysmenorrhea, renal colic, urinary retention
Drugs: abrupt discontinuation of antispasmodic drugs, malfunction of intrathecal pump
Skin: pressure ulcers, ingrown toenails, rash, cellulitis
Environmental: improper seating, poorly fit orthotics, extremes of temperature
Others: physical or emotional trauma/stress; DVT, infections

6.5.2 *Nonpharmacologic Management of Spasticity*

While evidence is lacking to support passive manual stretching as management of spasticity, it is often recommended as part of a home management regimen to maintain flexibility and prevent permanent contractures. Furthermore, passive stretching two to three times per day serves to limit the amount of antispasmodic agents utilized in the management of the spasticity. Education of both patient and caregivers by physical and occupational therapists can occur in the home. There is weak evidence to support the use of rigid or Lycra-based splints to simulate a prolonged stretch to spastic limbs; however, some criticize that splinting holds the joint in only one position and does not provide the dynamic movement as with manual stretching. Regardless, splinting can reduce skin breakdown and infection, especially in patients with spasticity in their wrist and finger, ankle, and toe flexors.

Postural management involves devices or maneuvers to ensure proper alignment when sitting, standing, or laying in a bed. Standing frames may be customized to allow people to stand for prolonged periods of time by providing support for the affected limbs. Collaboration with physical or occupational therapists is necessary, as well as with involved caregivers. Small trials of postural management in patients with SCI and MS showed reduced spasticity in lower extremities.

Exercises to strengthen core muscle groups such as the pelvic, trunk, and shoulder girdle or treadmill training has been shown in small studies to improve strength and stability and control over affected distal muscle groups. Physical therapy should be consulted and a patient should be evaluated for general ability to exercise, with caution in patients with severe osteoporosis and severe limitation in passive range of motion or those who are in the immediate postoperative period.

6.5.3 *Pharmacologic Treatments of Spasticity*

Oral antispasmodic agents, with baclofen as the first line and tizanidine and dantrolene as the second line, have been used for several decades and are a mainstay in management, despite lack of robust trials to provide evidence for these agents' effectiveness. Benzodiazepines, such as clonazepam (0.25–1 mg at bedtime or BID), can also be used, but the dose may be limited due to drowsiness. Timing of dosing should be tailored to a patient's lifestyle and function; for example, patients who are somewhat ambulatory should take lower doses during the daytime to allow spasticity and to provide stability. Bedtime dosing and immediately after awakening may be helpful as spasticity often increases with position change and reduced spasticity may facilitate personal care, respectively. Doses of these medications should be started at the lowest dose, especially in those who are still walking, as risk for falls can increase if spasticity unmasks underlying muscle weakness. For some, muscle spasticity provides some postural stability and reduction of spasticity may result in increased weakness or falls right after starting treatment. There is no evidence for combination therapy with oral antispasmodics and should only be reserved for patients who can only tolerate small doses of one drug and with little improvement in symptoms with one drug.

Cannabinoids, the pharmacologically active compound in marijuana, are available as oromucosal sprays in some countries and have been shown in multiple trials to result in subjective improvement in spasticity in up to 30–40% of patients (without objective improvement in spasticity measures). There is a long side effect profile, and long-term effects on cognition, mental health, and behavior are unknown.

Botulinum toxin injections into selected skeletal muscles result in focal reduction in spasticity without systemic side effects of weakness or sedation, though usually no improvement in function. Its use is recommended for patients with focal spasticity and should be performed only by trained physicians. Botulinum toxin injections are considered a first-line treatment, and patients do not need to try any oral medications prior to authorization with most insurance plans. Therapeutic effect is seen within 1 week of administration, with peak effect in 4–6 weeks and duration of effect about 12 weeks. If effective, planned injections every 12 weeks are appropriate.

If a patient with severe spasticity does not respond to adequate doses of oral antispasmodic drugs, they should be referred and evaluated for an intrathecal baclofen pump. When administered intrathecally, a small dose of baclofen can result in effective muscle relaxation without the systemic side effects.

6.5.4 Management of Sphincter Dysfunction

Bowel dysfunction: After a traumatic brain injury or spinal cord injury, constipation, impaction, and fecal incontinence due to overflow often occur. In addition, the decrease in mobility of the patient exacerbates this issue. It is important for the patient's quality of life that stool regularity is re-established. Increased dietary fiber and fluid can help ambulatory patients, but for less ambulatory patients, these interventions can exacerbate the problem. For those patients, medications are often necessary (see Table 6.10) [29]. Initial treatment is often with stool softeners and stimulant laxatives with the addition of a suppository, osmotic agents, and enemas. Determining the best regimen for each patient that is acceptable often takes a while to determine with trial of multiple agents till the preferred regimen is found. A visiting nurse with as needed medication orders can be especially helpful in this process. These nurses can see the patient frequently for a period of time to help determine the best medication and help teach how to administer a suppository or enema.

Urinary dysfunction: Most spinal cord or traumatic brain injury patients have urinary retention ("neurogenic bladder") which can lead to overflow incontinence. Urinary continence requires complex control of the brain, brain stem, spinal cord, and peripheral nerves where any injury to the brain or spinal cord can cause dysfunction. The most important decision is the drainage mechanism. Clean intermittent catheterization every 4–6 h is recommended [30], but requires manual dexterity that, depending on the type of injury, some patients do not have. For these patients, chronic urethral or suprapubic catheterization may be necessary. Clean intermittent

Table 6.10 Pharmacological treatment for constipation for patients with spinal cord injury

Suppositories	Bisacodyl suppository 10 mg PR daily Glycerin suppository
Stool softeners	Docusate 100 mg orally twice a day, can increase to 500 mg per day
Stimulant laxatives	Sennosides 17.2 mg orally at night, max 34.4 mg twice daily Bisacodyl 5–10 mg orally daily
Osmotic	Polyethylene glycol 1 capful orally as needed Lactulose 15–30 mL orally daily, may increase to twice daily
Enemas	Saline enema Mineral oil enema

catheterization has the same rates of infection as sterile technique and thus is recommended [31]. However, indwelling catheters can lead to more urinary tract infections, especially in the home setting where it may be more difficult for the patient to follow evidence-based recommendations to minimize the risk of infection. Patients with bladder and sphincter spasms can benefit from any of the many anticholinergic medications that exist for urinary urgency, but need to be aware of the side effects such as dry eyes, dry mouth, confusion, falls, and constipation.

Crede's method is the application of suprapubic pressure to cause bladder drainage. It also can be enhanced with Valsalva at the same time. It can lead to high intravesicular pressures and reflux, so monitoring by the provider is needed if complications occur [30].

Overflow incontinence causes skin maceration and breakdown, and the distended bladder can stimulate autonomic dysreflexia [30] with hypertension, sweating, and flushing. The hypertension is severe and can lead to cardiac problems. In addition, long-term urinary retention leads to hydronephrosis, urine reflux, and urinary tract infections [30].

6.6 Amyotrophic Lateral Sclerosis

ALS is a progressive neurodegenerative disease that is seen by most home-based primary care clinicians at the later stages of the disease. Annually, 5000 people are diagnosed with ALS in the United States, with age of onset between 40 and 60 years [32]. Most patients die of ALS within 2–5 years [33] of the diagnosis, and the home-based clinicians need to be able to manage symptoms and end-of-life care. Approximately, 10–20% of patients survive more than 10 years [34]. Patients suffer from progressive weakness without sensory symptoms [32] with bulbar, upper motor neuron, and lower motor neuron signs and symptoms. Patients presenting with bulbar signs such as dysphagia, dysarthria, and sialorrhea often have a shorter life expectancy [32]. There is no cure for ALS; therefore, treatments are directed at improvement of quality of life (QOL).

Most home-based clinicians will not be diagnosing ALS, and thus the focus in this section will be evaluation and management of symptoms related to more advanced stages of ALS.

6.6.1 General Management

Specialized multidisciplinary clinics have improved outcomes, including increased survival and less hospitalizations [33] for the care of patients with ALS. However, as the disease progresses, it may become difficult or impossible to access these clinics. Home-based medical providers should have relationships with these clinics to identify recommendations that can be implemented without bringing the patient into the office.

Riluzole is the only medication that is FDA approved for ALS treatment [35]. It has been shown to increase tracheostomy-free survival, possibly by 2–3 months. It is expensive but generally well-tolerated and should be offered to all patients as an option to prolong survival [36].

Most deaths from ALS are the result of respiratory failure and noninvasive ventilation with BiPAP prolongs survival [36]. Close monitoring of respiratory function and symptoms is necessary. Forced vital capacity (FVC) declines at a consistent individual rate [32] and should, therefore, be assessed every 3 months. Once the FVC is less than 50% predicted value, the patient should be considered for BiPAP or invasive ventilation [32]. When the BIPAP is ordered for the home, respiratory therapists can assess in the home for the right mask type and adjust the machine to the right settings with orders from the provider.

Most patients also develop dysphagia and dysarthria as weakness in muscles of the throat and mouth develop. They have an increased risk of aspiration and weight loss. Changes in a patient's speech may be the first sign of weakness [32] and should prompt a speech therapy consultation. Speech therapists can help work to improve speech and recommend assistive devices such as communication devices (alphabet boards, electronic communication devices). Gastrostomy tubes have been shown to prolong survival in ALS and should be considered in the context of the patient's overall condition and goals of care. The timing of the procedure can be challenging, as it can be difficult when the respiratory status is compromised [35]; it is therefore best to have the PEG placed before the patient's FVC is less than 50% predicted value [32].

Mobility deteriorates as muscle weakness and spasticity in the limbs progress. Referrals to physical therapists and occupational therapists through a home care agency can be helpful. There are many assistive devices that can be of use to patients and the home-based medical provider is uniquely able to assess for the need. These include canes, ankle foot orthoses, walkers, wheelchair, headrests, and eating utensils.

Caregiver support is an important aspect of the management of a patient with ALS especially when they are homebound. If possible, an interdisciplinary approach with social workers can help the caregiver identify and access support groups and other community resources.

One of the most important interventions for any provider who cares for patients with ALS is to address goals of care and other advanced directives. These issues need to be readdressed often, as choices may change and patients may not be able to fully address on the first conversation. Especially important are discussions regarding respiratory and nutritional choices.

6.6.2 Symptom Management in ALS

Sialorrhea is a common embarrassing symptom. It is also associated with aspiration pneumonia. Home suction machines are helpful and are covered by most insurances at least partially. Aides, funded through Medicare (Home Health Aides) or state Medicaid programs, usually cannot operate the machine, but private help or family can. First-line treatments include anticholinergic medications (see Table 6.11). Injections of botulinum toxin or radiation to the parotid and submandibular glands are often helpful at reducing or eliminating the drooling in refractory cases [32]. These injections are usually done in the ALS multidisciplinary clinic or neurology office.

- Pseudobulbar effect is characterized as laughter or crying devoid of emotionality. It affects 20–50% of patients with ALS. Antidepressants are often employed, but fixed-dose combination of dextromethorphan/quinidine reduced symptoms but can cause side effects of dizziness, nausea, and somnolence [33] (see Table 6.11).
- Fatigue is very common in patients with ALS, and some of the medications including riluzole can contribute. Fatigue can also be a symptom of depression, immobility, or respiratory dysfunction [33].
- Spasticity is a painful symptom and it impairs mobility. There are few studies of spasticity treatments in ALS, but it can be treated with benzodiazepines and baclofen [33] (see Table 6.11).

Table 6.11 Symptomatic treatments in amyotrophic lateral sclerosis

Symptom	Treatment
Spasticity	Baclofen 5–10 mg orally two to three times daily, can titrate to 20 mg four times daily
	Tizanidine 2–4 mg three times daily, can titrate to 24 mg daily
Pseudobulbar affect	Dextromethorphan/quinidine (20 mg/10 mg) orally once daily, can increase to two times daily
	Sertraline 50–100 mg orally at bedtime
	Amitriptyline 10–75 mg orally at bedtime
Sialorrhea	Atropine eye drops 0.4 mg orally every 4–6 h
	Glycopyrrolate 1–2 mg orally four times daily
	Scopolamine 0.125 mg SC three times daily
Depression	Sertraline 50–100 mg orally at bedtime
	Paroxetine 10–40 mg orally daily

- Pain is usually related to spasticity or neuropathy, but patients may have contractures or arthritis as well. Position change, padding, stretching, and massage are all nonpharmacological treatments. Otherwise treatments should include NSAIDS, acetaminophen, and then escalation to opioids [37].
- Cognitive impairment and behavioral disorders are common in later stages of ALS, occurring in 10–75% of patients [33]. Therefore, screening for cognitive issues through neurocognitive testing and caregiver interviews may be warranted based on the clinical circumstances.
- Depression is common in ALS patients and should be assessed by the home care provider. Many of the common screening tools can be used. Pharmacological treatment is mostly with selective serotonin reuptake inhibitors (see Table 6.11).

6.6.3 Referral to Hospice

- ALS patients are not routinely enough referred to hospice. Many who do not meet hospice criteria die within 6 months. The US-based ALS Peer Workgroup [38] has suggested specific criteria for referral of these patients to hospice (see Table 6.12).

Chronic neurological conditions can be debilitating for patients at a physical, cognitive, and psychiatric level. Understanding the manifestation of these conditions—their progression and the influence that other medical problems and medications can have on them—builds an integral foundation for a home-based clinician to exact a treatment plan. The management of these conditions oftentimes requires a multidisciplinary team who can work in synergy to address the varied symptom spectrum of these conditions. The home-based clinician's ability to conceptualize the neurologic sequelae of the conditions discussed in this chapter will enable them to orchestrate the necessary diagnostic and management plan efficiently and effectively, giving homebound patients and their caregivers the best achievable quality of life.

Table 6.12 Amyotrophic lateral sclerosis peer workgroup hospice referral triggers [37]

1. Forced vital capacity (FVC): 60% predicted (or rapid decline in FVC (more than 20%)) over 2–3 months
2. Clinical signs or clinical symptoms of respiratory insufficiency
3. Respiratory weakness requiring noninvasive positive pressure ventilation
4. Nutritional decline requiring enteral feeding
5. Severe pain or psychosocial distress requiring intensive palliative care interventions (including opioid medication)
6. Rapidly progressive paralysis (over 2–3 months) in two body regions

References

1. Tsao CW, Aday AW, Almarzooq ZI, Anderson CAM, Arora P, Avery CL, Baker-Smith CM, Beaton AZ, Boehme AK, Buxton AE, Commodore-Mensah Y, Elkind MSV, Evenson KR, Eze-Nliam C, Fugar S, Generoso G, Heard DG, Hiremath S, Ho JE, Kalani R, Kazi DS, Ko D, Levine DA, Liu J, Ma J, Magnani JW, Michos ED, Mussolino ME, Navaneethan SD, Parikh NI, Poudel R, Rezk-Hanna M, Roth GA, Shah NS, St-Onge MP, Thacker EL, Virani SS, Voeks JH, Wang NY, Wong ND, Wong SS, Yaffe K, Martin SS, American Heart Association Council on Epidemiology and Prevention Statistics Committee and Stroke Statistics Subcommittee. Heart disease and stroke statistics-2023 update: a report from the American Heart Association. Circulation. 2023;147(8):e93–e621. https://doi.org/10.1161/CIR.0000000000001123. Epub 2023 Jan 25. Erratum in: Circulation. 2023 Feb 21;147(8):e622. PMID: 36695182.
2. Amin HP, Madsen TE, Bravata DM, Wira CR, Johnston SC, Ashcraft S, Burrus TM, Panagos PD, Wintermark M, Esenwa C, American Heart Association Emergency Neurovascular Care Committee of the Stroke Council and Council on Peripheral Vascular Disease. Diagnosis, workup, risk reduction of transient ischemic attack in the emergency department setting: a scientific statement from the American Heart Association. Stroke. 2023;54(3):e109–21. https://doi.org/10.1161/STR.0000000000000418. Epub 2023 Jan 19. PMID: 36655570.
3. Ovbiagele B, Goldstein LB, Higashida RT, Howard VJ, Johnston SC, Khavjou OA, Lackland DT, Lichtman JH, Mohl S, Sacco RL, Saver JL, Trogdon JG, American Heart Association Advocacy Coordinating Committee and Stroke Council. Forecasting the future of stroke in the United States: a policy statement from the American Heart Association and American Stroke Association. Stroke. 2013;44(8):2361–75. https://doi.org/10.1161/STR.0b013e31829734f2. Epub 2013 May 22. Erratum in: Stroke. 2015 Jul;46(7):e179. PMID: 23697546.
4. Mackey J, Yamal JM, Parker SA, Silnes K, Rajan SS, Jacob AP, Wang M, Singh N, Jones WJ, Spokoyny I, Navi BB, Saver JL, Grotta JC, BEST-MSU Study Group. Golden hour treatment with tPA (tissue-type plasminogen activator) in the BEST-MSU study. Stroke. 2023;54(2):415–25. https://doi.org/10.1161/STROKEAHA.122.039821. Epub 2023 Jan 23. PMID: 36689579.
5. Jadhav AP, Desai SM, Jovin TG. Indications for mechanical thrombectomy for acute ischemic stroke: current guidelines and beyond. Neurology. 2021;97(20 Suppl 2):S126–36. https://doi.org/10.1212/WNL.0000000000012801. PMID: 34785611.
6. Powers WJ, Rabinstein AA, Ackerson T, Adeoye OM, Bambakidis NC, Becker K, Biller J, Brown M, Demaerschalk BM, Hoh B, Jauch EC, Kidwell CS, Leslie-Mazwi TM, Ovbiagele B, Scott PA, Sheth KN, Southerland AM, Summers DV, Tirschwell DL, American Heart Association Stroke Council. 2018 guidelines for the early management of patients with acute ischemic stroke: a guideline for healthcare professionals from the American Heart Association/American Stroke Association. Stroke. 2018;49(3):e46–110. https://doi.org/10.1161/STR.0000000000000158. Epub 2018 Jan 24. Erratum in: Stroke. 2018 Mar;49(3):e138. Erratum in: Stroke. 2018 Apr 18. PMID: 29367334.
7. Rehman AU, Mohsin A, Cheema HA, Zahid A, Rehman MEU, Ameer MZ, Ayyan M, Ehsan M, Shahid A, Rehman MAU, Shah J, Khawaja A. Comparative efficacy and safety of tenecteplase and alteplase in acute ischemic stroke: a pairwise and network meta-analysis of randomized controlled trials. J Neurol Sci. 2023;445:120537. https://doi.org/10.1016/j.jns.2022.120537. Epub 2022 Dec 29. PMID: 36630803.
8. Roaldsen MB, Lindekleiv H, Mathiesen EB. Intravenous thrombolytic treatment and endovascular thrombectomy for ischaemic wake-up stroke. Cochrane Database Syst Rev. 2021;12(12):CD010995. https://doi.org/10.1002/14651858.CD010995.pub3. PMID: 34850380; PMCID: PMC8632645.
9. Hariharan P, Tariq MB, Grotta JC, Czap AL. Mobile stroke units: current evidence and impact. Curr Neurol Neurosci Rep. 2022;22(1):71–81. https://doi.org/10.1007/s11910-022-01170-1. Epub 2022 Feb 7. PMID: 35129761.

10. Adams HP, Bendixen BH, Kappelle LJ, Biller J, Love BB, Gordon DL, Marsh EE. Classification of subtype of acute ischemic stroke: definitions for use in a multicenter clinical trial: TOAST: Trial of Org 10172 in Acute Stroke Treatment. Stroke. 1993;24:35–41. https://doi.org/10.1161/01.str.24.1.35.
11. Kleindorfer DO, Towfighi A, Chaturvedi S, Cockroft KM, Gutierrez J, Lombardi-Hill D, Kamel H, Kernan WN, Kittner SJ, Leira EC, Lennon O, Meschia JF, Nguyen TN, Pollak PM, Santangeli P, Sharrief AZ, Smith SC Jr, Turan TN, Williams LS. 2021 guideline for the prevention of stroke in patients with stroke and transient ischemic attack: a guideline from the American Heart Association/American Stroke Association. Stroke. 2021;52(7):e364–467. https://doi.org/10.1161/STR.0000000000000375. Epub 2021 May 24. Erratum in: Stroke. 2021 Jul;52(7):e483–4. PMID: 34024117.
12. Belagaje SR. Stroke rehabilitation. Continuum (Minneap Minn). 2017;23(1, Cerebrovascular Disease):238–53. https://doi.org/10.1212/CON.0000000000000423. PMID: 28157752.
13. Boaden E, Burnell J, Hives L, Dey P, Clegg A, Lyons MW, Lightbody CE, Hurley MA, Roddam H, McInnes E, Alexandrov A, Watkins CL. Screening for aspiration risk associated with dysphagia in acute stroke. Cochrane Database Syst Rev. 2021;10(10):CD012679. https://doi.org/10.1002/14651858.CD012679.pub2. PMID: 34661279; PMCID: PMC8521523.
14. Dizon MAM, De Leon JM. Effectiveness of initiating deep vein thrombosis prophylaxis in patients with stroke: an integrative review. J Neurosci Nurs. 2018;50(5):308–12. https://doi.org/10.1097/JNN.0000000000000385. PMID: 30138153.
15. Zubkov AY, Wijdicks EF. Deep venous thrombosis prophylaxis in cerebral hemorrhage. Rev Neurol Dis. 2009;6(1):21–5. PMID: 19367220.
16. Rothwell P, Giles M, Flossmann E, Lovelock C, Redgrave J, Warlow C, Mehta ZA. A simple tool to identify individuals at high early risk of stroke after a transient ischaemic attack: the ABCD score. Lancet. 2005;366(9479):29–36.
17. DeJean D, Giacomini M, Vanstone M, Brundisini F. Patient experiences of depression and anxiety with chronic disease: a systematic review and qualitative meta-synthesis. Ont Health Technol Assess Ser. 2013;13(16):1–33. PMID: 24228079; PMCID: PMC3817854.
18. Acciarresi M, Bogousslavsky J, Paciaroni M. Post-stroke fatigue: epidemiology, clinical characteristics and treatment. Eur Neurol. 2014;72(5–6):255–61. https://doi.org/10.1159/00036.
19. Harrison RA, Field TS. Post stroke pain: identification, assessment, and therapy. Cerebrovasc Dis. 2015;39(3–4):190–201. https://doi.org/10.1159/000375397. Epub 2015 Mar 5. PMID: 25766121.3763. Epub 2014 Sep 24. PMID: 25277765.
20. Linsenmeyer TA. Post-CVA voiding dysfunctions: clinical insights and literature review. NeuroRehabilitation. 2012;30(1):1–7. https://doi.org/10.3233/NRE-2012-0721. PMID: 22349836.
21. Hughes AJ, Daniel SE, Kilford L, Lees AJ. The accuracy of clinical diagnosis of idiopathic Parkinson's disease: a clinicopathological study. J Neurol Neurosurg Psychiatry. 1992;55(3):181–4.
22. Stamelou M, Bhatia KP. Atypical parkinsonism: diagnosis and treatment. Neurol Clin. 2015;33(1):39–56. https://doi.org/10.1016/j.ncl.2014.09.012.
23. Antonini A, Moro E, Godeiro C, Reichmann H. Medical and surgical management of advanced Parkinson's disease. Mov Disord. 2018;33(6):900–8.
24. Armstrong MJ, Okun MS. Diagnosis and treatment of Parkinson disease: a review. JAMA. 2020;323(6):548–60.
25. McGinley M, Goldschmidt CH, Rae-Grant AD. Diagnosis and treatment of multiple sclerosis. JAMA. 2021;325(8):765–10.
26. Thompson AJ, Toosy AT, Ciccarelli O. Pharmacological management of symptoms in multiple sclerosis: current approaches and future directions. Lancet Neurol. 2010;9:1182–99.
27. Strupp J, Romotzky V, Paed D, Galushko M, Golla H, Voltz R. Palliative care for severely affected patients with multiple sclerosis: when and why? Results of a Delphi survey of health care professionals. J Palliat Med. 2014;17:1128–36.

28. Lorenzl S, Nubling G, Perrar KM, Voltz R. Palliative treatment of chronic neurologic disorders (Chapter 10). In: Bernat JL, Beresford R, editors. Handbook of clinical neurology, vol. 118. 3rd ed. Amsterdam: Elsevier; 2013.
29. Tramonte S, Brand MB, et al. The treatment of chronic constipation in adults. J Gen Intern Med. 1997;12:15–24.
30. Francis K. Physiology and management of bladder and bowel continence following spinal cord injury. Ostomy Wound Manage. 2007;53:18–27.
31. Shekelle PG, Morton SC, Clark KA, Pathak M, Vickrey BG. Systematic review of risk factors for urinary tract infection in adults with spinal cord dysfunction. J Spinal Cord Med. 1999;22:258–72.
32. Davis M, Lou J. Management of amyotrophic lateral sclerosis (ALS) by the family nurse practitioner: a timeline for anticipated referrals. J Am Acad Nurse Pract. 2011;23:464–72.
33. Miller RG, Jackson JC, et al. Practice parameter update: the care of the patient with amyotrophic lateral sclerosis: multidisciplinary care, symptom management, and cognitive/behavioral impairment (an evidence-based review). Neurology. 2009;73:1227–33.
34. Eisen A, Schulzer M, MacNeil M, et al. Duration of amyotrophic lateral sclerosis is age dependent. Muscle Nerve. 1993;16:27.
35. Bensimon G, Lacomblez L, Meininger V. A controlled trial of riluzole in amyotrophic lateral sclerosis. N Engl J Med. 1994;330:585–91.
36. Bedlack R. Amyotrophic lateral sclerosis: current practice and future treatments. Curr Opin Neurol. 2010;23:524–9.
37. Blackhall L. Amyotrophic lateral sclerosis and palliative care: where we are, and the road ahead. Muscle Nerve. 2012;45:311–8.
38. Mitsumoto H. Promoting excellence in end-of-life care in ALS. Amyotroph Lateral Scler. 2005;6:145–54.

Chapter 7
Adult Psychiatric Care in the Home

Peter A. Boling, Lyons T. Hardy, Ericka L. Crouse, Kathryn A. Brennan, and Kathryn M. Rackson

7.1 Introduction

The home-based medical practitioner and treatment team often encounter psychiatric issues in the home-based primary care (HBPC) setting. These include the common problems of anxiety, depression, and grief that are prevalent in longitudinal medical practices, plus the need to help manage what are called serious mental illnesses (SMI) such as schizophrenia, bipolar disorder, and major depressive disorder, often for individuals who lack access to regular health or psychiatric care and become increasingly homebound and isolated by virtue of their mental health problems. This chapter will take a practical approach to guiding practitioners in this work. Dementia with behavioral disturbance is discussed in Chap. 5.

P. A. Boling (✉) · K. M. Rackson
Division of Geriatric Medicine, Virginia Commonwealth University School of Medicine, Richmond, VA, USA
e-mail: peter.boling@vcuhealth.org

L. T. Hardy
Virginia Commonwealth University School of Nursing, Richmond, VA, USA

E. L. Crouse
Department of Pharmacotherapy and Outcomes Science, Virginia Commonwealth University School of Pharmacy, Richmond, VA, USA

K. A. Brennan
Virginia Commonwealth University School of Medicine, Veterans Health Administration, Richmond, VA, USA

J. L. Colburn et al. (eds.), *Geriatric Home-Based Medical Care*,
https://doi.org/10.1007/978-3-031-68786-0_7

7.2 Patient Population, Screening, and Assessment

Mental health disorders are common. Lifetime prevalence is approximately 4% for bipolar disease, 0.5–1% for schizophrenia, 15% for anxiety disorders, and 5–10% for major depression. In those who are home limited, these conditions are more common. Depression is particularly pervasive with 10–12% of patients with chronic physical illness experiencing depression and prevalence of depression greater than 25% in the home-limited population [1].

The United States Preventive Services Task Force (USPSTF) recommends screening for depression in the general adult population [2]. Given the high prevalence of depression in homebound older adults, universal depression screening in this population is especially important. Providers in the home can use standardized screening tools such as the PHQ-2 [3] and PHQ-9 [4]. The PHQ-2 consists of the first two questions of the PHQ-9 and is often used as a "pre-screening" test. If a patient screens positive (by answering "yes" to either of these questions or scoring >/= 3 on a scale of 0–6), a more in-depth screening such as the PHQ-9 can be administered. The PHQ-9 is shown in Table 7.1. An alternate option for screening for depression in older adult populations is the Geriatric Depression Scale. This has a similar sensitivity and specificity as the PHQ-9. It is also discussed in Chap. 5, Table 5.4.

Comprehensive assessment of patients in home-based medical care should include inquiry about prior episodes of SMI such as schizophrenia and bipolar disorder. Clues that might indicate the presence of one of these disorders include

Table 7.1 PHQ-9

Over the *last 2 weeks*, how often have you been bothered by any of the following problems?	Not at all	Several days	More than half of the days	Nearly every day
1. Little interest or pleasure in doing things	0	1	2	3
2. Feeling down, depressed, or hopeless	0	1	2	3
3. Trouble falling or staying asleep, or sleeping too much	0	1	2	3
4. Feeling tired or having little energy	0	1	2	3
5. Poor appetite or overeating	0	1	2	3
6. Feeling bad about yourself—or that you are a failure or have let yourself or your family down	0	1	2	3
7. Trouble concentrating on things, such as reading the newspaper or watching television	0	1	2	3
8. Moving or speaking so slowly that other people could have noticed? Or the opposite—being so fidgety or restless that you have been moving around a lot more than usual	0	1	2	3
9. Thoughts that you would be better off dead or of hurting yourself in some way	0	1	2	3
(For coding: Total score ____=____+____+____)				

inpatient psychiatric care by history, history of suicidal ideation or suicide attempts, history of psychosis, multiple psychiatric medications, antipsychotic or anticonvulsant medications, or tardive dyskinesia on physical exam. Obtaining collateral information from family members and others is important as some patients with SMI may have poor insight into or memory of their psychiatric history.

An unfortunate consequence of electronic record use is that it can lead to the accumulation of inaccurate diagnostic labels that may not be well-substantiated or may be outdated. For example, a person may have been started on quetiapine or haloperidol during an acute hospitalization to treat delirium or agitation, but then are inaccurately labeled as being treated for schizophrenia. In cases such as this, it is important to clarify the details of a patient's psychiatric history and update any inaccuracies in the electronic health record accordingly.

The physical exam is important. Observe for tears shed, withdrawn or flattened affect, bizarre or unusual behavior or comments, and inattention to self-care or hygiene. Start with open-ended approaches and allow time for patients to answer. Sometimes taking an indirect angle is helpful, asking about the family, the new caregiver, life in general, and about the things the patient would like to do, rather than asking specifically about depressed mood and using diagnostic terms that may connote "mental health" problems.

7.3 Family and Social History as Part of the Assessment

Family history Many mental illnesses are known to have a genetic component. Conditions such as depression, schizophrenia, and bipolar disorder are more common in people with a family history of psychiatric disorders. Assessing family history of drug and alcohol use is also important, as these behaviors may become normalized within a family, and living with those under the influence can lead to traumatic experiences.

Social History In older age, as health declines and as death and loss of family members increases, depression and prolonged grief disorder all become more common. Moving from home, loss of a caregiver, or loss of function and independence can be major stressors.

Patients with mental health disorders are better able to manage their symptoms when they are active and have something that brings meaning to their lives. While this can be difficult for patients who are homebound, there are many ways they can still find joy in the day-to-day. This can be as simple as performing housework, spending time with family, and staying involved in a religious community.

7.4 Trauma-Informed Care

Traumatic events can result in long-standing psychiatric symptoms including post-traumatic stress disorder, depression, and anxiety. Trauma reactions are by no means limited to people who have served in the military. A traumatic event is defined as an event or circumstance that is experienced to be physically or emotionally harmful. The Adverse Childhood Experiences study showed a correlation between childhood trauma and mental and physical health conditions in later life [5]. A simple question that can be used to assess trauma is "In your life, have you ever had any experience that was extremely frightening, horrible, or upsetting?" It should be noted that it is not necessary to screen for prior trauma and even if they answer no to this question, it does not mean they have not experienced trauma in their lives.

Trauma-informed care (TIC) is an approach to medical care that acknowledges the importance of maintaining an awareness that many patients may have experienced trauma in their pasts. TIC advocates a "universal precautions" approach in which clinicians apply TIC principles to all patients, whether or not there is a known history of trauma. Since many patients may not feel comfortable disclosing past traumas, a universal precautions approach is warranted. Clinicians should always ask permission before conducting a physical exam, explain to the patient what to expect, maintain open communication about the patient's experience during the exam, and avoid extensive questioning about past traumatic events. Patients should be asked if they have any special preferences during physical exams and routine physical care. Pelvic and genital exams may be particularly traumatic for patients who have a history of sexual abuse or assault. Applying the TIC approach, further outlined by the Substance Abuse and Mental Health Services Administration, includes recognition of the traumatic event and the person's individual experience with the event, as well as the lasting effects that can occur. The "four R's" provide a framework for evaluation and management of past trauma: realization of the potential impact of trauma, recognition of signs and symptoms, responding with appropriate resources and interventions, and avoiding retraumatization [6].

7.5 Major Depression and Generalized Anxiety

Major depression is commonly found in the homebound population. A recent study estimated rates of depression in the semi- and fully homebound population to be 26.5–59.3% [7]. Social isolation, medical comorbidities, loss of independence, and functional limitations are risk factors for development of depression, which may explain the significantly higher rates of depression in this population. The DSM-5 defines major depressive disorder (MDD) as having five or more depressive symptoms over the same 2-week period: depressed mood, anhedonia, weight loss or gain, insomnia or hypersomnia, psychomotor agitation or retardation, fatigue, feeling worthless or excessive guilt, decreased concentration, or thoughts of death or suicide. In order to be considered MDD, symptoms must cause clinically significant distress or impairment in social or occupational functioning and must not be better explained by another medical condition or effects of a substance. Patients should be asked about their history of manic or hypomanic episodes to distinguish major depressive disorder from bipolar disorder. The PHQ-9, discussed in detail in Sect. 7.2, is an effective screening tool for MDD. The goal of treatment for MDD is remission of symptoms and restoration of baseline functioning. Treatment typically consists of a combination of pharmacotherapy and psychotherapy. Pharmacotherapy options for treatment of depression are discussed in further detail in Sect. 7.12. Cognitive behavioral therapy (CBT) and interpersonal psychotherapy are the most common types of psychotherapy used for treatment of MDD [8].

Anxiety disorders are also common in the homebound population. Anxiety symptoms among the homebound population have also been found to be correlated with cognitive impairment [9]. Generalized anxiety disorder (GAD) is the most common anxiety disorder in the general population. GAD is more frequently found in women and is often comorbid with major depression. The DSM-5 defines GAD as excessive anxiety or worry occurring more days than not for at least 6 months. The individual must find it difficult to control the worry, and the anxiety must be associated with at least three of the following symptoms: restlessness, easily fatigued, difficulty concentrating, irritability, muscle tension, or sleep disturbance. The GAD seven-item (GAD-7) scale can be used to help quantify the severity of symptoms [10]. The mainstay of treatment for GAD is pharmacotherapy and cognitive behavioral therapy. Pharmacologic options are discussed in further detail in Sect. 7.11. Complementary treatments such as mindfulness exercises and yoga have also been studied.

7.6 Psychosis, Hallucinations, Delusions, and Paranoia

Hallucinations are common in severe mental illnesses, but they also accompany other conditions and are not necessarily diagnostic of a primary psychosis. Auditory hallucinations that are related to a primary psychiatric disorder are often experienced as voice talking or whispering. These may or may not be intelligible or recognizable to the individual. Often the content is very upsetting and disturbing. Auditory hallucinations such as hearing a song playing may be more likely related to neurological conditions. Visual hallucinations can reflect drug side effects, Lewy body dementia, and delirium due to medical illness. Charles Bonnet syndrome, or visual hallucinations in patients with severe visual loss who otherwise lack psychiatric diagnoses, is also common in the elderly population. Some hallucinations are unique and specific such as seeing cats in patients with late stage Parkinson's disease who take dopaminergic medication. Paranoia and delusions occur in primary psychotic disorders such as schizophrenia but are also common in dementia and delirium. Major depressive disorder can be associated with psychosis. Rapid intervention is indicated in the case of psychotic depression.

7.7 When Medical and Psychiatric Illness Symptom Overlap

Consider both physical health problems and mental health conditions in your differential diagnosis and assessment (see Table 7.2). Medical problems can simulate mental health disorders and vice versa; and in a given case, symptoms and signs that suggest medical illness and those that indicate psychiatric illness often intermingle. Delusions and hallucinations may result from medications, delirium, and encephalopathy or from dementias such as Lewy body disease rather than mood disorders and psychoses. Weight loss, sleep cycle changes, and cognitive function changes often indicate depression in older patients. Fatigue, lethargy, and anhedonia can be related to anemia, hypothyroidism, sleep apnea, or diabetes. Somatic complaints such as abdominal pain or chest pain may resolve when patients are treated for depression. Chronic pain can also lead to psychiatric symptoms such as depression and anxiety. Persons with sleep concerns may be screened for sleep apnea or restless legs syndrome. Narcolepsy is rare but should be considered if there is excessive, overwhelming sleepiness during the day and may respond to psychostimulant medication. Neurosyphilis is rare in advanced old age but is a treatable cause of neuropsychiatric disease in middle-aged adults.

Table 7.2 Medical conditions that can mimic mood disorders

Medication side effects
Uncontrolled pain
Constipation
Infection
Hyperthyroidism and hypothyroidism
Electrolyte disturbance
Uremia
Liver dysfunction
Severe anemia (hemoglobin <8)
Hypoxia
Sleep disorders (sleep apnea and/or restless legs syndrome)
Hyperglycemia and hypoglycemia (blood sugars >400, <60)
Subclinical seizures
Brain lesions (tumor, stroke, subdural hematoma)
CNS infection (i.e., neurosyphilis, abscess)

7.8 Social Isolation

Older homebound adults are at increased risk of social isolation and loneliness compared to younger adults. Even before the COVID-19 pandemic, a survey from the Commonwealth Fund found that 37% of high-needs adults—those with two or more chronic medical conditions and physical or cognitive limitations—reported feeling socially isolated, lacking companionship, and feeling left out, lonely, or isolated from others, compared with 15% of other adults [11]. Physical distancing measures implemented to reduce the transmission of COVID-19 beginning in 2020 has further exacerbated the problem of loneliness and social isolation in this population. Feelings of loneliness are associated with adverse physical and mental health outcomes [12]. There are several different tools that can be used to screen for loneliness and social isolation including the UCLA Loneliness Scale and the Revised Social Support Questionnaire (SSQ6) [13]. Home-based primary care clinicians should work together with their interdisciplinary team to identify patients at risk for social isolation or loneliness and implement interventions aimed at increasing social support and finding opportunities for social interaction.

There are also individuals in every community who have gradually and intentionally separated themselves from society and keep to themselves. Some have mental illness and many have unusual ways of dressing, grooming, and keeping house. They may hoard items and belongings and are careless about personal hygiene or dress. Many are cognitively intact and have no defined mental health disorder. Some may have personality disorders as defined by the DSM-5-TR (Diagnosis and Statistical Manual, Edition 5, Text Revision). One of the more difficult dimensions in mental health is the category of personality disorders (ten of them in DSM-5-TR) that share as common features (1) distorted thinking patterns, (2) problematic emotional responses, (3) over- or under-regulated impulse control, and (4) interpersonal difficulties. Among "cluster A" or the odd, eccentric clusters are paranoid personality disorder, schizoid personality disorder, and schizotypal personality disorder. Individuals with these personality disorders are less likely to seek psychiatric care but may be identified in home-based interventions. Hoarding behaviors are important for the home-based primary care provider to address as excess clutter can increase risk of falls, pose fire hazard risks, and further contribute to feelings of social isolation. It is important to approach this topic thoughtfully, as some patients may have insight into the negative effects of their hoarding behavior, while others may not feel it is a problem.

7.9 Concurrent Chemical Dependency and Mental Illness

Dependency on or heavy misuse of alcohol, cocaine, and other chemical substances may complicate treatment and diagnosis of mental illness. Often the chemical dependency must be addressed before progress can be made with depression, anxiety, or other mental illness. This usually requires the help of specialists in addiction disorders and psychiatric care resources. There has been an upward trend in alcohol use in older adults in the USA. Data from the National Survey on Drug Use and Health indicate that approximately 11% of adults over age 65 report drinking 4–5 alcoholic beverages per day [14]. Patients should be asked specifically about commonly used names for street drugs and various alcoholic beverages. Performing comprehensive urine drug screen testing may also be indicated. Patients may abuse prescription drugs that they obtain from others or from their own prescriptions.

Cannabis use is also increasingly prevalent in older adults, likely due to increased legalization and availability. Pain, insomnia, and anxiety have been the most common reasons cited for cannabis use. A study in the *Journal of the American Geriatrics Society* in 2020 found that 15% of older adults surveyed had used cannabis in the past 3 years. About half of these older adults reported using cannabis regularly on a daily or weekly basis, whereas 46% reported using cannabinoid-only products such as CBD [15]. Cannabidiol (CBD) is a cannabinoid compound found in the cannabis plant that does not produce a euphoric effect because it does not contain tetrahydrocannabinol (THC). It is important to note that the effects of cannabis and cannabinoids when combined with specific medications are not well understood, and more research is needed to better understand the efficacy and safety of different cannabis formulations in treating some of these common conditions in older adults. While use is increasing, there is not a clear connection in older adults between cannabis use and worsening mental illness.

7.10 Managing Controlled Medications in Home-Based Medical Care

In the setting of concurrent mental illness and chronic medical conditions, a frequent challenge is management of controlled medications. Because of diversion and accidental deaths, this is a national focus. Many patients at home experience chronic pain or anxiety, for which opioids and other controlled medications may be needed and should be prescribed if indicated. Careful documentation about diagnosis, numbers of pills that are prescribed, pill counts, patient contracts related to controlled substances, and in some cases regular use of urinary drug screens are all important. Reviewing a patient's profile in your state's prescription drug monitoring program (PDMP) database prior to prescribing a controlled substance can help identify patients who may be misusing controlled substances or at risk of overdose. Keep track of current local and national regulations and remain compliant. Diversion is illegal and a form of elder abuse. Providers must be thorough in determining the appropriateness of medication use. If there is concern for diversion or misuse, providers must ultimately decline to continue prescribing controlled medicines. This may be difficult, particularly when there is a genuinely painful condition and concern about elder abuse and neglect, yet the older patient refuses to leave the situation for what we would consider to be a safer alternative. Lock boxes and other strategies may allow the prescriber to continue providing medications that are truly indicated for the patient.

7.11 Managing Mental Health Problems Using Non-pharmacologic Resources

Managing conditions without medications is always a good initial goal when possible. In some conditions, such as depression, there is evidence that cognitive behavioral therapy (CBT) is equivalent to or better than antidepressant medication. Many older individuals respond well to CBT and other forms of psychotherapy. For patients who have experienced trauma, trauma-focused psychotherapy may be indicated. One of the problems in home care is finding a mobile resource for this kind of treatment, but when resources exist, clinicians should offer them. Typically, ongoing psychotherapy is provided by licensed clinical social workers (LCSW) and psychologists. Licensed professional counselors (LPC) are licensed to provide psychotherapy but are not credentialed by Medicare so would not be available to see patients with Medicare. Psychiatrists and advanced practice psychiatric nurses provide psychiatric care that often incorporates medication treatment. The rise of telehealth and telepsychiatry in the 2020s has increased access to mental health services for the homebound population, as many of these patients now no longer need to leave the home to seek this type of care. Some episodes of depression are situational and transient and should not result in medication management. Improved socialization may help, as may reassurance and effective management of concurrent symptoms such as pain that can lead to depression [16]. Another intervention that has good research support is the use of relaxation techniques such as deep breathing, progressive muscle relaxation, and guided imagery. These can be taught to patients in 10–15 min and can be very beneficial for managing pain, anxiety, and depression [17].

Physical activity and exercise are also important components of improving mental health. Even those who have mobility limitations can usually perform chair exercise or a stretching program. The importance of adequate sleep to mental and physical health cannot be overstated. Many patients who complain of difficulty sleeping will benefit from basic sleep hygiene interventions such as adhering to routine bedtime and wake-up times, increasing activity level during the day, removing TVs and electronics from the bedroom, avoiding any electronic devices for at least an hour before bedtime, and keeping the bedroom cool and dark. In addition, bright light therapy using a light box has good evidence to support its use in treating depressive disorders [18]. Recommended parameters are using the light box for 30 min as soon as possible after waking up (prior to 10 a.m.) and placing the box slightly above the head. Patients can read or do other activities during light therapy. For those who may have limited resources, spending time outside in the morning can be a good alternative if mobility permits.

7.12 Medications for Psychiatric Disorders

Assuming that non-pharmacologic strategies have failed, use of medications for mental illness is a key skill in home-based medical care. A comprehensive discussion is beyond the scope of this chapter but general guidelines follow.

When starting new psychiatric medications in older adults, caution should be taken with dosing, but symptoms should not be undertreated. Some older patients do not improve until doses are raised to therapeutic ranges. When prescribing, also take into consideration concurrent medical conditions, drug-drug interactions, and whether dosage adjustments are needed for renal impairment or hepatic impairment.

In depression, antidepressant medications are used as the first-line pharmacologic strategy. These include selective serotonin reuptake inhibitors (SSRIs), serotonin norepinephrine reuptake inhibitors (SNRIs), and several atypical antidepressants such as bupropion and mirtazapine. Among SSRIs, paroxetine is relatively more anticholinergic. Tricyclic antidepressants (TCAs) are still used in some cases; however, they have anticholinergic properties and should be used with caution in the elderly. If a TCA is used, nortriptyline is preferred over amitriptyline; and therapeutic drug monitoring (levels) may be indicated. TCA overdose can be fatal, so they should not be given to patients with active suicidal ideation. Because of drug interactions and required diet restrictions, monoamine oxidase inhibitors (MAOIs) are used infrequently for treatment-resistant depression. When tapering or switching medications, give consideration to potential for duplication of neurotransmitter effects (serotonin toxicity) or re-emergence of depression, and keep a careful watch during these transitions, checking on patients every few weeks.

When selecting an antidepressant medication, be mindful of other symptoms that may benefit from that particular medication. For example, chronic neuropathic pain or migraine headaches may also respond to SNRIs or TCAs. Bupropion is also used for smoking cessation. Mirtazapine and TCAs may benefit those who have difficulty with insomnia. Mirtazapine may also increase appetite. Antidepressants that are commonly used in older patients include escitalopram, citalopram, mirtazapine, and sertraline. Side effect profiles and potential for drug interactions should be taken into consideration in medication selection. All antidepressants may increase the risk of falls, and elderly patients may be more susceptible to antidepressant-induced hyponatremia, particularly with serotonergic agents (SSRI, SNRI, others) and when used in combination with thiazide diuretics—thus sodium level should be monitored after starting these drugs.

Patients usually require at least a 4–6-week trial on a given antidepressant to determine benefit. Doses must be increased to a therapeutic range before concluding the drug is not effective. It is helpful to target and quantify the specific symptoms being treated and evaluate those systematically when deciding whether a medication is effective. While the patient's subjective experience is important, simply asking patients if they feel "better" may provide an inaccurate assessment. Additionally, with major depression a treatment period of 6–12 months or longer is usually needed. Early withdrawal of medication is not advisable unless there are adverse drug effects.

In active bipolar disorder, patients usually have a psychiatric care provider involved. If the nonpsychiatric home-based medical care provider is the only provider involved, continuing maintenance medications is important to prevent manic and depressive episodes. Commonly used treatments are the anticonvulsants such as valproic acid, carbamazepine, and lamotrigine. Lithium is another effective mood stabilizer but may be less often preferred due to the side effects, drug interactions, and a narrow therapeutic window. Second-generation antipsychotics (SGAs) are also effective as mood stabilizers for patients with bipolar disorder. The depressive phase of bipolar disorder is managed differently than major depression. Often patients with significant bipolar disorder are taking multiple medications, and in these cases, psychiatric providers are an important part of the treatment team.

In disorders such as schizophrenia and schizoaffective disorder, there is a subpopulation of older individuals whose psychiatric disease has stabilized and who are now able to function with less intensive psychiatric interventions. There may be chronic fixed delusions or hallucinations that are not particularly disturbing to the patient, and these can be managed by acknowledging the existence of symptoms, tracking them, and maintaining the patient on some medications to limit exacerbations. Nonpharmacological techniques such as distraction can also be very helpful. These patients can remain stable in the community for years without many changes to their regimen. If the problems are less stable or more complex, psychiatrically trained providers should be involved. Regular review for the development of tardive dyskinesia should be performed for any patient on long-term antipsychotic medication therapy.

7.13 Psychiatric Medication Pharmacology and Prescribing

Table 7.3 provides information and guidelines regarding the more commonly used prescription medications.

Among the first rules of prescribing for geriatric patients is to minimize anticholinergic burden, particularly in those with dementia. First-generation TCAs such as amitriptyline should be avoided. TCAs may occasionally be used when SSRI or SNRI medications have failed and the patient still has significant depressive symptoms. If a TCA is used, *N*-demethylated versions such as desipramine and nortriptyline are less anticholinergic and are preferred. Because TCA overdose can be fatal, they should not be given to patients with active suicidal ideation. Among SSRIs, paroxetine is relatively more anticholinergic.

Prescribers should assess liver and kidney function and adjust doses based on organ function and drug clearance properties.

For insomnia and anxiety, sedating agents such as benzodiazepines and nighttime sedative hypnotics should be limited, and patients should be informed about

Table 7.3 Pharmacology, cautions and side effects of common psychotherapeutic medications

	Initial dose for elderly (per day)	Dose range in elderly	Timing	Half-life (h)	Clearance/ elimination	Adverse effects	Additional considerations
Antidepressants							
Citalopram	10 mg	10–20 mg	Daily	35–50% higher in elderly	Primarily hepatic	Nausea, insomnia, sedation, sexual dysfunction, QTc prolongation, hyponatremia; occasionally tremors and some fall risk	Maximum dose in elderly 20 mg due to QTc prolongation; and in hepatic impairment or if combined with CYP2C19 inhibitors May be sedating due to histaminic activity
Escitalopram	5 mg	5–10 mg	Daily	27–32 50% higher in elderly	Primarily hepatic	Nausea, insomnia, sedation, sexual dysfunction, hyponatremia, less QTc effect than citalopram	
Sertraline	25 mg	25–200 mg	Daily	26	Primarily hepatic	N/V, insomnia, sedation, sexual dysfunction, hyponatremia, more diarrhea than other SSRIs	Less drug interactions than other SSRIs
Fluoxetine	10 mg	10–40 mg	Daily	24–72 (acute use) 96–144 (chronic use)	Primarily hepatic	Activating SSRI, weight loss, nausea, insomnia, sexual dysfunction, hyponatremia	Prolonged half-life in elderly Active metabolites' half-life is longer than parent drug CYP 2C19 + 2D6 inhibitor

Paroxetine	10 mg	10–40 mg	Daily	21	Primarily hepatic, metabolites cleared by kidneys	Sedation, weight gain, hyponatremia, more anticholinergic than other SSRIs	Levels can be elevated: (2×) if hepatic or (4×) if renal impairment; withdrawal syndrome can occur when stopping med CYP 2D6 inhibitor
Venlafaxine XR	37.5 mg daily	37.5–225 mg	Daily	3–7	Primarily hepatic, metabolites cleared by kidneys	Dose-dependent hypertension, nausea, sexual dysfunction, insomnia	Withdrawal syndrome can occur when stopping med
Duloxetine	20–30 mg daily	30–120 mg	1–2×/day	12	Primarily hepatic, metabolites cleared by kidneys	Nausea, insomnia, sexual dysfunction, less QTc prolongation than venlafaxine [19]	Not recommended if Cr Cl<30 mL/min Also FDA approved for pain syndromes
Mirtazapine	7.5–15 mg at bedtime	7.5–45 mg	Bed	20–40	Both hepatic and renal	Sedation and weight gain	45 mg should be dosed in the morning; reduce dose in renal impairment
Bupropion	100–150 mg	100–450 mg daily	IR: TID SR: BID XL: daily	12–30	Primarily hepatic, metabolites cleared by kidneys	Insomnia, anxiety, tremor, weight-neutral	SR or XL preferred over IR. Do not use in bulimia, anorexia, seizure disorders Reduce dose in renal disease CYP 2B6 and D6 inhibitor
Trazodone	25–50 mg at bedtime	25–150 mg	Bed	7–10	Primarily hepatic	Sedation, orthostasis, priapism (rare)	Used primarily off-label to treat insomnia

(continued)

Table 7.3 (continued)

	Initial dose for elderly (per day)	Dose range in elderly	Timing	Half-life (h)	Clearance/ elimination	Adverse effects	Additional considerations
Nortriptyline	10 mg	10–100 mg	Bed	23.5–79	Primarily hepatic, metabolites cleared by kidneys. Half-life at longer end of spectrum in older adults	Sedation, weight gain, orthostasis	Drug levels, target 50–150 ng/mL
Second-generation antipsychotics							
Risperidone	0.25–0.5 mg	0.5–2 mg	1–2×/ day	3–20	Primarily hepatic, metabolites cleared by kidneys	Metabolic, orthostasis, EPS, sedation, high prolactin level, dysphagia, osteoporosis, sedation	

Quetiapine	12.5–25 mg	12.5–300 mg	1–3×/day	6	Primarily hepatic, metabolites cleared by kidneys	Orthostasis, sedation, metabolic, QTc prolongation, less EPS, constipation	May be considered in persons with Parkinson's disease Lower doses more sedating—histaminic properties
Olanzapine	2.5 mg	2.5–10 mg	Bed	21–54	Primarily hepatic, metabolites cleared by kidneys	Metabolic (more than other agents in class), sedation, dysphagia, anticholinergic, constipation	Smoking can reduce olanzapine concentration
Aripiprazole	2 or 2.5 mg	Not clear adults: 2–15 mg	Daily	75	Primarily hepatic, metabolites cleared by kidneys	More activating, insomnia, akathisia	Dose reduction required if on concurrent CYP2D6 or CYP3A4 inhibitors
Clozapine	12.5 mg	12.5–200 mg	Bed—BID	4–12	Primarily hepatic, metabolites cleared by kidneys	Agranulocytosis, seizures, constipation, orthostasis, sedation, QTc prolongation, drooling, weight gain, cardiomyopathy	Monitor ANC (absolute neutrophil count) weekly for 6 months; every 2 weeks next 6 months; and then monthly Seizure risk is dose-dependent If misses more than 48 h return to initial dose and retitrate. May be preferred in movement disorders Smoking can reduce clozapine concentration

(continued)

Table 7.3 (continued)

	Initial dose for elderly (per day)	Dose range in elderly	Timing	Half-life (h)	Clearance/ elimination	Adverse effects	Additional considerations
Pimavanserin	34 mg	10–34 mg	Daily	57	Hepatic	Peripheral edema, QTc prolongation, nausea, confusion	Approved only for Parkinson's disease psychosis Lacks dopamine antagonist activity Lower rates of orthostasis or EPS than other antipsychotics Reduce dose with CYP3A4 inhibitors Half-life of active metabolite is 200 h
First-generation antipsychotics							
Haloperidol	0.5 mg	0.5–4 mg	1–3×/ day	18	Primarily hepatic, metabolites cleared by kidneys	EPS, sedation	Avoid in Parkinson's disease
Mood stabilizers							
Valproic acid/ divalproex (VPA)	250–375 mg	500–2000 mg	SR: BID ER: QD IR: TID	9–19	Primarily hepatic, metabolites cleared by kidneys	Sedation, hyponatremia, falls, low platelet count, elevated ammonia, diarrhea, increased LFTs, pancreatitis, alopecia, edema, weight gain	Elderly patients using VPA for behavior may respond at low levels Malnourished, end-stage renal disease, or low albumin, levels may not reflect an accurate level and a free VPA level may be indicated

Lithium	150–600 mg[a]	150–1200 mg Based on serum level	1–3×/day IR + ER forms avail	24 Extended in elderly	Renal	Weight gain, nausea, nocturia, psoriasis, hypothyroidism, hyperparathyroidism, nephrogenic diabetes insipidus	Hydration is important Narrow therapeutic range, blood levels must be monitored regularly Early signs of toxicity n/v, tremor, slurred speech, ataxia, AMS, lethargy Monitor renal function and adjust lithium dosage accordingly Target lower end of dose range in elderly Drug interactions (e.g., NSAIDs, ACE-I, ARBs, thiazide diuretics)
Carbamazepine	100–200 mg	200–800 mg based on serum level	BID-TID	25–65 (initial use) 12–17 (chronic use)	Primarily hepatic, metabolites cleared by kidneys	Hyponatremia, increased LFTs, agranulocytosis, aplastic anemia, rash	Potent inducer of CYP1A2, 2B6, 2C19, 2C8, 2C9, 3A4
Lamotrigine	25 mg[b]	25–400 mg	IR: BID XR: Daily	Depends on interacting medications	Hepatic and renal	Nausea, rash, edema, insomnia, sedation, dizziness	Risk of adverse effects increased with rapid titration and when taken concurrently with divalproex sodium. Follow strict slow titration schedule to minimize risk of rash

IR immediate release, *SR* sustained release, *XL* extended release, *OH* orthostatic hypotension, *EPS* extrapyramidal symptoms, *N/V* nausea and vomiting, *metabolic* weight gain, diabetes, increased cholesterol, *LFTs* liver function tests, *NSAID* nonsteroidal anti-inflammatory, *ACE-I* angiotensin-converting enzyme inhibitors, *AMS* altered mental status, *ARB* angiotensin receptor blockers, *h* hour

[a] Lithium initial doses should be based on renal function and drug interactions; elderly patients require lower doses than healthy young adults

[b] Initial lamotrigine dose depends on concurrent meds. As monotherapy 25 mg daily; with concurrent valproic acid 25 mg every other day; with concurrent carbamazepine, phenytoin, or phenobarbital 50 mg daily

risks. Falls and related injuries are common side effects. Research links long-term use of benzodiazepines and hypnotics to the development of dementia [20]. Additionally, the combination of benzodiazepines and opioid pain medications increases risk of overdose and should be avoided if possible. Benzodiazepines are highly habit-forming and may paradoxically increase anxiety when the effects wear off, leading to a cycle of requiring more and more medication to obtain the same effect. If benzodiazepines must be used, choose agents with a shorter half-life such as lorazepam (6–8 h) and limit the duration of use. SSRIs and SNRIs are considered the first-line pharmacological treatment for anxiety disorders; however, it takes time to obtain a therapeutic benefit. At bedtime, trazodone has become a preferred medication to promote sleep, though without much evidence. Sedation is a side effect of trazodone, and while it is relatively safe to use for sleep, it is important to be aware that trazodone can cause orthostasis in older adults. Given chronic insomnia is not particularly responsive to medication, the author's general practice is to use non-pharmacologic measures first. As discussed previously, sleep hygiene interventions can be very effective. If medication is indicated, consider melatonin or melatonin receptor agonists (i.e., ramelteon). The newest class of insomnia medications, the orexin antagonists (e.g., suvorexant, lemborexant), are beginning to be studied in older adults including those with Alzheimer's disease.

When prescribing psychiatric medications, attention is needed to emerging pharmacologic problems, including serotonin syndrome, neuroleptic malignant syndrome, hyponatremia, and QT prolongation. Serotonin syndrome is a serious but rare condition that involves a serotonergic crisis which may be related to a combination of several serotonergic agents. Presenting symptoms include mental status changes, nausea, vomiting, malaise, and autonomic instability. More advanced symptoms may include hyperreflexia, muscle rigidity, and myoclonus. Caution should be exercised when combining serotonergic antidepressants with linezolid. Neuroleptic malignant syndrome is most commonly related to antipsychotic medications and may include mental status changes, autonomic instability (especially hyperthermia), and eventually muscular rigidity. Hyponatremia is a side effect to antidepressant medications that occurs more commonly in the elderly. Monitor patients for mental status changes after starting an antidepressant, particularly if they take other agents that can put them at risk for hyponatremia (e.g., thiazide diuretics) [21].

When newly prescribing medications or when nonspecific but potentially significant side effects such as nausea, altered mentation, weakness, falls, or constipation are reported, check for relatively common problems such as hyponatremia, caused by inappropriate secretion of antidiuretic hormone (SIADH) due to the medication. If present, confirm the diagnosis with a concurrent urine osmolality and serum osmolality—in SIADH the urine osmolality will be higher than serum. Be aware that use of diuretics invalidates this testing algorithm.

QTc prolongation is an increasing focus, particularly with certain agents and combinations, such as antipsychotics (e.g., quetiapine, ziprasidone, haloperidol) and some antidepressants (e.g., citalopram). The Food and Drug Administration (FDA) suggests a maximum dose of citalopram 20 mg in patients 60 years and older. Guidelines suggest concern when QTc intervals exceed 460 ms, serious, and even fatal; arrhythmias may be the first indication of this problem. Usually the dangerous arrhythmias occur in patients with underlying heart disease or with greater increases in QTc (500 ms or more). The best practice is to monitor the QTc by ECG after starting and periodically, ensure electrolytes (i.e., potassium and magnesium) are within normal limits, take appropriate precautions, and weigh burden and benefit. Important here is that these rhythm problems are known to occur but are relatively rare. Sometimes the stability of the psychiatric condition outweighs the unknown risk of a potential rhythm problem.

In some cases of refractory psychosis or nonadherence, injectable depot medications are effective. These situations should involve a psychiatrically trained person, at least for periodic review. Injectable medications given without an incapacitated patient's permission should be established on the basis of well-documented authority (guardian, POA). Haloperidol, fluphenazine, risperidone, paliperidone, aripiprazole, and olanzapine are available in a long-acting formulation. Also, electroconvulsive therapy can be effective in severe cases where drugs are not adequate.

7.14 Home-Based Services Covered by Insurance (Medicare Part A Home Health Agency Psychiatric Care)

An underused resource in psychiatric home care is the home health agency. In part this is because many agencies have not developed the needed team, which includes nurses with special qualifications in psychiatric care and licensed clinical social workers. When the teams exist, Medicare covers psychiatric diagnoses for skilled home healthcare episodes, and there is evidence of improved outcomes such as in patients with more severe forms of depression [22]. Inquire among local agencies to see if these resources exist. In addition, for patients who have had at least one psychiatric hospitalization in their lifetime, who have a serious mental illness, who have the potential to improve functioning, and who have Medicaid, mental health skill building is an available service. This benefit provides up to 12 h per week of in-home mental health support provided by trained personnel who are supervised by licensed mental health professionals.

7.15 Patient Selection for In-Home Psychiatric Care

If patients with psychiatric disorders are chronically homebound, or in some cases homeless, it is appropriate to see them in the community (at home) rather than in an office. Mental health conditions can be the cause of homebound status. Just as when medical diagnoses lead to inability to visit the office, seeing psychiatrically incapacitated patients at home improves access to care and gives more insight to providers and can increase efficacy of treatment. Examples of home-limiting psychiatric conditions are severe agoraphobia, severe depression, psychoses, and dementia. Conversely, home-based medical care providers should not inadvertently foster dependency or reduce autonomy. In some cases, short-term in-home care for psychiatric conditions is all that the patients need, just as is the case for some medical home-based medical care conditions.

7.16 Community Resources

One solution to alleviate impacts of psychiatric conditions are adult day programs. They help alleviate home caregiver responsibilities. The other participants should be at a similar level of cognitive function, staff should be well trained, and activities should be suited to the patient's needs and preferences. Orienting the patient to the care setting and making sure they are comfortable is a key part of the initial process—think about the first day of school for children as an analogy. Unfortunately, the right resource may not exist and after some attempts adult day care may not work. Short-term respite care, in adult group homes or in nursing homes, can also be important when caregivers need a break.

The community mental health clinic or public health department in your community may offer a crisis intervention team who will provide in-home assessments and treatments either urgently or chronically depending on local funding. When placement into a facility appears necessary, either voluntary or involuntary, these mobile teams often play a central role. Engaging law enforcement may also be a last-resort intervention when community resources do not support the use of crisis intervention services in the home.

Many communities have mobile psychological or psychiatric care practices. Experience suggests that these often focus on group care settings such as assisted living and nursing homes for reasons of efficiency, but sometimes these clinicians will visit private homes and apartments.

In the 1980s and 1990s, there were numerous studies, including many randomized trials of small, intensive community-focused teams, with the acronyms assertive community treatment (ACT), mental health intensive care management (MHICM), and program of assertive community treatment (PACT). This literature is summarized by Mueser [23]. Notably, caseloads in these intensive models were in the 10–30 patient range and enrolled subjects numbered fewer than 100, predominantly individuals with schizophrenia, bipolar disorder, and schizoaffective disorder. Teams functioned as a sort of "virtual hospital" with services as intensive as nurses administering medications in the home on a daily basis if needed. These models of home-based care are both effective and cost-effective and the studies are quite robust. However, this work requires funding and a team that includes staff with training to care for this very complex population. Typically, these teams include a psychiatrist or psychiatric advanced practice nurse, social workers, psychiatric nurses, and case managers. In many states, Medicaid provides funding for PACT team services. Some PACT teams are provided by private agencies and some are provided by community mental health clinics. If psychiatric home care is a special interest, there is evidence that integrating mobile psychiatric home care with housing can be effective [24].

7.17 Patient and Provider Safety

The key issues here are abuse and neglect, risk of self-harm in patients with impaired cognition, and suicidal or homicidal concerns. Providers have a mandate to report known or suspect abuse or neglect. Abuse and neglect are subjects for an entire book and are briefly addressed in Chap. 12 : "Common Social and Ethical Issues in Home-Based Medical Care."

A suicidal or homicidal patient is an emergency situation. In general, calling 911 or 988 is the best course, unless there is another resource such as an emergency response behavioral health team. Older white males have a higher rate of suicide than other groups. Depression, bipolar disorder, substance use disorders, and schizophrenia are all associated with higher rates of suicide. Patients who make brief references to suicidal ideation, without a plan or frequent perseveration are at lower risk than those who dwell on the subject, have severe depression, or are able to describe an intent and a plan. In any case, all firearms and other obvious weapons should be removed, and dangerous medicines should be secured.

Safety and de-escalation training are important for home-based medical providers. It is important to recognize the potential for aggression, which may include such signs as pacing, tone and volume of voice, staring, and erratic behavior. De-escalation techniques can include calm, clear communication, nonconfrontational body language, setting boundaries, and addressing underlying issues. That said, home-based medical care providers should remove themselves from situations that are volatile, particularly when drugs and alcohol are involved, and should arrange a chaperone or withdraw from a case if need be. The presence of weapons in the home should be assessed for provider safety as well.

Other than suicidal or homicidal thinking, circumstances that require psychiatric hospital admission typically relate to depression, mania, or psychosis that are severe enough to prevent the patient from caring for themselves at their baseline level of functioning. Common indications are weight loss, behaviors that are unmanageable, and hallucinations or delusions that cannot be controlled with outpatient medication adjustment. Prior to a psychiatric admission, evaluate for medical instability that would require initial management. Laws regarding criteria and process for involuntary hospitalization vary by state, so it is important to be familiar with regulations in your locality.

7.18 Capacity Determination and Competence

A common decision point in home-based medical care for patients with psychiatric problems is whether the patient has capacity to make decisions, which is something determined by experienced clinicians. Capacity comes into play when deciding about treatment, living situation, or use of resources. For a detailed discussion of capacity determination, please see Chap. 12, "Common Social and Ethical Issues in Home-Based Medical Care."

References

1. Davitt JK, Gellis ZD. Integrating mental health parity for homebound older adults under the Medicare home health care benefit. J Gerontol Soc Work. 2011;54:309–24.
2. Siu AL, US Preventive Services Task Force (USPSTF). Screening for depression in adults: US Preventive Services Task Force recommendation statement. J Am Med Assoc. 2016;315(4):380–7.
3. Kroenke K, Spitzer RL, Williams JB. The patient health questionnaire-2: validity of a two-item depression screener. Med Care. 2003;41(11):1284–92.
4. Kroenke K, Spitzer RL, Williams JB. The PHQ-9: validity of a brief depression severity measure. J Gen Intern Med. 2001;16(9):606–13.
5. Felitti VJ, Anda RF, Nordenberg D, Edwards V, Koss MP, Marks JS. Relationship of childhood abuse and household dysfunction to many of the leading causes of death in adults. Am J Prev Med. 1998;14(4):245–58.
6. Substance Abuse and Mental Health Services Administration. SAMHSA's concept of trauma and guidance for a trauma informed approach. HHS Publication No. [SMA] 14-4884. Rockville, MD: Substance Abuse and Mental Health Services Administration; 2014.
7. Ornstein KA, Leff B, Covinsky K, Ritchie C, Federman A, Roberts L, Kelley A, Siu A, Szanton SL. The epidemiology of homebound in the United States. JAMA Intern Med. 2015;175(7):1180–6.
8. American Psychiatric Association. Practice guideline for the treatment of patients with major depressive disorder. 3rd ed. 2010. http://psychiatryonline.org.proxy.library.vcu.edu/guidelines.aspx.
9. Petkus AJ, Gum AM, Wetherell JL. Anxiety and cognitive impairment in homebound older adults. Int J Geriatr Psychiatry. 2013;28(9):989–90.
10. Spitzer RL, Kroenke K, Williams JB, Löwe B. A brief measure for assessing generalized anxiety disorder: the GAD-7. Arch Intern Med. 2006;166(10):1092–7.
11. Ryan J, Abrams MK, Doty MM, Shah T, Schneider EC. How high-need patients experience health care in the United States: findings from the 206 commonwealth fund survey of high-need patients. Issue Brief (Commonw Fund). 2016;43:1–20.
12. Sakurai R, Yasunaga M, Nishi M, Fukaya T, Hasebe M, Murayama Y, Fujiwara Y. Coexistence of social isolation and homebound status increase the risk of all cause mortality. Int Psychogeriatr. 2019;31(5):703–11.
13. Veazie S, Gilbert J, Winchell K, et al. Addressing social isolation to improve the health of older adults: a rapid review. Rockville, MD: Agency for Healthcare Research and Quality (US); 2019. Appendix F, Social Isolation and Loneliness Definitions and Measures. https://www.ncbi.nlm.nih.gov/books/NBK537897/.

14. Breslow RA, Castle IP, Chen CM, Graubard BI. Trends in alcohol consumption among older Americans: national health interview surveys, 1997-2014. Alcohol Clin Exp Res. 2017;41(5):976–86.
15. Yang KH, Kaufmann CN, Nafsu R, Lifset ET, Nguyen K, Sexton M, Han BH, Kim A, Moore AA. Cannabis: an emerging treatment for common symptoms in older adults. J Am Geriatr Soc. 2020;69(1):91–7.
16. England MJ, Butler AS, Gonzalez ML. Psychosocial intervention for mental and substance use disorders: a framework for evidence-based standards. Washington, DC: Institute of Medicine of the National Academies Press; 2015. http://books.nap.edu/openbook.php?record_id=19013&page=R1.
17. Hofmann SG, Gómez AF. Mindfulness-based interventions for anxiety and depression. Psychiatr Clin North Am. 2017;40(4):739–49. https://doi.org/10.1016/j.psc.2017.08.008. Epub 2017 Sep 18.
18. Tao L, Jiang R, Zhang K, Qian Z, Chen P, Lv Y, Yao Y. Light therapy in non-seasonal depression: an update meta-analysis. Psychiatry Res. 2020;291:113247.
19. Rochester MP, Kane AM, Linnebur SA, Fixen DR. Evaluating the risk of QTc prolongation associated with antidepressant use in older adults: a review of the evidence. Ther Adv Drug Saf. 2018;9(6):297–308.
20. Tseng L, Huang S, Peng L, Chen L, Hsiao F. Benzodiazepines, z-hypnotics, and risk of dementia: special considerations of half-lives and concomitant use. Neurotherapeutics. 2020;17(1):156–64.
21. Jacob S, et al. Hyponatremia associated with selective serotonin reuptake inhibitors in older adults. Ann Pharmacother. 2006;40:1618–22.
22. Bruce ML, Raue PJ, Reilly CF, Greenberg RL, Meyers BS, Banerjee S, Pickett YR, Sheeran TF, Ghesquiere A, Zukowski DM, Rosas VH, McLaughlin J, Pledger L, Doyle J, Joachim P, Leon AC. Clinical effectiveness of integrating depression care management into Medicare home health: the depression CAREPATH randomized trial. JAMA Intern Med. 2015;175(1):55–64.
23. Mueser KT, Bond GR, Drake RE, Resnick SG. Models of community care for severe mental illness: a review of research on case management. Schizophr Bull. 1998;24(1):37–74.
24. Stergiopoulos V, Hwang SW, Gozdzik A, Nisenbaum R, Latimer E, Rabouin D, Adair CE, Bourque J, Connelly J, Frankish J, Katz LY, Mason K, Misir V, O'Brien K, Sareen J, Schütz CG, Singer A, Streiner DL, Vasiliadis HM, Goering PN, At Home/Chez Soi Investigators. Effect of scattered-site housing using rent supplements and intensive case management on housing stability among homeless adults with mental illness: a randomized trial. JAMA. 2015;313(9):905–15.

Chapter 8
Functional Assessment and Common Functional Problems

Robert M. Zimbroff and Mattan Schuchman

8.1 Assessing Function at Home

Understanding and measuring functional status is a cornerstone of a comprehensive home-based assessment. Most home-based primary care (HBPC) practices use functional status as a criterion for eligibility to receive care. Accurate assessment is therefore important to determine enrollment, and a screening assessment may occur by phone before the first home visit is scheduled.

Functional status refers to the ability of an individual to complete activities. Function will fluctuate with disease course, rehabilitation, environmental and task modifications, and with availability of caregiving. Clinicians commonly refer to two subgroups of functional activities: tasks necessary for basic daily living (ADLs) and instrumental activities of daily living (IADLs) necessary to maintain a household. Requiring assistance to complete ADLs or IADLs has been associated with adverse health outcomes including hospitalization, depression, nursing home placement, social isolation, and shorter lifespan. Dependence with ADLs can help estimate prognosis in advanced illness [1]. In a high-quality HBPC practice, ADLs and IADLs are assessed at every new patient visit and reassessed annually and after significant events such as a hospitalization.

Common tools for assessing function include the Barthel, Katz, and Lawton indices listed in Table 8.1 [2]. The Barthel index is a ten-item measure of ADLs and mobility: feeding, bathing, grooming, dressing, bowel and bladder continence, toileting, chair transfer, ambulation, and stair climbing. The Katz index measures six realms of independence in ADLs: bathing, dressing, toileting, continence,

R. M. Zimbroff (✉)
Division of Geriatric Medicine, University of California, San Francisco, San Francisco, CA, USA

M. Schuchman
Division of Geriatric Medicine and Gerontology, Johns Hopkins University School of Medicine, Baltimore, MD, USA

J. L. Colburn et al. (eds.), *Geriatric Home-Based Medical Care*,
https://doi.org/10.1007/978-3-031-68786-0_8

Table 8.1 Commonly used tools to assess ADLs and IADLS

Katz Index of Independence in Activities of Daily Living (ADLs)	Lawton Instrumental Activities of Daily Living Scale (IADLs)
Bathing	Telephone use
Dressing	Shopping
Toileting	Food preparation
Continence	Housekeeping
Transferring	Laundry
Feeding	Transportation
	Medication management
	Financial management

transferring, and feeding. The Lawton index incorporates eight items to measure independence in IADLs, which are considered "higher-order" processes: telephone use, shopping, food preparation, housekeeping, laundry, transportation, medication management, and managing finances.

In the home setting, we favor the Katz and Lawton tools, as they are simple, are widely used, and help track changes over time in functional status. These two indices can also be modified for greater specificity to reflect how patients adapt to functional challenges. For instance, instead of using binary yes/no responses to independence in ADLs or IADLs, alternates could include "independent, modified independent (i.e., can perform independently with use of assistive device), minimal assistance (i.e., supervision, contact guard), and moderate assistance, fully dependent." In the case of bathing, for example, a person may maintain modified independence by washing up at the sink with a cloth rather than showering.

A person's environment has a significant impact on their ability to perform functional tasks. Limitations in function are not necessarily intrinsic, rather they stem from the gap between personal capability and environmental demand. A person's ability to rise from a chair depends upon the type of chair as much as it does a person's strength or coordination. An HBPC provider's ability to observe how an individual performs tasks in their home environment offers deeper insight into ADLs and IADLs than in a traditional office visit. The provider can observe both the layout of the home and the patient demonstrating an activity in their typical setting. For example, asking a person to demonstrate walking and transferring is an essential part of the physical exam in HBPC. Furthermore, clues during a home assessment, such as how medications are stored, the condition of the kitchen, and the presence of stacks of old papers and bills, can give a clinician insight into whether IADLs such as shopping, medication management, and financial management are being completed.

Another way to quantify function is life-space mobility. Life-space comprises the area in which a person lives. It ranges from staying in bed, to a single room, floor, home, street, community, and so forth. By asking key questions of a patient before enrolling, such as "in the past month have you left your house?", "when were you last in a car, bus, or taxi?", and "how do you do your shopping?", HBPC staff can assess life-space to assess eligibility of the patient for the practice and to develop appropriate care plans for patients [3].

8.2 Falls

8.2.1 Prevalence

The World Health Organization defines a fall as "an event which results in a person coming to rest inadvertently on the ground or floor or other lower level." Nearly one-third of older adults will fall once or more on an annual basis. In 2018, the Centers for Disease Control (CDC) found that in the prior year, 27.5% of adults aged over 65 reported at least one fall. In 2018 adults aged over 65 years experienced 8.4 million fall-related injuries, and approximately 32,000 resulted in death [4].

Falls exact a toll both in terms of morbidity and mortality, leading to decreased physical function, loss of independence, and subsequent institutionalization. Each year, approximately 3 million older adults are treated in the emergency department for a fall-related injury, accounting for up to 6% of hospitalizations and 10% of all emergency department visits from older adult patients. The cost of falls to the healthcare system is upwards of $50 billion annually [5]. Furthermore, falls engender a vicious cycle; the majority of older adults who have fallen or are at high risk for falls experience a fear of falling that may lead to restricted activity, a further decline in independence, and increased future fall risk.

8.2.2 Risk Factors

The strongest risk factors for falls include a history of two or more falls in the prior year, difficulty walking or climbing steps, and difficulty with bathing or dressing. These each confer a three- to fourfold increase in risk. Sensory impairment, including diminished proprioception and feeling in the feet (e.g., diabetic neuropathy), equilibrium, and vision, is a major risk factor. Autonomic dysfunction and dysregulation of blood pressure also increase the risk of falls. Other risk factors include decreased strength, gait and balance impairment, incontinence, pain, diabetes, dementia, male sex, living alone, and low body mass index [6].

Medications are also implicated in fall risk. Polypharmacy, most commonly defined as routinely taking five or more medications, is associated with an increased falls risk [7]. Particular classes of medications commonly prescribed to older adults increase risk of falls, including antihypertensives, anticholinergics, and medications that impact the central nervous system such as antidepressants, antipsychotics, antiepileptics (including gabapentinoids), opioids, benzodiazepines, and skeletal muscle relaxants.

Homebound status increases risk for falls, and conversely, falls increase likelihood of becoming homebound. Prevention and treatment for recurrent falls are an important aspect of HBPC [8].

8.2.3 Prevention and Treatment

Given the high risk of falls in the HBPC patient population, *all* patients should be considered at risk for falls, and a plan for fall prevention should be developed regardless of whether the individual had falls in the previous year. If a patient has fallen or had a near fall in the past year, elucidate the circumstances of the fall and any contributing risk factors, such as new medications. Physical examination should focus on identifying physical risk factors, such as visual, cognitive, proprioceptive, and strength deficits. Orthostatic blood pressure should be measured for those able to change positions (lying to sitting, sitting to standing). Laboratory tests should be limited to those that might uncover a suspected risk factor, such as determining the underlying causes of neuropathy.

The home environmental assessment is a critical component of assessing and treating falls and has been shown in randomized trials to reduce falls [9]. The home-based medical clinician can conduct a visual inspection of the home during an initial visit, with attention to common sites of falls such as the bedroom and bathroom. Environmental recommendations to reduce fall risk include adequate lighting (especially night lights, motion sensors); removing loose mats and rugs; removing trip hazards, such as toys from grandchildren; using nonslip bath mats and shower chairs; installing grab bars; installing handrails on both sides of a stairwell; using close-toed, rubber-soled footwear; and using chairs with arms. The provider can also identify patient-level barriers to implementing recommendations such as willingness to modify the home environment or funds to do so. In some communities, grants may be available to help subsidize home modification costs to promote "aging in place." The Community Aging in Place, Advancing Better Living for Elders (CAPABLE) model is one such program in which patient-directed home modifications have been shown to reduce falls and increased confidence in performing household tasks without fear of falling [10]. Furthermore, it is important to follow up on whether patients made the suggested modifications, which, similar to other behavior change interventions, often requires repeated motivational conversations.

Providers' approach to preventing falls on an individual level should be multifactorial. Patients who are at high risk should be referred for physical and occupational therapy, if they can participate in therapy, as this intervention has been shown to be effective with a USPSTF grade of "B." Exercise programs that can be taught and performed in the home have demonstrated effectiveness in decreasing falls and fall-related injuries, though the interventions have not specifically been studied in the homebound population [11]. In addition to a home exercise regimen, providers should assess high-risk patients for individual-level risk factor modification. Providers should review medication lists and eliminate medications whose benefit may be outweighed by the additional risk of falls. Orthostasis and hyponatremia should be corrected if possible. Pain should be adequately controlled, ideally with local treatments, since both pain itself and pain medications are implicated in fall risk. Vision should be optimized when possible. Of note, use of bifocals or transitional lenses is discouraged because they require neck mobility to look down for hazards on the ground. When appropriate, the treatment of osteoporosis reduces the risk of hip fracture, as 95% of hip fractures are caused by falls [4]. Encourage people at high risk for falls who live alone to have a phone or personal emergency response system at hand in case they are unable to get up to call for help after a fall. Recent technological advances including Amazon's Alexa or other virtual assistance technologies have been helpful in providing emergency support for patients who are cognitively intact. Interventions to improve function and fall risk are listed in Table 8.2.

Table 8.2 Ways to address functional impairment in homebound older adults

Place referrals to physical and occupational therapy
Create tailored exercise programs for gait, strength, balance as tolerated
Provide mobility aids (cane, walker, transfer board, etc.)
Review medications, especially for fall-risk-increasing drugs
Modify the home environment to eliminate hazards and add enabling modifications
Refer to CAPABLE
Address orthostasis and cardiac issues (e.g., atrial fibrillation)
Correct sensory impairments (vision, hearing)
Treat underlying movement disorders (e.g., Parkinson's disease)
Ensure appropriate footwear
Control pain, ideally with localized treatments
Treat urinary incontinence

8.3 Conclusion

A functional assessment is integral to an HBPC evaluation and can help address the risk of falls, a common problem in HBPC patients. A methodical approach of assessing ADLs and IADLs will help identify patients appropriate for HBPC and develop an effective treatment plan. Prevention of falls is multidisciplinary and relies on home medical providers, nurses, and physical and occupational therapists.

References

1. Shi SM, Olivieri-Mui B, McCarthy EP, Kim DH. Changes in a frailty index and association with mortality. J Am Geriatr Soc. 2021;69(4):1057–62. https://doi.org/10.1111/jgs.17002.
2. Roedl KJ, Wilson LS, Fine J. A systematic review and comparison of functional assessments of community-dwelling elderly patients. J Am Assoc Nurse Pract. 2016;28(3):160–9. https://doi.org/10.1002/2327-6924.12273.
3. Liu M, Xue QL, Gitlin LN, Wolff JL, Guralnik J, Leff B, Szanton SL. Disability prevention program improves life-space and falls efficacy: a randomized controlled trial. J Am Geriatr Soc. 2021;69(1):85–90. https://doi.org/10.1111/jgs.16808. Epub 2020 Sep 20. PMID: 32951215; PMCID: PMC8344360.
4. Moreland BKR, Henry A. Trends in nonfatal falls and fall-related injuries among adults aged ≥65 Years—United States, 2012–2018. MMWR Morb Mortal Wkly Rep. 2020;69:875–81. https://doi.org/10.15585/mmwr.mm6927a5.
5. Florence CS, Bergen G, Atherly A, Burns E, Stevens J, Drake C. Medical costs of fatal and nonfatal falls in older adults. J Am Geriatr Soc. 2018;66(4):693–8. https://doi.org/10.1111/jgs.15304. Epub 2018 Mar 7. PMID: 29512120; PMCID: PMC6089380.
6. Zhao YL, Alderden J, Lind B, Stibrany J. Risk factors for falls in homebound community-dwelling older adults. Public Health Nurs. 2019;36(6):772–8. https://doi.org/10.1111/phn.12651. Epub 2019 Aug 12. PMID: 31407384.
7. Masnoon N, Shakib S, Kalisch-Ellett L, et al. What is polypharmacy? A systematic review of definitions. BMC Geriatr. 2017;17:230. https://doi.org/10.1186/s12877-017-0621-2.
8. Liu M, Peng W, Miyawaki CE, Mo C, Luo Y, Gong N. The bidirectional relationship between homebound status and falls among older adults: a longitudinal study. BMC Geriatr. 2022;22(1):923. https://doi.org/10.1186/s12877-022-03588-1. PMID: 36457078; PMCID: PMC9714142.
9. Cumming RG, Thomas M, Szonyi G, et al. Home visits by an occupational therapist for assessment and modification of environmental hazards: a randomized trial of falls prevention. J Am Geriatr Soc. 1999;47(12):1397–402. https://doi.org/10.1111/j.1532-5415.1999.tb01556.x.
10. Spoelstra SL, Sikorskii A, Gitlin LN, Schueller M, Kline M, Szanton SL. Dissemination of the CAPABLE model of care in a Medicaid waiver program to improve physical function. J Am Geriatr Soc. 2019;67(2):363–70. https://doi.org/10.1111/jgs.15713. Epub 2018 Dec 13. PMID: 30548594.
11. Tricco AC, Thomas SM, Veroniki AA, Hamid JS, Cogo E, Strifler L, Khan PA, Robson R, Sibley KM, MacDonald H, Riva JJ, Thavorn K, Wilson C, Holroyd-Leduc J, Kerr GD, Feldman F, Majumdar SR, Jaglal SB, Hui W, Straus SE. Comparisons of interventions for preventing falls in older adults: a systematic review and meta-analysis. JAMA. 2017;318(17):1687–99. https://doi.org/10.1001/jama.2017.15006. Erratum in: JAMA. 2021 Apr 27;325(16):1682. PMID: 29114830; PMCID: PMC5818787.

Chapter 9
Common Medical Conditions in Home-Based Medical Care

Linda Paniszyn, Robert M. Zimbroff, Mattan Schuchman, and Won Lee

9.1 Unintentional Weight Loss

Unintentional weight loss is clinically defined as more than a 5% reduction in body weight within 6–12 months. It is common among homebound patients and is associated with increased morbidity and mortality. Studies have reported that as many as 27% of community-dwelling frail older adults and 50–60% of nursing home residents are affected, and the incidence among homebound older adults probably falls somewhere within this range [1]. In the homebound population, unintentional weight loss may be associated with functional decline in the activities of daily living, increased risk of institutionalization, in-hospital morbidity, increased risk of hip fracture in women, decreased quality of life, and increased overall mortality. At the extreme, cachexia has been associated with increased infections, pressure ulcers, poor wound healing, and failure to respond to medical treatments. Weight loss is an expected part of disease trajectory in dying patients with multiple chronic conditions; thus, a clinician should work up possible causes in the context of the patient's overall medical condition and their goals of care.

L. Paniszyn (✉) · W. Lee
Section of Geriatrics, Department of Medicine,
Boston University Chobanian & Avedisian School of Medicine, Boston, MA, USA
e-mail: Linda.Paniszyn@bmc.org

R. M. Zimbroff
Division of Geriatric Medicine, University of California, San Francisco,
San Francisco, CA, USA

M. Schuchman
Division of Geriatric Medicine and Gerontology, Johns Hopkins University School of Medicine, Baltimore, MD, USA

J. L. Colburn et al. (eds.), *Geriatric Home-Based Medical Care*,
https://doi.org/10.1007/978-3-031-68786-0_9

9.1.1 Etiology

Weight loss among community-dwelling older adults is common with approximately one-third losing 4% or more over 1 year in one study [2]. However, substantial weight loss should not be attributed to the normal aging process. Several important age-associated physiologic changes do predispose an older adult to weight loss, such as declining chemosensory function (smell and taste), reduced efficiency of chewing, slowed gastric emptying, and alterations to the neuroendocrine axis, which are associated with decreased appetite.

In homebound older adults, the causes of unintentional weight loss are often diverse and complex, with psychiatric and socioeconomic factors playing an important part. A majority of homebound older adults have multiple chronic illnesses, take a variety of medications, and have impaired cognition and mobility, all of which predispose them to weight loss. Poverty and social isolation also commonly contribute to weight loss resulting from limited access to nutritious and preferred foods [3].

Medication adverse effects are a common but often overlooked causative factor for weight loss. Many medications alter taste and can cause anorexia. Additionally, polypharmacy can lead to satiety owing solely to the number of medications consumed. Drugs such as sedatives and opiate analgesics may interfere with cognition and affect the patient's ability to eat. Many medications used in older adults are also constipating which can lead to decreased appetite and early satiety. Any medication temporally related to the development of involuntary weight loss should be suspected.

Depression is a common underdiagnosed and undertreated contributor to weight loss in older adults. Individuals with cognitive impairments and dementia who are agitated or have a tendency to wander can expend significant energy in pacing. Others may lose the skills to cook and feed themselves or simply forget that they have not eaten.

9.1.2 Evaluation

It is important to first establish the extent of weight loss. Serial measurements of body weight offer the simplest screening tool but may not always be possible, especially for frail patients who are no longer able to stand. If it is not possible to measure weight directly, change in clothing size, visual comparison to old photos, or serial measurements of mid-arm and mid-thigh circumference can be helpful. Questions about appetite may help elucidate whether the weight loss is caused by inadequate energy intake or has occurred despite an adequate intake. Several screening tools exist for identifying older adults at risk for poor nutrition [4].

Previous and current medical history can identify conditions that can lead to weight loss and drugs that may contribute via their side effects. A history that is attentive to the gastrointestinal symptoms is essential, e.g., oral pain, xerostomia, dysgeusia, nausea, vomiting, abdominal pain, constipation, and diarrhea. A broad review of systems may elicit additional symptoms that might direct further investigation. Older adults with weight loss should undergo screening for dementia and depression using standardized assessment tools; both can be associated with weight loss. A detailed social history should include questions about how the patient obtains and prepares food and what help they receive in doing so. Home-based medical providers have a unique opportunity to obtain this information firsthand by speaking with the caregivers during home visits, and with permission observing the refrigerator, pantry, and home environment.

A physical examination may help exclude major cardiovascular and respiratory illnesses as well as abdominal masses, organomegaly, prostate enlargement, and breast masses that may indicate cancer. Evaluation of the oral cavity may reveal causes of difficulty with chewing or swallowing.

Initial workup should include complete blood count, basic metabolic panel, liver function tests, thyroid function tests, inflammatory markers, and urinalysis. Chest radiography and abdominal ultrasonography can also be considered if history and exam suggest pulmonary or gastrointestinal involvement, respectively. Age-appropriate cancer screening may be considered; however, many home-limited patients do not have a life expectancy that justifies the risks of routine cancer screening. If baseline test results are normal, continued watchful waiting with periodic repeat physical examination is a reasonable strategy, and undirected pan-body scanning is not recommended. Conversations regarding risks/burdens vs. benefits of further testing and goals of care should be ongoing.

9.1.3 *Treatment*

If a correctable cause for weight loss can be identified in the evaluation, treatment should focus on the issue at hand. If no cause can found or if the cause is not treatable, common strategies to address unintentional weight loss in homebound older adults include dietary changes and environmental modifications listed below in Table 9.1.

When weight loss becomes resistant to nutritional intervention at the end of life, it is important to focus on the comfort measures that are consistent with a person's goals of care. These measures can include careful hand feeding for pleasure eating while minimizing aspiration risk, treating pain and nausea aggressively, and proper oral care. Home hospice referral can provide patients and families with necessary support.

If patients start having difficulty swallowing or no longer care to eat, feeding tubes are a way to provide nutrition. The benefit of feeding tubes varies in different medical conditions, and the discussion of artificial nutrition and hydration is complex and often emotionally charged. Evidence shows that feeding tubes do not provide adequate nutrition, prolong life, prevent aspiration, or improve comfort in

Table 9.1 Dietary and environmental strategies

Minimize dietary restrictions and liberalize diet to enhance the palatability of the food
Maximize intake of high-energy foods at the best meal of the day. Many older adults consume most of their daily energy intake at breakfast
For those with dementia, eat smaller meals more often, eat favorite foods and snacks, provide finger foods, and eat together with others
Avoid gas-producing foods that may cause early satiety
Optimize and vary dietary texture
Use flavor enhancers to counteract age-related decrease in smell and taste thresholds
Add fats to usual foods to increase calorie totals
Ensure adequate oral health
Take high-energy and nutritionally dense supplements between meals to minimize appetite suppression and compensatory decreased intake of foods
Get assistance with grocery shopping and food preparation
Utilize community nutritional support services, such as meal on wheels
Reconcile medications regularly to reduce polypharmacy

patients with advanced dementia [5]. In these difficult situations, home-based clinicians can provide important guidance to allow patients and families to make decisions that reflect their preferences and goals.

Evidence to recommend pharmacotherapy for appetite stimulation is sparse. Available evidence does not show improvement in quality of life, morbidity, or mortality. Furthermore, the side effect profile of appetite stimulants (e.g., sedation) is not trivial. Thus, appetite stimulants to treat unintentional weight loss are not generally recommended.

Megestrol acetate, a progesterone derivative, has been used to stimulate appetite initially approved for AIDS cachexia. A 2018 systematic of data shows a mean weight increase of approximately 2 kg; however, there is no change in quality of life or mortality [6]. Data in older patients are limited, and adverse effects and risk are significant. Adverse effects of megestrol include gastrointestinal upset, insomnia, impotence, hypertension, thromboembolic events, and adrenal insufficiency.

Mirtazapine, a serotonin antagonist used to treat depression, is another medication sometimes used for unintentional weight loss in older patients due to the fact that weight gain is a common side effect. Systematic data on use in unintentional weight loss is not available. Dizziness and orthostatic hypotension are possible adverse effects of mirtazapine; caution is warranted in patients at risk of falls. It may be appropriate to use mirtazapine in the context of treatment of comorbid depression and weight loss.

Dronabinol and medical cannabis has been shown to improve appetite in patients with AIDS [7] but is associated with adverse effects, particularly central nervous system toxicity (sedation, fatigue, hallucination). Data demonstrating change in quality of life or life expectancy is lacking.

9.2 Urinary Incontinence

Urinary incontinence (UI) is among the top ten principal diagnoses among individuals receiving home health services. Approximately 30% of women aged 70 or greater experience some involuntary urine loss [8]. Persons who are incontinent may experience anxiety, embarrassment, depression, and social isolation. People may not volunteer their symptoms due to embarrassment or the belief that UI is a normal part of aging. UI increases caregiver stress due to changing wet clothing and bedding, urine odor, increased laundry needs, time and effort toileting the patient, and the cost of briefs and pads. UI often coexists along with other conditions and thus is correlated with frailty, longer length of hospital stay, and reduced lifespan in community-dwelling older adults [9]. UI also contributes to skin breakdown, including pressure ulcers and fungal infection.

9.2.1 Etiology/Differential Diagnosis

The major types of UI are divided into stress, urge, functional, and overflow incontinence (see Table 9.2). The types of UI are distinguished by their characteristic signs, symptoms, and underlying causes. In many patients, more than one mechanism exists. Urge incontinence is characterized by a sudden urge to void which results in involuntary urine loss. Patients often report that they cannot make it to the bathroom in time. Stress incontinence is characterized by an inability to hold urine during coughing or sneezing and is associated with impaired sphincter function and pelvic floor weakness. Mixed incontinence is a combination of both stress and urge incontinence and is the most predominant type of UI in older women. Overflow incontinence occurs when the bladder is full yet does not empty normally, resulting in periodic leakage of urine and a large post-void residual (PVR) volume of urine in the bladder. Overflow incontinence may be caused by prostatic enlargement or neurogenic bladder, which occurs when the central nervous system does not initiate bladder contraction in conditions such as spinal cord injury, multiple sclerosis, stroke, or Parkinson's disease. Functional incontinence is the result of physical, cognitive, or psychiatric disabilities and a common type of UI in homebound persons. Lastly, other medical conditions can be associated with UI, including fecal

Table 9.2 Types of urinary incontinence

	Common symptoms	Common causes
Stress	Leakage with intraabdominal pressure	Pelvic floor weakness
Urge	Sudden need to void	Overactive bladder
Mixed	Components of both urge and stress incontinence	
Functional	Inability to self-toilet	Functional limitation
Overflow	Intermittent urine leakage with increased post-void residual	Neurogenic bladder or outlet obstruction

impaction, pelvic organ prolapse, medication side effects (especially diuretics), atrophic vaginitis, hyperglycemia, volume overload, alcohol use disorder, delirium, and excess fluid intake, including of caffeinated beverages.

Many age-related changes in the physiology of the lower urinary tract can contribute to UI in older adults. These changes include detrusor overactivity, with or without impaired bladder contractility, decreased bladder sensation, decreased bladder capacity, pelvic floor dysfunction, urogenital atrophy, decreased urethral closure pressure, and prostatic obstruction in men. Age-related changes in neurons that regulate bladder function may predispose older adults to neurogenic bladder dysfunction.

9.2.2 Assessment

All homebound adults should be screened for UI. Assessing the ability to toilet is part of the ADL assessment described above. Home-based medical care providers are positioned to recognize signs of UI that may not be evident in a primary care office visit by noting the smell of urine, disposable pads on furniture, or boxes of pads, diapers, or pull-ups. History should focus on acute versus chronic onset of symptoms, timing, frequency, associated symptoms such as dysuria or coughing, awareness of urination, and amount of leakage. A voiding diary may help the patient or caregiver explain the circumstances and severity of UI episodes. Review all medications for their impact on mental status, urinary retention, cough, polyuria, constipation, and other contributing factors to UI. Nonprescription substances, such as alcohol and some supplements, can also affect UI.

When appropriate and with the presence of a chaperone, a physical exam can confirm the presence of pelvic organ prolapse, atrophic vaginitis, and/or weakened pelvic floor muscles. A rectal exam can confirm fecal impaction or prostatic hypertrophy. Distended bladders can be palpated and percussed just over the pubic symphysis. Lower extremity edema increases the risk of nocturia, since some of the fluid is mobilized into the intravascular space when legs are elevated at night. In people with UI, the buttocks, genital areas, and low back may show signs of skin breakdown, pressure ulcers, or fungal infections as a result of sitting or lying in wet clothing or diapers.

An assessment of the home environment can aid in the diagnosis and formulation of an effective treatment plan. Observe the patient in a "walk-through" of the steps in toileting, if feasible, including use of assistive devices and assistance from a caregiver. Observe transfers, ambulation, and ability to manipulate clothing. Assess the accessibility of the toilet and any trip hazards present. Assess caregivers and their behaviors, including hours of availability, willingness and ability to help with toileting, and any physical and cognitive limitations. Other clinicians, notably occupational therapists, can contribute to a thorough assessment of both the home environment and a patient's ability to toilet.

Further testing may be needed in some situations. Bladder post-void residual volume (PVR) measurement can diagnose urinary retention associated with the neurogenic bladder or the bladder outlet obstruction of BPH or prior prostate surgery. PVR can be measured in the home with a portable bladder scanner or by catheterization. Post-void volumes between 50 and 100 mL may be acceptable for persons over 65 years of age [10].

9.2.3 Treatment

Improvement in continence is possible for many patients, including those with cognitive and/or physical impairments and multiple comorbidities. Lifestyle and behavioral treatments for UI include pelvic floor muscle training, prompted voiding, limiting intake of bladder irritants, and limiting nighttime fluid consumption. These conservative techniques should be tried for 8–12 weeks and then assessed for success [8].

9.2.3.1 Nonpharmacologic Management

Pelvic floor muscle training (PFMT) , or "Kegels," can reduce incontinence in cognitively intact homebound adults with stress, urge, or mixed UI and in patients with OAB; men with post-prostatectomy incontinence may also benefit, if more modestly. Patients can practice isolating the pelvic floor muscles aiming to stop urination midstream. Patients can do 10–15 muscle contractions 3 times a day. Once the patient is comfortable with the technique, they can utilize the contractions to suppress both urge and stress incontinence, employing the technique at a strong urge to void or during a stress incontinence activity such as sneezing or coughing. Patients with urge incontinence should be encouraged to repeat the contractions until the acute urge subsides rather than trying to run to the bathroom in time. Some physical therapists are trained in pelvic floor physical therapy and can assist in teaching important techniques to assist with stress incontinence.

Prompted voiding, a potentially effective strategy for cognitively impaired patients, is a method in which the caregiver asks the patient if they are wet or dry every 2 h while awake, or the patient sets a timer themselves. Then the caregiver asks the patient if they would like to use the toilet and encourages the patient to do so. For this strategy to be effective, a willing and able caregiver must be available for most of the patient's waking hours. The time intervals can be adjusted to accommodate competing demands on caregivers or patients. In one study of cognitively impaired homebound older adults with an available caregiver, prompted voiding reduced the number of daytime incontinence episodes by about 25% [11]. For nocturia, strategies include limiting fluids in the evening, adjusting the timing of diuretics, and treating dependent lower extremity edema by elevating the legs for several hours before bedtime.

Physical or occupational therapists can address functional incontinence and environmental barriers through gait, balance, and strength training. Therapists can assess the need for and order assistive devices, such as walkers, canes, Hoyer lifts, raised toilet seat, and grab bars, and can train patients and caregivers in their use [12].

"Contained incontinence" using pads, pull-ups, diapers, or catheters may be the most realistic option for some patients for whom other treatments are not effective or possible. A patient may be able to achieve the "social presentation of continence" and thus maintain quality of life and avoid complications such as skin breakdown and infection.

Intermittent or indwelling catheterization may be required to treat neurogenic bladder causing overflow incontinence. Intermittent catheterization, usually performed every 4 h, requires a willing and able patient or caregiver. A 2013 Cochrane review found no evidence to create guidelines for choosing among intermittent, external, indwelling, or suprapubic catheterization [13], so clinicians should base their decisions on urologist recommendations, patient preferences, and goals of care. Catheterization is sometimes necessary to treat other forms of incontinence but is usually reserved for end-of-life symptom palliation and for promoting the healing of stage III or IV pressure sores.

9.2.3.2 Pharmacologic Management

The main pharmacological treatments for UI are anticholinergics and the beta-3 adrenoceptor agonist mirabegron. A review by the Agency for Healthcare Research and Quality (AHRQ) found that medications are more effective than placebo in treating adult women but that overall effectiveness is low. Complete continence was achieved less than 20% of the time for all medications reviewed, although reductions in frequency of UI episodes were often higher [14].

Patients with urge neurogenic bladder, urge UI, and/or OAB may find relief with anticholinergics that improve urine flow, lower bladder pressure, and prevent detrusor overactivity. Anticholinergics may also reduce urine leakage between intermittent catheterizations in patients with neurogenic bladder. When selecting an anticholinergic, an extended release preparation may be preferred over an immediate-release formula due to lower side effect profile. Providers should weigh the risk of anticholinergic side effects, which include notably dry mouth, risk for falls, confusion, orthostatic hypotension, constipation, and blurred vision, and heed recommendations for geriatric and renal dosing. Mirabegron has a similar rate of effectiveness compared to anticholinergics at reducing incontinence episodes in persons with urge UI and OAB but with lower rates of dry mouth and constipation. Postmenopausal women with stress UI may benefit from low-dose vaginal estrogen.

For patients who report that UI has a significant impact on their quality of life and have not attained acceptable outcomes using the strategies above, referral to urology or urogynecology may provide additional treatment options. These treatments include the use of bladder wall botulinum toxin for OAB, pessary placement for organ prolapse, or posterior tibial nerve or sacral electrical stimulation. In nursing home patients, a population functionally similar to HBPC, prostate reduction surgery has been shown to be ineffective in reducing dependency on catheters. It should be noted that for fully homebound patients, getting to specialists can be a challenge and may unfortunately limit access to some of these specialist-based interventions.

9.3 Polypharmacy

Optimal medication prescribing is a mainstay of medical practice but is significantly important in the care of the older adult. Polypharmacy in older adults is associated with an increase in adverse drug events, impaired cognition, functional decline, falls, and decreased quality of life. Polypharmacy is associated with long-term care placement and increased use of the healthcare system [15].

Definitions of polypharmacy vary, but it is commonly defined as the use of more than five medications [16]. Over-the-counter, herbal, and nutritional supplements are included in this tally. An estimate of Medicare beneficiaries shows 50% of older adults receive five or more medications [17]. Risk factors for polypharmacy include older age, cognitive impairment, frailty, multiple chronic conditions, transitions of care, and automated refill systems [18]. Common health conditions (e.g., heart failure or diabetes) are typically treated with a combination of therapeutics to follow the latest evidence-based guidelines or adhere to disease-specific quality metrics which can quickly compound polypharmacy. Increased numbers of prescribed medications lead to more medication nonadherence.

Polypharmacy is associated with an increase in adverse drug events [19]. An adverse drug event is an injury resulting from medication use—including physical harm, mental harm, or loss of function. These adverse drug events may occur due to a decrease in drug clearance seen in the aging process. Drug-drug interactions are a frequent cause of preventable adverse drug events, and prevalence of drug-drug interactions can be seen in a range of 15–40% in frail older adults [20]. Prescribing cascades occur when an adverse drug event is mistakenly identified as a symptom of a de novo medical condition and another medication is then prescribed to treat this perceived condition rather than discontinuation of the offending drug. Adverse drug events account for 30% of all hospital admissions and adverse drug events are common after hospital discharges and are often preventable [21].

9.3.1 Evaluation

One of the benefits of performing home-based medical visits is the ability to do a detailed medication review in the patient's home setting. In conjunction with the patient and caregiver, the medical team member has an opportunity to identify what medications are or are not being taken and whether these medications are being taken correctly and as prescribed. Many times, patients do not consider over-the-counter medications or nutritional supplements to be medications, so home visits are an opportunity to check in the cabinets and drawers for a full medication reconciliation. In addition to prescription and nonprescription pills, there may be topical ointments, ophthalmic drops, transdermal patches, and injectable medications that patients may neglect bringing to the office for a medication review. Often one can find expired or discontinued medications that the patient may still be taking inadvertently. Evaluating how the patient organizes their medications and assessing the patient's understanding of each medication and how they should be taking it are instrumental in a comprehensive medical assessment. One way to commonly do this is to ask the patient to show us their medications, what each is for, and how often they take it.

Once it is ascertained which medications the patient is taking, use of an assessment tool can provide a framework for considering what medications should be continued or discontinued [16]. One example is the American Geriatrics Society Beers Criteria which provides guidance regarding medications that should be avoided by most older adults, medications that should be avoided in older adults with certain conditions, medications that should be used with caution, medication interactions, and changes in dosing based on kidney function [22]. Decision support tools using Beers criteria are now incorporated into many electronic health records, and there are decision support tools that can be used in handheld devices while on home visits.

Screening Tool of Older Persons' Prescriptions (TOPP) and Screening Tool to Alert to Right Treatment (START) include criteria for potentially inappropriate prescribing in older adults and potential prescribing omissions [23]. These criteria are developed by an expert panel with the purpose of minimizing inappropriate prescribing in older adults by way of up-to-date literature reviews and consensus validation. A Cochrane review in 2018 did not reveal any one tool to show significant superiority in clinical outcomes [16], but these tools can be a helpful starting place. The practice of managing polypharmacy includes regular and systematic medication reviews to identify potential inappropriate medications or supplements and ongoing therapeutic benefit of current treatment.

9.3.2 Prescribing

When evaluating a new symptom or condition and before starting a new medication, there are many things to contemplate. Consider any underlying causes for the symptoms—could this symptom be an effect of a current medication? Are there effective alternative nonpharmacologic treatments available? What are the risks and benefits of medication? Will this medication be short or long term? What are potential drug-drug or dietary interactions? Will the patient be able to adhere to this medication regimen? Will the patient or caregiver be able to administer this medication

Table 9.3 Steps for prescribing (adapted from the WHO Guide to Good Prescribing [24])

Step 1	Identify the patient's or caregiver's concern or issue: symptoms, diagnosis, and patient characteristics and values
Step 2	Identify the therapeutic objective: Is it curative, symptomatic, and preventive, and how long will it be prescribed?
Step 3	Identify the treatment choice: Is it the standard of treatment based on available evidence, is it suitable for the patient, and are there contraindications or interactions?
Step 4	Start the treatment with clear language and avoiding abbreviations
Step 5	Educate patients and caregivers about instructions for use, potential common and serious side effects, and review of expected outcomes
Step 6	Monitor treatment based on effect with a systematic medication review and determine if the medication should be continued or adjusted or stopped
Step 7	Factor in drug cost when prescribing. Clinicians often overlook cost of prescriptions, and in one study two-thirds of older patients planned to underuse their medications due to cost [25]. Patients may not fill a prescription due to cost but may not reveal this to the medical team
Step 8	Use electronic health records and computer-based tools to reduce prescribing errors [26]. Many electronic health records share prescription information across health systems and pharmacy networks and can inform the team about health conditions, medication allergies, and other medications that have been prescribed or discontinued

reasonably and safely? All of questions should be asked within the context of the patient's and caregiver's goals of care, level of function, values, and preferences.

Appropriate prescribing involves a systematic approach as advocated by the World Health Organization [24] and can readily be applied during a home-based medical visit (see Table 9.3).

9.3.3 *Deprescribing*

One component of good prescribing is deprescribing. Deprescribing is defined as a systematic approach of adjusting medications down to minimum effective dosage and stopping them when the potential for harm outweighs the benefit of the medication. Each home-based visit is an opportunity to identify and prioritize medications that can be decreased in dose or frequency or discontinued all together within the context of the patient's goals, life expectancy, functional status, values, and preferences. Patients do not necessarily bring up their desire to take medications to their medical team, and often deprescribing is a process that evolves through ongoing conversations with patients and caregivers [27]. These conversations can center around any adverse effects that the patient may be experiencing from a medication or identifying "legacy prescribing" which is when medications meant to be prescribed for a finite duration are continued indefinitely (e.g., benzodiazepines or proton pump inhibitors) [28].

An initial step to deprescribing is first identifying potentially inappropriate medications, followed by determining if it is safe and reasonable to reduce, taper, or stop a medication. Classes of medications that have high potential to be inappropriate include central nervous system acting medications, benzodiazepines, antihistamines, anticholinergics, muscle relaxants, opioid analgesics, and sedative hypnotics. It is important to counsel the patient about potential discontinuation symptoms and document any potential positive or negative outcomes after reducing or stopping the medication [29]. Focusing on one medication at a time will ensure any effects can be correctly attributed to that medication.

Patients or caregivers may express reluctance to a dose reduction or discontinuation of a medication for several reasons such as the length of time on the medication, any perceived benefits of the medication, or concern for a negative outcome after stopping the medication. Therefore, it is prudent to prioritize which medications to target (e.g., medications with highest risk of adverse effects) and consider tapering the doses incrementally while monitoring and supporting the patient and caregiver.

9.3.4 Promoting Medication Adherence

Many patients feel they spend a significant portion of their day taking their medications. Complex and multidose medication schedules decrease adherence and increase risks for errors and adverse drug events. Multidose medication schedules can contribute to caregiver burden and stress. Low health literacy and cognitive impairment increase the chance of error in taking medications as prescribed [30].

One of the most straightforward ways to improve the likelihood of a patient being able to adhere to a regimen is to consolidate and streamline the dosing schedule. High-frequency dosing or non-daily regimens such as every other day or every Monday, Wednesday, and Friday increase room for error. Constructing a visual tool such as an easy-to-understand medication chart or schedule with pill pictures can be a helpful reference guide for patients and caregivers.

Beyond tradition pill bottles, there is a variety of medication systems available. Blister packs and pillboxes have shown better medication adherence than pill bottles alone. A basic pill organizer can be set up by a patient or caregiver on a weekly basis and can be labeled as a visual cue to patients. The patient can see when the medications were taken which is also helpful to caregivers and clinicians. These pillboxes can be daily or multidose organizers. Easy-open organizers may include features like buttons which can make it easier to open for those with dexterity issues. Automatic pill dispensers may be an option for those who would benefit from automated reminders. Some models can be prefilled with 4 weeks of medications and can be equipped with blinking lights, audio alarms, and be linked to a computer or mobile device with notifications about missed doses. Several automated pill dispensing systems and "smart" pill containers have been developed to remind patients to take their medications, but little evidence exists to support one technology over another.

Prefilled medication packaging is a system with many advantages. They are widely available, can often be delivered to the home, and often are covered by the patient's insurance plan. Medications can be packaged into blister packets with individually sealed compartments containing tablets, and patients can access the medication by pushing through the foil seal. Calendar blister packaging includes labeling of the date and description of the contents. Some pill packaging systems are dosed by frequency (e.g., morning, afternoon, evening doses) and dispensed on a roll that unspools over 4 weeks. Patients can tear off a packet dose from the roll when it is time to take the medications and the packets are labeled with the date and contents. Prefilled pill packaging can be extremely helpful to organize medications, track adherence, and remove the need to manage multiple different pill bottles. Disadvantages to this form of packaging include difficulty opening the packages, challenges following a calendar format, and limited use for medications that are prescribed to be taken "as needed." This style of packaging is usually set up for a month at a time so adjusting, removing, or adding a medication in the middle of a cycle may prove impossible.

Pharmacist-led comprehensive medication assessments are a way to identify polypharmacy and potentially inappropriate medication use. Pharmacists are often members of the interdisciplinary home-based medical team. Pharmacists can conduct home visits, telemedicine visits, or independent reviews of patient medication lists. Additionally, comprehensive pharmacist assessments can help to identify barriers to adherence, provide guidance and education, suggest cost-effective alternatives, and recommend solutions to improve medication adherence [31].

9.4 Sleep Disturbances

Sleep disorders are common in homebound older adults, often underdiagnosed, worsen quality of life, and increase dementia and mortality risk. Nearly half of older adults report poor sleep symptoms. While there are sleep pattern changes that occur as a part of normal aging, bothersome sleep patterns require careful investigation to identify and address any reversible factors contributing to poor sleep. Evaluating for primary sleep disorders, such as obstructive sleep apnea or restless leg syndrome, is also necessary [32].

9.4.1 Sleep Changes in Normal Aging

Total sleep time, nocturnal sleep time, and deep sleep time decrease with aging, while the frequency of daytime naps and nocturnal awakenings increases with aging. These sleep pattern changes occur independent of many factors including medical comorbidities and medications [33].

It has been found that there is an approximately 10–12-min reduction of total sleep time per decade of life from childhood until sleep time plateaus after 60 years of age [34].

Older adults also often experience a shift of sleep schedule to earlier hours. Compared to younger adults, older adults are about 1 h advanced in sleep-wake cycle, body temperature rhythm, and timing of secretion of melatonin and cortisol [35]. It has been thought that the decreasing function of the suprachiasmatic nucleus—the central endogenous pacemaker that regulates 24-h circadian rhythms—is associated with the disruption of circadian rhythm with increasing age [36].

It can be helpful to know about these normal changes when counseling older adults and their caregivers. If a change in sleep behavior is noted by an older adult or caregiver but the change is neither bothersome to the older adult nor interfering with their function, it is not recommended to pursue treatment. In these cases, education about sleep changes in normal aging may be needed.

9.4.2 *Causes of Disrupted Sleep*

9.4.2.1 Poor Sleep Hygiene

Home care provides the unique opportunity to see and experience the environment in which the older adult sleeps. Questions to consider that may cause disrupted sleep include the following: Is it very hot or cold in the bedroom? Is the older adult sleeping on an old recliner with shot supports in front of a television? Is there clutter preventing access to the bedroom? Is the older adult sharing a cramped bed? Is the street outside very noisy? Is there adequate sunlight into the living spaces during the day and adequate darkness at night? These environmental observations can provide the basis of the sleep hygiene assessment.

Further history must be obtained to assess behavioral factors as well. Irregular bedtime, lack of daytime stimulation, daytime napping, lack of exercise, late screen time use, and late caffeine or alcohol consumption are all examples of behavioral factors that contribute to poor sleep. If the older adult or caregiver can keep a sleep diary recording bedtime and nighttime disturbance, this may also be helpful in identifying contributing causes of poor sleep. Sleep hygiene evaluation is the cornerstone of addressing sleep disturbance in the home care setting.

9.4.2.2 Medications/Drugs

Older adults are prone to unwanted side effects due to physiologic changes with aging that affect drug clearance. During the home visit medication review, it is important to ask to see all the over-the-counter medications and supplements in addition to all the prescribed medications. Sometimes asking the older adult or caregiver, "Anything else?" two or three times is necessary to obtain all the medications from various locations in the home. In addition to prescribed medications, over-the-counter as well as illicit substances can impair sleep. In Table 9.4 are several drug classes known to negatively affect sleep quality.

Table 9.4 Commonly used drug classes and their effect on sleep

Alcohol	Though sometimes used to self-medicate for help with falling asleep, alcohol actually reduces REM sleep duration and increases sleep disruptions [37]
Alpha-agonists	For example, ephedrine and pseudoephedrine—Used for weight loss orally or nasal congestion intranasally and unfortunately found in many over-the-counter medications and supplements. Drugs in this class can increase heart rate and restlessness
Antidepressants	Selective serotonin reuptake inhibitors (SSRIs), serotonin-norepinephrine reuptake inhibitors (SNRIs), tricyclic antidepressants (TCAs), and monoamine oxidase inhibitors (MAOIs) have been found to reduce REM and have variable effect on sleep continuity [38]. If sleep disturbance occurs after starting once of these medications, any benefit must be balanced against this side effect on an individual basis
Benzodiazepines, barbiturates, and non-benzodiazepine receptor modulators	Historically used to treat anxiety and insomnia though not recommended for sleep disturbance in older adults as the potential for adverse events outweigh any short-term benefit. Although these medications are associated with modest improvements in sleep latency and sleep duration, they also suppress deep sleep which compromises sleep's restorative effects [39]. It is recommended to trial a slow taper of these medications to improve sleep even if initially prescribed for insomnia
Beta-blockers	Used for arrhythmias and chronic heart failure. Beta-blockers reduce melatonin production and may increase risk of insomnia [40]
Caffeine-containing supplements	For example, green tea—Caffeine has long been known to cause wakefulness and has been found to specifically reduce total sleep time and sleep efficiency and worsen perceived sleep quality [41]
Cholinesterase inhibitors	For example, donepezil—Activation of the cholinergic nervous system by donepezil has been shown to increase REM sleep [42], but in some older adults, cholinesterase inhibitors have also been linked to sleep disturbances and nightmares [43]
Diuretics	Can cause nocturia and muscle cramping that disturb sleep
H1-blockers, first generation	For example, diphenhydramine—Antihistamines are found in many over-the-counter medicines with the designation "PM." while this class of medication is commonly used as a sleep aid, they are not recommended in older adults since there is poor evidence of effectiveness and no systematic data addressing harms [44]. These medications are known to cause drowsiness and increase risk of falls
Nicotine	Causes sleep fragmentation and decreased slow wave sleep with reduced sleep efficiency and increased daytime sleepiness. It can also cause vivid dreams [45]
Steroids	May cause sleep disturbance through three possible pathways: Activating the hypothalamic-pituitary axis, decreasing melatonin production, and hyperarousal caused by modification in neuroinhibitory pathways [46]

9.4.2.3 Medical and Psychiatric Conditions

Many sleep disturbances are secondary to underlying medical or psychiatric conditions; see Table 9.5. Therefore, it is worthwhile reviewing chronic medical issues and evaluating for potential new conditions if new sleep difficulties are reported in order to optimize symptoms. For example, if an older adult has uncontrolled pain, focusing on addressing their pain may also help their sleep.

9.4.2.4 Primary Sleep Disorders

There are seven major categories of primary sleep disorders in the third edition of the International Classification of Sleep Disorders (ICSD-3): insomnia disorders, sleep-related breathing disorders, central disorders of hypersomnolence, circadian rhythm sleep-wake disorders, sleep-related movement disorders, parasomnias, and other sleep disorders [47]. These categories are then further categorized into 60 specific diagnoses, and we will not review all possible primary sleep diagnoses in this chapter. Instead, we will highlight a few distinct features of each category that may change management in home care.

Insomnia—Primary insomnia disorders are broken down into chronic or short-term insomnia and require a report of a sleep initiation or sleep maintenance problem, adequate opportunity and circumstances to sleep, and daytime consequences as the result of the insomnia symptoms. Since these symptoms can be a component of many medical and psychiatric conditions, a diagnosis of insomnia disorder should be considered only when the insomnia is prominent and requires further management.

Sleep-related breathing disorders—This category is divided into four major groups: central sleep apnea syndromes, obstructive sleep apnea (OSA) disorder,

Table 9.5 Commonly encountered medical and psychiatric conditions that affect sleep

Anxiety	Difficulty falling asleep
Chronic heart failure	Orthopnea, paroxysmal nocturnal dyspnea
Chronic lung disease	Coughing, dyspnea
Delirium	Disrupted sleep-wake cycle, fluctuating mental status
Dementia	Disrupted sleep-wake cycle; increased risk of coexisting primary sleep disorder with Parkinson's disease and Lewy body dementia
Depression	Difficulty falling asleep
Diabetes	Nocturia, polyuria, polydipsia
GERD	Nocturnal cough, heartburn worse when supine
Pain	Difficulty falling asleep, nocturnal awakenings
Post-traumatic stress disorder	Nightmares
Renal disease	Restless legs, daytime fatigue
Substance use disorder	Daytime fatigue or irritability, other symptoms depending on substance
Thyroid disease	Hot flashes, nocturnal awakenings, daytime fatigue
Urinary frequency/incontinence	Nocturia

sleep-related hypoventilation disorders, and sleep-related hypoxemia disorder. The most common sleep-related breathing disorder in older adults is OSA. Clinicians must maintain a high degree of clinical suspicion to screen for the condition and order appropriate diagnostic testing. The snoring, tiredness, observed apnea, blood pressure, body mass index, age, neck size, gender (STOP-Bang) questionnaire is a concise and validated tool to screen for OSA [48]. While laboratory polysomnography (PSG) is the gold standard for OSA diagnosis, it is often costly, involves lengthy wait times, and is difficult for older adults receiving home care to access. Home sleep apnea testing (HSAT) is an acceptable alternative and is increasing in accessibility, so HSAT should be considered if OSA is suspected and the test is available.

Central disorders of hypersomnolence—These are disorders in which the primary complaint is daytime sleepiness that is not due to another sleep disorder, including disturbed sleep or misaligned circadian rhythms. This category includes narcolepsy and hypersomnia which are usually not first diagnosed in older adulthood.

Circadian rhythm sleep-wake disorders—This category is characterized by a chronic or recurrent sleep disturbance due to alteration of the circadian system or misalignment between the environment and an individual's sleep-wake cycle. Advanced sleep-wake phase disorder is a specific diagnosis seen in older adults marked by sleep and wake times that are habitually early compared with conventional times. This change in sleep may be due to normal sleep changes with aging and may not need intervention if not bothersome to the older adult or interfering with their function.

Parasomnias—Parasomnias are undesirable complex physical events or experiences (e.g., nightmares) that occur during entry into sleep, within sleep, or during arousals from sleep. These disorders occur most commonly in childhood.

Sleep-related movement disorders—Sleep-related movement disorders are characterized by simple, stereotypic movements that disturb sleep. Restless leg syndrome is included in this category and is marked by the urge to move the legs and/or the presence of uncomfortable sensations that occur primarily with rest, and these symptoms are at least partially relieved with movement and have a circadian aspect in that the symptoms occur primarily at night. There are medications known to help with these symptoms and should be considered if symptoms are very bothersome (see "Pharmacologic Management" section).

Other sleep disorders—This category includes sleep disorders that cannot be appropriately classified elsewhere either because the disorder overlaps with more than one category or when insufficient data has been collected to firmly establish another diagnosis.

9.4.3 Nonpharmacologic Management

The mainstays of intervention for most sleep disturbances center around nonpharmacologic strategies with good sleep hygiene at the forefront (see Table 9.6). Addressing any potentially reversible factors contributing to poor sleep due to underlying comorbidities is also a key step.

Table 9.6 Behavioral and environmental recommendations to improve sleep

Environmental recommendations	• Maintain comfortable room temperature • Optimize bed for accessibility and sleep—adjust bed height, use bed railings, use supportive mattress • Minimize noise—turn off television/try white noise machine • Keep living areas well lit and bedroom dark • Trial separation of bed partners if a partner may be causing disruptions • Keep pets out of the bedroom if causing disruptions
Behavioral recommendations	• Get into bed at a regular time every day • Keep a regular pattern of eating • Limit fluid intake before bedtime/keep commode or urinal within reach if nocturia is an issue • Avoid daytime napping • Exercise during the day • Avoid screen time before bed • Avoid late caffeine/alcohol consumption • Avoid smoking

The best evidence for treatment of sleep disturbances is cognitive behavioral therapy for insomnia (CBT-I) [49]. CBT-I is a multipronged intervention that uses cognitive and behavioral techniques like stimulus control therapy, sleep restriction therapy, relaxation training, cognitive restructuring, and sleep hygiene education to replace maladaptive thoughts and sleep habits and to reduce arousal associated with sleep. It can be helpful for both secondary sleep disturbances and primary sleep disorders. A systematic review in 2012 comparing CBT-I to medications found low- to moderate-grade evidence that CBT-I has superior effectiveness to benzodiazepine and non-benzodiazepine drugs in the long term and suggests CBT-I as first-line treatment for insomnia [50]. If CBT-I is accessible, referral is recommended.

Bright light therapy has also been found to be helpful although the evidence is less robust. For older adults with sleep disturbance, there is no consensus on the optimum treatment protocol for bright light therapy, but it may help not only with sleep quality but also with unwanted behavioral and cognitive symptoms associated with dementia and depression [51]. For homebound older adults who do not have windows in their home, ensuring bright lighting during the day may be helpful.

9.4.4 *Pharmacologic Management*

If sleep disturbance remains bothersome despite feasible nonpharmacologic management, pharmacologic management should be considered. As previously noted, the first pharmacologic intervention should be careful review and optimization of the existing medication list, and then any potential sleep offenders should be deprescribed or decreased in accordance with the older adult's priorities. As previously noted in this section, there are several medications that have been used historically to treat insomnia in older adults but can actually worsen sleep quality—benzodiazepines, barbiturates, non-benzodiazepine receptor modulators, and first-generation H1 blockers. There are also numerous supplements that are marketed as sleep aids though lack sufficient evidence to recommend use and are not regulated by the U.S. Food and Drug Administration (FDA). Older adults and caregivers may ask about valerian root, cannabidiol (CBD), or other cannabis derivatives, but there is insufficient evidence of effectiveness and substantial evidence of possible adverse effects in older adults, so these are not recommended. As is unfortunately the case with most drug studies, there are few studies evaluating effectiveness and safety of specifically in older adults. In Table 9.7 are medications that may be reasonable to try in the appropriate clinical setting.

Table 9.7 Pharmacologic management for poor sleep

Drug name	Mechanism of action	Starting dose
Melatonin	A hormone produced by the pineal gland that is a known regulator of circadian rhythm, and its production decreases with age. Oral melatonin is a supplement and not FDA regulated; however, there is evidence of its efficacy and is considered safe in older adults. In a systematic review of melatonin use in older adults, sleep efficiency and total sleep time improved, and sundowning in patients with Alzheimer's disease was reduced [52]. Older adults should be instructed to take at 2 h before anticipated bedtime for best effect	3 mg
Ramelteon	Melatonin receptor agonist. Unlike melatonin, ramelteon is a medication that requires a prescription and is FDA regulated. In one randomized controlled trial specifically including older adults, ramelteon significantly reduced patient reports of sleep latency over 5 weeks of treatment with no significant rebound insomnia or withdrawal effects [53]. It also has a favorable side effect profile	8 mg
Mirtazapine	Antidepressant with a dual mode of action of noradrenergic and serotonergic properties. It is approved to treat depression, panic disorder, and tension headaches, though it is increasingly used for sleep disturbance in older adults given its favorable side effect profile. It has been found to be safe and effective for long-term use, and use should be considered if the older adult has concurrent depressive symptoms [54]. It should be administered at least 1 h before bedtime	7.5 mg
Trazodone	Antidepressant that has serotonergic properties as well as significantly blocks H1 and alpha-1 receptors. It is FDA approved to treat insomnia as well as depression and behavioral disturbance in dementia though based on limited data. It has been found to be effective in the treatment of sleep-maintenance insomnia, especially in patients with comorbid mental health disorders, and it increases the duration of deep sleep. It should also be administered at least 1 h before bedtime	25 mg

(continued)

Table 9.7 (continued)

Drug name	Mechanism of action	Starting dose
Dopamine agonists, e.g., pramipexole	FDA approved to treat the primary sleep disorder restless leg syndrome. These medications can also be used treat Parkinson's disease. Their use for sleep disturbance outside these scenarios are not recommended	0.125 mg—Pramipexole
Prazosin	Primarily blocks alpha-1 receptors. This medication lowers blood pressure and has off-label use to treat PTSD-related nightmares and sleep disruption. Its efficacy for PTSD symptoms has been supported in at least ten clinical studies [55]. In older adults with PTSD who do not have orthostasis, prazosin should be considered	0.5 mg
Antipsychotics, e.g., quetiapine	Antipsychotics are not recommended to treat sleep disturbance in older adults despite their widespread use. Due to serious potential adverse effects of antipsychotics, guidelines for the treatment of insomnia have recommended their use only in older adults with specific comorbid psychiatric disorders, and even then, their use should be limited to the shortest duration possible	12.5 mg—Quetiapine

References

Weight Loss

1. Alibhai SM, Greenwood C, Payette H. An approach to the management of unintentional weight loss in elderly people. CMAJ. 2005;172(6):773–80. https://doi.org/10.1503/cmaj.1031527.
2. Ritchie CS, Joshipura K, Silliman RA, Miller B, Douglas CW. Oral health problems and significant weight loss among community-dwelling older adults. J Gerontol A Biol Sci Med Sci. 2000;55(7):M366–71. https://doi.org/10.1093/gerona/55.7.m366. PMID: 10898252.
3. Fischer J, Johnson MA. Low body weight and weight loss in the aged. J Am Diet Assoc. 1990;90(12):1697–706. PMID: 2131340.
4. Rolland Y, Perrin A, Gardette V, Filhol N, Vellas B. Screening older people at risk of malnutrition or malnourished using the Simplified Nutritional Appetite Questionnaire (SNAQ): a comparison with the Mini-Nutritional Assessment (MNA) tool. J Am Med Dir Assoc. 2012;13(1):31–4. https://doi.org/10.1016/j.jamda.2011.05.003. Epub 2011 Jun 23. PMID: 21700503.
5. American Geriatrics Society Ethics C, Clinical P, Models of Care C. American Geriatrics Society feeding tubes in advanced dementia position statement. J Am Geriatr Soc. 2014;62(8):1590–3. https://doi.org/10.1111/jgs.12924.
6. Ruiz-García V, López-Briz E, Carbonell-Sanchis R, Bort-Martí S, Gonzálvez-Perales JL. Megestrol acetate for cachexia-anorexia syndrome. A systematic review. J Cachexia Sarcopenia Muscle. 2018;9(3):444–52. https://doi.org/10.1002/jcsm.12292. Epub 2018 Mar 14. PMID: 29542279; PMCID: PMC5989756.
7. Beal JE, Olson R, Laubenstein L, Morales JO, Bellman P, Yangco B, Lefkowitz L, Plasse TF, Shepard KV. Dronabinol as a treatment for anorexia associated with weight loss in patients with AIDS. J Pain Symptom Manage. 1995;10(2):89.

Urinary Incontinence

8. Wu JM, Vaughan CP, Goode PS, Redden DT, Burgio KL, Richter HE, Markland AD. Prevalence and trends of symptomatic pelvic floor disorders in U.S. women. Obstet Gynecol. 2014;123(1):141–8. https://doi.org/10.1097/AOG.0000000000000057. PMID: 24463674; PMCID: PMC3970401.
9. Lukacz ES, Santiago-Lastra Y, Albo ME, Brubaker L. Urinary incontinence in women: a review. JAMA. 2017;318(16):1592–604. https://doi.org/10.1001/jama.2017.12137.
10. Gratzke C, Bachmann A, Descazeaud A, et al. EAU guidelines on the assessment of non-neurogenic male lower urinary tract symptoms including benign prostatic obstruction. Eur Urol. 2015;67(6):1099–109. https://doi.org/10.1016/j.eururo.2014.12.038.
11. Engberg S, Sereika SM, et al. Effectiveness of prompted voiding in treating urinary incontinence in cognitively impaired homebound older adults. J WOCN. 2002;29(5):252–65. https://doi.org/10.1067/mjw.2002.127207.
12. McDowell BJ, Engberg S, Sereika S, et al. Effectiveness of behavioral therapy to treat incontinence in homebound older adults. J Am Geriatr Soc. 1999;47(3):309–18. https://doi.org/10.1111/j.1532-5415.1999.tb02994.x.
13. Jamison J, Maguire S, McCann J. Catheter policies for management of long term voiding problems in adults with neurogenic bladder disorders (review). Cochrane Library. 2013. http://www.ncbi.nlm.nih.gov/pubmed/24249436. Accessed 20 Feb 2015.
14. Shamliyan T, Wyman J, Kane RL. Nonsurgical treatments for urinary incontinence in adult women: diagnosis and comparative effectiveness. AHRQ Publication No 11(12)-EHC074-EF. 2012. https://doi.org/10.5489/cuaj.1224832.

Polypharmacy

15. Doumat G, Daher D, Itani M, Abdouni L, El Asmar K, Assaf G. The effect of polypharmacy on healthcare services utilization in older adults with comorbidities: a retrospective cohort study. BMC Prim Care. 2023;24(1):120. https://doi.org/10.1186/s12875-023-02070-0. PMID: 37237338; PMCID: PMC10214698.
16. Rankin A, Cadogan CA, Patterson SM, et al. Interventions to improve the appropriate use of polypharmacy for older people. Cochrane Database Syst Rev. 2018;(9):CD008165.
17. National Center for Health Statistics. Health, United States, 2016. Hyattsville, MD: Centers for Disease Control and Prevention; 2017. p. 25. https://www.cdc.gov/nchs/data/hus/hus16.pdf#01. Accessed 20 Oct 2018.
18. Wastesson JW, Morin L, Laroche ML, Johnell K. How chronic is polypharmacy in old age? A longitudinal nationwide cohort study. J Am Geriatr Soc. 2019;67(3):455–62. https://doi.org/10.1111/jgs.15717. Epub 2018 Dec 21. PMID: 30575952.
19. Field TS, Gurwitz JH, Avorn J, McCormick D, Jain S, Eckler M, Benser M, Bates DW. Risk factors for adverse drug events among nursing home residents. Arch Intern Med. 2001;161(13):1629.
20. Bjorkman IK, Fastbom J, Schmidt IK, et al. Drug-drug interactions in the elderly. Ann Pharmacother. 2002;36:1165–71.
21. Kanaan AO, et al. Adverse drug events after hospital discharge in older adults: types, severity, and involvement of beers criteria medications. J Am Geriatr Soc. 2013;61:1894–9.
22. American Geriatrics Society. 2019 updated AGS Beers criteria® for potentially inappropriate medication use in older adults [published ahead of print January 29, 2019]. J Am Geriatr Soc. https://onlinelibrary.wiley.com/doi/abs/10.1111/jgs.15767. Accessed 22 Feb 2019.

23. O'Mahony D, O'Sullivan D, Byrne S, O'Connor MN, Ryan C, Gallagher P. STOPP/START criteria for potentially inappropriate prescribing in older people: version 2. Age Ageing. 2015;44(2):213–8.
24. De Vries TPGM, Henning RH, Hogerzeil HV, Fresle DA, WHO Action Programme on Essential Drugs et al. Guide to good prescribing: a practical manual/authors: T. P. G. M. de Vries et al.; with contributions from F. M. Haaijer-Ruskamp and R. M. van Gilst. World Health Organization; 1994. https://apps.who.int/iris/handle/10665/59001.
25. Piette JD, Heisler M, Wagner TH. Cost-related medication underuse: do patients with chronic illnesses tell their doctors? Arch Intern Med. 2004;164:1749–55.
26. Abramson EL, Barrón Y, Quaresimo J, Kaushal R. Electronic prescribing within an electronic health record reduces ambulatory prescribing errors. Jt Comm J Qual Patient Saf. 2011;37(10):470–8. https://doi.org/10.1016/s1553-7250(11)37060-2. PMID: 22013821.
27. Reeve E, Wiese MD, Hendrix I, Roberts MS, Shakib S. People's attitudes, beliefs, and experiences regarding poly-pharmacy and willingness to deprescribe. J Am Geriatr Soc. 2013;61(9):1508–14.
28. Mangin D, Lawson J, Cuppage J, et al. Legacy drug-prescribing patterns in primary care. Ann Fam Med. 2018;16(6):515–20.
29. Jansen J, Naganathan V, Carter SM, et al. Too much medicine in older people? Deprescribing through shared decision making. BMJ. 2016;353:i2893.
30. Wolf MS, Curtis LM, Waite K, Bailey SC, Hedlund LA, Davis TC, Shrank WH, Parker RM, Wood AJ. Helping patients simplify and safely use complex prescription regimens. Arch Intern Med. 2011;171(4):300.
31. Nightingale G, Hajjar E, Swartz K, Andrel-Sendecki J, Chapman A. Evaluation of a pharmacist-led medication assessment used to identify prevalence of and associations with polypharmacy and potentially inappropriate medication use among ambulatory senior adults with cancer. J Clin Oncol. 2015;33(13):1453–9. Epub 2015 Mar 23.

Sleep Disturbances

32. Robbins R, Weaver MD, Barger LK, Wang W, Quan SF, Czeisler CA. Sleep difficulties, incident dementia and all-cause mortality among older adults across 8 years: findings from the National Health and Aging Trends Study. J Sleep Res. 2021;30(6):e13395. https://doi.org/10.1111/jsr.13395. Epub 2021 Jun 2. PMID: 34080234; PMCID: PMC9204609.
33. Li J, Vitiello MV, Gooneratne NS. Sleep in normal aging. Sleep Med Clin. 2018;13(1):1–11. https://doi.org/10.1016/j.jsmc.2017.09.001. Epub 2017 Nov 21. PMID: 29412976; PMCID: PMC5841578.
34. Ohayon MM, Carskadon MA, Guilleminault C, Vitiello MV. Meta-analysis of quantitative sleep parameters from childhood to old age in healthy individuals: developing normative sleep values across the human lifespan. Sleep. 2004;27(7):1255–73. https://doi.org/10.1093/sleep/27.7.1255. PMID: 15586779.
35. Kripke DF, Elliott JA, Youngstedt SD, Rex KM. Circadian phase response curves to light in older and young women and men. J Circadian Rhythms. 2007;5:4. https://doi.org/10.1186/1740-3391-5-4. PMID: 17623102; PMCID: PMC1988787.
36. Mattis J, Sehgal A. Circadian rhythms, sleep, and disorders of aging. Trends Endocrinol Metab. 2016;27(4):192–203. https://doi.org/10.1016/j.tem.2016.02.003. Epub 2016 Mar 3. PMID: 26947521; PMCID: PMC4808513.
37. Ebrahim IO, Shapiro CM, Williams AJ, Fenwick PB. Alcohol and sleep I: effects on normal sleep. Alcohol Clin Exp Res. 2013;37(4):539–49. https://doi.org/10.1111/acer.12006. Epub 2013 Jan 24. PMID: 23347102.
38. Wichniak A, Wierzbicka A, Walęcka M, Jernajczyk W. Effects of antidepressants on sleep. Curr Psychiatry Rep. 2017;19(9):63. https://doi.org/10.1007/s11920-017-0816-4. PMID: 28791566; PMCID: PMC5548844.

39. Holbrook A, Crowther R, Lotter A, Endeshaw Y. The role of benzodiazepines in the treatment of insomnia: meta-analysis of benzodiazepine use in the treatment of insomnia. J Am Geriatr Soc. 2001;49(6):824–6. https://doi.org/10.1046/j.1532-5415.2001.49161.x. PMID: 11454123.
40. Tikhomirova OV, Zybina NN, Kozhevnikova VV. Vliyanie dlitel'nogo priema beta-adrenoblokatorov na sekretsiyu melatonina, kachestvo sna i sosudistoe porazhenie golovnogo mozga [The effect of long-term beta-blockers on melatonin secretion, sleep quality, and vascular brain damage]. Zh Nevrol Psikhiatr Im S S Korsakova. 2021;121(8):7–12. https://doi.org/10.17116/jnevro20211210817. PMID: 34481429.
41. Clark I, Landolt HP. Coffee, caffeine, and sleep: a systematic review of epidemiological studies and randomized controlled trials. Sleep Med Rev. 2017;31:70–8. https://doi.org/10.1016/j.smrv.2016.01.006. Epub 2016 Jan 30. PMID: 26899133.
42. Mizuno S, Kameda A, Inagaki T, Horiguchi J. Effects of donepezil on Alzheimer's disease: the relationship between cognitive function and rapid eye movement sleep. Psychiatry Clin Neurosci. 2004;58(6):660–5. https://doi.org/10.1111/j.1440-1819.2004.01317.x. PMID: 15601392.
43. Ross JS, Shua-Haim JR. Aricept-induced nightmares in Alzheimer's disease: 2 case reports. J Am Geriatr Soc. 1998;46(1):119–20. https://doi.org/10.1111/j.1532-5415.1998.tb01033.x. PMID: 9434681.
44. Sateia MJ, Buysse DJ, Krystal AD, Neubauer DN, Heald JL. Clinical practice guideline for the pharmacologic treatment of chronic insomnia in adults: an American Academy of Sleep Medicine clinical practice guideline. J Clin Sleep Med. 2017;13(2):307–49. https://doi.org/10.5664/jcsm.6470. PMID: 27998379; PMCID: PMC5263087.
45. Jaehne A, Loessl B, Bárkai Z, Riemann D, Hornyak M. Effects of nicotine on sleep during consumption, withdrawal and replacement therapy. Sleep Med Rev. 2009;13(5):363–77. https://doi.org/10.1016/j.smrv.2008.12.003. Epub 2009 Apr 2. PMID: 19345124.
46. Cole JL. Steroid-induced sleep disturbance and delirium: a focused review for critically ill patients. Fed Pract. 2020;37(6):260–7. PMID: 32669778; PMCID: PMC7357890.
47. Sateia MJ. International classification of sleep disorders-third edition: highlights and modifications. Chest. 2014;146(5):1387–94. https://doi.org/10.1378/chest.14-0970.
48. Chung F, Yegneswaran B, Liao P, Chung SA, Vairavanathan S, Islam S, Khajehdehi A, Shapiro CM. STOP questionnaire: a tool to screen patients for obstructive sleep apnea. Anesthesiology. 2008;108(5):812–21. https://doi.org/10.1097/ALN.0b013e31816d83e4. PMID: 18431116.
49. Alessi C, Martin JL, Fiorentino L, Fung CH, Dzierzewski JM, Rodriguez Tapia JC, Song Y, Josephson K, Jouldjian S, Mitchell MN. Cognitive behavioral therapy for insomnia in older veterans using nonclinician sleep coaches: randomized controlled trial. J Am Geriatr Soc. 2016;64(9):1830–8. https://doi.org/10.1111/jgs.14304. Epub 2016 Aug 22. PMID: 27550552; PMCID: PMC5351772.
50. Mitchell MD, Gehrman P, Perlis M, Umscheid CA. Comparative effectiveness of cognitive behavioral therapy for insomnia: a systematic review. BMC Fam Pract. 2012;13:40. https://doi.org/10.1186/1471-2296-13-40. PMID: 22631616; PMCID: PMC3481424.
51. Gammack JK. Light therapy for insomnia in older adults. Clin Geriatr Med. 2008;24(1):139–49, viii. https://doi.org/10.1016/j.cger.2007.08.013.
52. Olde Rikkert MG, Rigaud AS. Melatonin in elderly patients with insomnia. A systematic review. Z Gerontol Geriatr. 2001;34(6):491–7. https://doi.org/10.1007/s003910170025. PMID: 11828891.
53. Roth T, Seiden D, Sainati S, Wang-Weigand S, Zhang J, Zee P. Effects of Ramelteon on patient-reported sleep latency in older adults with chronic insomnia. Sleep Med. 2006;7(4):312–8. https://doi.org/10.1016/j.sleep.2006.01.003. Epub 2006 May 18. PMID: 16709464.
54. Anttila SA, Leinonen EV. A review of the pharmacological and clinical profile of mirtazapine. CNS Drug Rev. 2001;7(3):249–64. https://doi.org/10.1111/j.1527-3458.2001.tb00198.x. PMID: 11607047; PMCID: PMC6494141.
55. Green B. Prazosin in the treatment of PTSD. J Psychiatr Pract. 2014;20(4):253–9. https://doi.org/10.1097/01.pra.0000452561.98286.1e. PMID: 25036580.

Chapter 10
Common Infections

June M. McKoy and Jennifer Rocio Delgado Felipa

10.1 Introduction

While the home can be a sanctuary, homebound individuals' risk for infections increases as care providers breach the home environment [1]. Furthermore, it has been reported that rates of infections in adults receiving home-based medical care have increased and account for 17% of unplanned hospitalizations [2, 3]. Several factors influence the risk of infection among homebound older adults, including frailty, prior infections, prior hospitalizations, and poor cognition. Furthermore, physiologic aging changes, atypical presentation of infectious diseases, provider behavioral practices, and variability in the physical structures of the home pose unique challenges. The COVID-19 pandemic underscored the importance of infection control in the home environment and the potential dire consequences for older adults. To be sure, common infections have also assumed an unparalleled urgency. This chapter focuses on physiologic aging changes and common infections impacting older adults who are aging in place.

10.2 Physiologic Changes with Aging

Age-related physiologic changes contribute to increased vulnerability to infections and prevent older adults from mounting a robust response to infections. Immunosenescence, an age-related dysfunction of the immune system that results in enhanced risk of infection, is the primary reason for the decreased response to

J. M. McKoy (✉) · J. R. D. Felipa
Division of Geriatric Medicine, Department of Medicine, Northwestern University Feinberg School of Medicine, Chicago, IL, USA
e-mail: j-mckoy@northwestern.edu

J. L. Colburn et al. (eds.), *Geriatric Home-Based Medical Care*,
https://doi.org/10.1007/978-3-031-68786-0_10

invading infections. There is a functional decline in both innate immunity and adaptive immunity that encompasses cell-mediated and humoral immunity. Furthermore, as the thymus involutes, there is a decline in the proportion of naïve T cells. Reduced production of B and T cells in the bone marrow and thymus and diminished function of mature lymphocytes in secondary lymphoid tissues occur. As a result, older adults do not respond to immune challenge as robustly as the young. The immune system becomes less able to identify foreign antigens, macrophages destroy bacteria more slowly, T cells respond less quickly to the antigens, there are fewer white blood cells capable of responding to new antigens, and older adults have smaller amounts of complement proteins and do not produce as many of these proteins as younger people in response to bacterial infections. Although the amount of antibody produced in response to an antigen remains about the same overall, the antibodies become less able to attach to the antigen. This change may partly explain why pneumonia, influenza, infective endocarditis, and tetanus are more common among older people and result in death more often. These changes may also partly explain why vaccines are less effective in older people and thus why it is important for older people to get booster shots (which are available for some vaccines).

10.3 Urinary Tract Infections

A urinary tract infection (UTI) is defined as significant bacteriuria in a person with urinary signs or symptoms and no alternate source of infection. UTIs are the most common types of infection in older adults. Traditionally, UTIs are categorized as either uncomplicated or complicated [1].

Uncomplicated UTIs occur in patients with a functionally and structurally normal urinary tract system. Conversely, complicated UTIs occur in patients with functionally or structurally abnormal urinary tract systems. Examples of functional abnormalities in the urinary tract system include ureteric reflux, incomplete bladder emptying, and chronic kidney disease. Examples of structural abnormalities include a cystocele, urethral stricture, an indwelling catheter, and prostatic hypertrophy; all of these abnormalities increase in frequency with age. Most UTIs in functionally impaired older adults (i.e., homebound geriatric patients) are considered complicated because most of these patients have some functional or structural issue with their urinary tract [1, 4].

In young, otherwise healthy adults, the diagnosis and treatment of a UTI are straightforward. The diagnosis can often be solely based on a patient's history of dysuria, urinary urgency, and urinary frequency; further evaluation that includes a physical exam and a urinalysis and culture may be utilized to confirm the diagnosis. Commonly, empiric antibiotic therapy is initiated based on self-reported symptoms [4]. In the homebound older adult with deficits in cognitive and physical function, medical providers are sometimes faced with challenges in diagnosing UTIs. Not only do some patients struggle to communicate their symptoms, but the symptoms might be atypical or might be in the setting of a long-standing history of baseline urinary issues that blurs acute physical changes, including a fever [1, 4].

10.3.1 Asymptomatic Bacteriuria (ASB)

It is well settled that asymptomatic UTI or bacteriuria should not be treated with antibiotics. By definition, asymptomatic bacteriuria is the obtaining of a positive urine culture from an appropriately collected urine specimen in a noncatheterized patient who has no urinary symptoms. Risk factors for ASB include female organs, advancing age, and being institutionalized. Prevalence of asymptomatic bacteriuria (ASB) for women over the age of 80 living in the community has been estimated to be as high as 20% [1, 5]. Importantly, the prevalence of ASB is higher among geriatric patients in long-term care facilities (25–50% in women and 15–40% in men) compared to ambulatory older patients. Homebound older adults are likely to have multiple comorbidities that can lead to impaired voiding or use of an indwelling catheter, which are usually associated with an increased prevalence of ASB [1, 5, 6]. The Infectious Disease Society of America (ISDA) recommends against treating ASB with antimicrobials, except in some very specific instances (i.e., pregnancy and prior to a urological procedure with a high likelihood of mucosal bleeding) [1, 5].

10.3.2 Etiology

In most cases, bacteria causing UTIs are gastrointestinal flora that have colonized the perineum and traveled up the urethra to the prostate, bladder, and/or kidney. Thus, patients with chronic-indwelling catheters or those who perform clean intermittent catheterization (CIC) for conditions such as neurogenic bladder are at an increased risk of both UTIs and ASB given the increased risk of introducing bacteria into the urethra. Furthermore, external catheters (i.e., condom catheters) also increase the risk of bacteriuria by increasing the pathogenic bacteria in the perineum. Less frequently, patients can develop a UTI from hematogenous spread of a pathogen causing a bacteremia from a nonurinary source.

Physiologic aging changes, such as a decrease in estrogen production with its attendant increase in pH in the genitourinary mucosa, can lead to vaginal colonization with uropathogens and decreased colonization with protective lactobacilli. Additionally, structural abnormalities in the genitourinary system of older women are more likely to result in the development of cystocele and an increase in UTIs. For older men, prostatic hypertrophy and urethral stricture increase leading to obstructive uropathies, urinary retention, and increased infection risks. In both older men and women, the increased development of bladder diverticulae is another risk factor for recurrent UTIs. Functionally, the bladder residual volume increases in older adults with age. This can be worsened by several neurologic illnesses, such as

Parkinson disease (PD), Alzheimer disease (AD), and strokes all of which can impair bladder emptying and thus increase the risk of UTIs [1]. In PD, the loss of dopamine and the resulting interruption of signals from the brain to the bladder can lead to impaired bladder emptying. Chronic bacterial prostatitis, an indolent type of UTI seen in older men, can be challenging to treat because of the poor penetration of antibiotics into the prostate. As such, the prostate in men with chronic prostatitis or those with prostatic calculi can become a reservoir for bacteria, resulting in frequent relapses of cystitis, sometimes with long periods of time between infections [1].

10.3.3 Differential Diagnosis

The differential diagnosis for homebound older adults who are suspected of having a UTI varies depending on the presenting signs and symptoms (see Table 10.1). The differential diagnosis for perineal discomfort includes bacterial and fungal vaginitis in women and chronic prostatitis in men. Urinary frequency can be seen in new-onset or poorly controlled diabetes mellitus. Gross hematuria is seen in patients with urological cancer, nephrolithiasis, nephritis, and trauma associated with placing an indwelling catheter. Pyelonephritis presents with the triad of fever, costovertebral pain, and tenderness. Malodorous urine can be seen in patients with UTIs, as well as those with volume depletion and those with urinary incontinence and poor hygiene [1, 5, 6]. An increase in agitation or confusion without accompanying urinary signs or symptoms in a patient with dementia may represent progression of dementia versus delirium. The differential for delirium is broad and includes medication, side effects, a UTI or other infection, or a change in the patient's environment. Families and patients may request that a urinalysis be done in the setting of agitation, but clinicians need to proceed cautiously and consider each presenting

Table 10.1 Differential diagnosis of UTI

Alternative diagnosis	Comments
Asymptomatic bacteriuria	Consider in patients presenting with delirium who lack the ability to give a urinary ROS
Volume depletion	Consider in patients presenting with malodorous urine without other urinary signs or symptoms
Poor hygiene	Patients presenting with malodorous urine
Urothelial cancer	Patients presenting with painless hematuria
Bacterial or fungal vaginitis	Patients presenting with perineal discomfort in older patients with vaginas
Chronic prostatitis	Patients presenting with perineal discomfort in older patients with prostates
Pyelonephritis	Technically a specific type of a complicated UTI, presenting with the triad of fever, costovertebral pain, and tenderness
Nephrolithiasis	Patients presenting with hematuria and pain

case on an individual basis. Increasingly, the anecdotal teaching point of checking a urinalysis (U/A) and urine culture on all older adults with delirium is being questioned. While it is appropriate, in the setting of delirium, to check a U/A and culture if there are signs and symptoms indicating a UTI or if the homebound older adult is unable to provide symptom information, anchoring on a UTI opens patients to the risk of unnecessary treatment [7].

10.3.4 Investigations at Home

Investigations at home should begin with a thorough history and physical examination. In homebound patients who may have cognitive impairment with or without urinary incontinence, this history may need to be obtained from the caregiver to reliably determine whether a patient is experiencing urinary frequency or dysuria. For functionally impaired patients, it may be challenging to ascertain whether a patient is experiencing urinary urgency. New or increased incontinence should prompt consideration of further workup as a possible symptom of a UTI [4–6]. Caregivers and patients can be asked about foul-smelling urine, with the caution to clinicians in interpreting the significance of this sign: not all malodorous urine is due to a UTI, and not all UTIs produce foul-smelling urine. Malodorous urine may be associated with bacteriuria, caused by the polyamine production of the bacteria. However, malodorous urine does not help the clinician to understand if the patient is experiencing a UTI or ASB or simply volume depletion or dehydration [1, 5, 6]. Caregivers and patients should also be asked about gross hematuria, fever, and suprapubic and costovertebral pain.

When a UTI in a homebound older adult is part of the differential diagnosis, the clinician should pay close attention to certain aspects of the physical exam, including level of consciousness, vital signs, and suprapubic and costovertebral tenderness. Urine dipstick testing for nitrite and leukocyte esterase (LE) can be done at home with results available within minutes. Nitrite is used as a surrogate for bacteriuria but has a low sensitivity. Notably, when nitrite is positive, the test does not distinguish between asymptomatic and symptomatic bacteriuria [4]. Leukocyte esterase is used as a surrogate for pyuria. Pyuria indicates an inflammatory process in the genitourinary tract, which can include, but is not limited to, a UTI. While a result of positive LE is not conclusive in making the diagnosis of a UTI, a negative LE has high specificity for excluding a UTI [1].

Urine can also be collected in the home and be analyzed in a lab for more extensive microscopic testing, with results within hours; the culture will result within days. Ideally, the urine sample collected for a urine culture should be a straight catheterization or clean catch sample to avoid contamination with perineal flora. Urine cultures should be obtained for all male patients with symptomatic UTIs and all women with presumed kidney involvement or underlying functional or anatomical GU abnormalities. Expert opinion and guidelines suggest that community-dwelling women with a history of recurrent uncomplicated cystitis who present with typical urinary symptoms can be treated empirically without a culture. However, if these patients present with atypical symptoms, have recently been on antibiotics, or have had a rapid recurrence of urinary symptoms following treatment for a presumed cystitis, a urine culture should be obtained to help guide diagnosis and appropriate therapy [4, 8].

Many homebound older adults have functional or structural impairment in their urinary tract system, causing their UTIs to be classified as complicated UTIs. Thus, homebound older adults with a suspected UTI should have a urine culture submitted and treatment deferred in most cases until the culture results. The decision to treat the patient empirically while waiting for culture results or to wait for culture results and then choose an antimicrobial is discussed below [4, 8]. In analyzing the urine sample, significant bacteriuria is defined as greater than or equal to 10^5 colony-forming units (CFU)/mL for noncatheterized patients. Since a clean catch specimen can be challenging to obtain in homebound older adults due to possible visual, cognitive, and dexterity impairments, as well as the possibility of incontinence, the gold standard for collection is clean intermittent catheterization (CIC) [1]. Most home-based practices obtain a culture by the CIC method when there is a high clinical suspicion for a UTI and when the culture results are likely to change management (i.e., a patient has previously had multidrug-resistant UTI). The procedure itself can lead to bacteriuria, cause some discomfort, and increase agitation in cognitively impaired individuals [1, 6]. Urine samples for culture should be sent to the laboratory as soon as possible to obtain accurate CFU counts. For patients who have external (condom) urinary catheters at baseline, the following procedure can be used to decrease the risk of contamination with perineal flora: (1) Clean the glans penis. (2) Apply a new external catheter, including a new collecting bag. (3) Collect the urine sample after voiding [4, 6]. Notably, there is insufficient evidence as to what constitutes "significant" bacteriuria for patients with condom catheters. For patients who have an indwelling urethral or suprapubic or intermittent catheterization, signs and symptoms compatible with a catheter-associated UTI include acute onset fever, rigors, delirium, malaise with no other identified cause, costovertebral angle pain, new onset hematuria, and pelvic discomfort. Patients who have had their catheters removed may experience urinary urgency, frequency, or dysuria [6]. Patients with spinal cord injuries may experience increased muscle spasticity, autonomic dysfunction, or malaise [6]. Significant bacteriuria is defined as greater than or equal to 10^3 colony-forming units (CFU)/mL for patients with chronic-indwelling urethral or suprapubic catheters. Further complicating the diagnosis of a UTI in patients with chronic-indwelling catheters, is the high rates of ASB found in these patients. In one study, ASB was found in 100% of patients with chronic-indwelling catheters [5, 6]. In a chronically catheterized patient suspected of having a UTI, if the catheter has been in place for more than 2 weeks, the catheter should be replaced, and the urine culture should be obtained from the newly placed catheter before initiating antibiotics [6].

The approach to diagnosis and treatment of UTIs in cognitively impaired, non-catheterized older adults with alteration in mental status must be a nuanced one. The clinician will need to depend on bystander information coupled with a urinalysis.

The clinician then must decide whether the bacteriuria represents ASB or a UTI. Given that ASB has a higher prevalence in the functionally impaired older adult, we caution healthcare providers to be careful in attributing delirium without urinary symptoms to a UTI [1, 5]. Repeatedly treating ASB with multiple courses of antibiotics leads to resistant UTIs and other infectious complications including *Clostridium difficile*. Other potential harms of antimicrobial treatment include acute kidney injury, noninfectious diarrhea, nausea, and cachexia [1, 5, 6].

10.3.5 Pharmacologic Therapy

When a patient is suspected of having a UTI, clinicians must decide whether to start antibiotics empirically or wait for urine culture results. We suggest that this decision be based on a combination of factors, including the severity of the patient's clinical presentation, whether the patient has a chronic-indwelling urinary catheter, and the clinician's index of suspicion for a UTI. For all patients with moderate to severe symptoms (fever defined as >37.9 °C or 1.5 °C above baseline temperature, costovertebral angle (CVA) tenderness, rigors, hypotension, tachycardia, suprapubic pain, or gross hematuria), empiric antibiotic therapy should be initiated while waiting for the results of the urine culture [8]. For patients (regardless of catheter status) with milder symptoms and lower clinical suspicion of a UTI, we suggest waiting for the culture results to return before starting antimicrobial therapy [8].

For noncatheterized patients, we generally favor empiric treatment with either nitrofurantoin monohydrate/macrocrystals (100 mg orally twice daily for 5 days) or trimethoprim–sulfamethoxazole (TMP–SMX) (160/800 mg orally twice daily for 3–7 days). For a patient with a sulfa allergy, TMP monotherapy can be used. Both nitrofurantoin and TMP–SMX are cost-effective drug treatments. Nitrofurantoin should be avoided in patients with renal impairment or those suspected of having pyelonephritis. There are increasing rates of TMP–SMX and fluoroquinolone resistance in the community, as well as multidrug-resistant vancomycin-resistant *Enterococci* and extended-spectrum beta-lactamase-producing *Escherichia coli* and *Klebsiella pneumoniae*. ISDA recommends using TMP–SMX as empiric treatment for a UTI only if local resistance patterns show a resistance rate of *E. coli* of less than 20% and it has not been used for this patient to treat a UTI in the past 3 months [1, 4]. The use of fluoroquinolones as empiric treatment for UTIs is controversial. Some studies have shown fewer adverse effects with ciprofloxacin use, while other guidelines advise against empirically using fluoroquinolones because of the risk of increasing uropathogen resistance. Moxifloxacin should not be used to treat UTIs as it has poor urinary excretion. Hyperglycemia is common with fluroquinolones, and although uncommon, hypoglycemia has been reported with all fluroquinolones and more frequently so in older adults with type 2 diabetes mellitus. The underlying mechanism appears to be blockage of adenosine 5′-triphosphate-sensitive potassium channels in pancreatic beta cell membranes. Amoxicillin can be effective as a targeted therapy for Gram-positive organisms, but it is *not* recommended as a first-line agent because of the high prevalence of Gram-negative bacteria resistance to this agent. Amoxicillin/clavulanic acid and cephalosporins can also be effective as targeted therapy but are also *not* recommended as empiric therapy because of their broad-spectrum activity and cost [9]. Given the physiologic aging changes of decreased glomerular filtration rate, clinicians must renally dose antibiotics (see Table 10.2). For patients on warfarin who require antibiotic therapy, we recommend that antibiotic initiation be guided by one of the following two strategies. The first option is to check an INR within 1 week of initiating antibiotic therapy, regardless of the class of antibiotics, and adjust the warfarin dose as needed. The second option is to preemptively decrease the dose of warfarin by 15–20% when antibiotics are initiated. There are insufficient data to recommend one strategy over the other [10, 11].

The American Urological Association recommends that vaginal estrogen be used to reduce the risk of recurrent UTIs in postmenopausal women, unless there is a contrandication. Vaginal estrogen can reduce cell shedding and urinary inflamatory scores, and increases the presence of lactobacillus, whose re-dominance in the vagina decreases the risk of recurrent UTIs. Pain and fever can be treated with acetaminophen [1].

10.3.6 Nonpharmacological Therapy

Oral hydration is recommended for UTIs, as well as for the isolated symptom of foul-smelling urine. Avoidance of unnecessary urinary catheterization, appropriate perineal hygiene, and incontinence care are recommended. The evidence for the use

Table 10.2 Antibiotic coverage of UTIs

Antibiotic	Comments
Nitrofurantoin monohydrate/ macrocrystals	Recommended empiric treatment for noncatheterized patients. Contraindicated for patients with renal impairment
Trimethoprim–sulfamethoxazole	Recommended empiric treatment for noncatheterized patients if local resistance patterns show resistance rate of *E. coli* of less than 20% and it has *not* been used for this patient to treat a UTI in the past 3 months
Trimethoprim	Alternative to TMP-SMX for patients with sulfa allergy
Ciprofloxacin	Controversial use as a first-line empiric agent. Fewer adverse reactions. Increasing uropathogen resistance to this agent
Levofloxacin	Controversial use as a first-line empiric agent. Fewer adverse reactions. Increasing uropathogen resistance to this agent. Glucose abnormalities in diabetic patients
Amoxicillin	*Not* recommended as an empiric treatment. Can be used as a targeted therapy for Gram-positive organisms
Amoxicillin/clavulanic acid	*Not* recommended as an empiric therapy. Broad spectrum. Expensive. Can be used as targeted therapy
Other cephalosporins	*Not* recommended as an empiric therapy. Broad spectrum. Expensive. Can be used as targeted therapy

of cranberry products for the prevention of UTIs in the homebound older adult remains inconclusive [1, 5, 6].

10.4 Pneumonia

Pneumonia is one of the most common diseases diagnosed and treated in the United States, and mortality rates for this infection remain high. The incidence of pneumonia increases with aging as does the impact of pneumonia on both mortality and morbidity. For older adults, age-related changes, a weakened immune system, and accompanying comorbid illnesses can affect lung function and predispose to development of pneumonia. Undoubtedly, multiple factors coalesce to cause the development of pneumonia, including impairment of mucociliary clearance, slower and less efficient clearance of secretions by the mucociliary system, decrease in chest wall compliance, and decrease in lung compliance because of osteoporotic changes and kyphosis. Defined as an acute infection of the pulmonary parenchyma, pneumonia can be caused by various pathogens including bacteria, viruses, or fungi that overcome the host's defense mechanisms. Most homebound patients will acquire pneumonia in the community (community-acquired pneumonia or CAP) or through aspiration (aspiration pneumonia) of bacterial content from the mouth or pharynx. Of note, CAP is defined as an acute infection of the pulmonary parenchyma acquired outside of the hospital or in patients admitted to the hospital for fewer than 48 hours.

Hospital-acquired pneumonia (HAP) is an acute infection of the pulmonary parenchyma that develops while patients are in the hospital, and healthcare associated pneumonia (HCAP) was defined as that acquired in other healthcare facilities such as nursing homes or other chronic care facilities and was meant to identify patients at risk for developing multi-drug resistant infections. HCAP is no longer used as this categorization was thought to have been overly sensitive and arguably led to increased use of inappropriately broad antibiotics. For the purposes of this chapter discussion, we will focus on CAP and aspiration pneumonia, the most commonly diagnosed penumonias in the homebound patient.

10.4.1 Differential Diagnosis and Etiology

As noted earlier, the incidence of pneumonia increases with chronic illness, debility, and advanced age as these conditions interact to impact pulmonary defense mechanisms and increase the risk of CAP. Specifically, conditions that increase the risk of CAP commonly seen in homebound individuals include the following:

- Alteration in normal level of consciousness, which predisposes to aspiration (i.e., dementia, stroke, seizures, medications, drug/alcohol use disorder).
- Tobacco or alcohol use.

- Hypoxemia related to chronic illnesses like chronic obstructive pulmonary disease (COPD), chronic heart failure, interstitial lung disease, and others.
- Malnutrition.
- Immunosuppression.
- ≥65 years of age
- Chronic obstructive pulmonary disease (COPD).
- Dysphagia of varying etiologies, including esophageal lesions and motility problems.
- Bronchial obstruction due to stenosis, tumor, or foreign body.
- Medications, including acid suppressive therapy, antipsychotic medications, and corticosteroids.

10.4.2 Differential Diagnosis for Bacterial Pneumonia

- Viral pneumonia.
- Asthma.
- Chronic obstructive pulmonary disease.
- Bronchitis.
- Pulmonary embolism.
- Aspiration pneumonitis/pneumonia.
- Chronic heart failure.
- Pleural effusion.
- Fungal pneumonia.

10.4.3 Investigations in the Home

Changes caused by infection in older adults are often subtle, and nonspecific complaints may be the only evidence of infection. It is therefore not surprising that pneumonia can present in a variety of ways in the older adult, especially in those who are homebound. Studies examining the diagnosis of pneumonia by history and physical examination using chest radiograph as a gold standard find no combination of signs and symptoms (i.e., cough, fever, tachycardia, or crackles) that reliably predict the diagnosis with acceptable sensitivity [12]. Symptoms usually present acutely with patients complaining of changes over a few days. Common clinical complaints that should trigger evaluation for possible pneumonia include dyspnea, cough, fever, chest pain with pleuritic features, and increased sputum production, especially purulent sputum as is sometimes seen with bacterial pneumonia. Atypical complaints like "not feeling like myself," gastrointestinal upset, and alteration in mental status can be the harbingers of a pneumonia diagnosis.

Given that many homebound patients are living with neurological disease and/or dementia, aspiration pneumonia deserves special consideration. Diseases that lead to reduced cognition or consciousness predispose to aspiration, as does dysphagia of any origin, esophageal disease, and the presence of a feeding tube. In one study, oropharyngeal dysphagia was strongly associated with CAP in older adults (occurring in 91% of patients with CAP) [2]. Any patient with these risk factors diagnosed with pneumonia in the community should be suspected of having either CAP or aspiration pneumonia, regardless of whether an aspiration event was witnessed. Aspiration can be silent or occur during sleep and may develop into pneumonia even without a known inciting event. Of note, it is important to distinguish aspiration pneumonitis from true aspiration pneumonia. Some aspiration events can result in a chemical pneumonitis with a pulmonary inflammatory response that presents as transient respiratory difficulty or distress but resolves quickly. If pneumonitis is suspected, there is no role for antibiotics in treatment. However, it is important that clinicians remain vigilant in their identification of aspiration pneumonia, as unlike in CAP, the organisms causing aspiration pneumonia are more likely to be oral or upper airway flora, including anaerobic bacteria or, much less commonly, Gram-negative bacilli or *Staphylococcus aureus*.

On physical examination, patients should be evaluated for fever, tachypnea, and tachycardia. In older adult patients, especially those with dementia, tachypnea may be the only sign, as fever is less likely. Counting the respiratory rate is an important component of the physical examination. If there is a consolidation, tactile fremitus will be increased, and there will be dullness to percussion. On pulmonary auscultation, rales are the most common abnormal finding [13], but wheezes, crackles, or rhonchi may be audible in many patients. Notably, pneumonia can be present with a normal lung exam. If the patient's history and physical examination do not clearly diagnose pneumonia, the gold standard in pneumonia diagnosis is plain chest radiograph. Utilization of portable x-ray machines for in-home chest radiographs can be invaluable in diagnosing pneumonia or other pulmonary pathology when history and physical examination are equivocal unrevealing. Chest radiograph can show lobar consolidation or interstitial infiltrate suggestive of different microbiological pathogens, but there are no pathognomonic chest radiographic findings for specific organisms. Of note, chest radiograph can be falsely negative, especially in dehydrated patients. One study found that approximately 11% of negative chest X rays later had positive CT scan findings consistent with pneumonia [14]. Routine laboratory testing is considered to have little value in determining the etiology of pneumonia. However, it may have prognostic significance in older adult patients and is therefore recommended. Most clinicians who provide home-based medical care will be able to collect blood for basic laboratories in a timely fashion looking primarily for leukocytosis with a leftward shift on differential. Other testing that may be helpful includes viral polymerase chain reaction (PCR), especially if influenza is suspected, as its early diagnosis may avoid unnecessary antibiotic use. Procalcitonin (PCT), a serum biomarker that can help to distinguish bacterial from other causes of infection or inflammation, is also considered to be a useful parameter for predicting the severity of CAP in older adults.

Microbiological testing, including sputum culture and blood culture can be done but is rarely helpful in the outpatient setting. Furthermore, obtaining adequate sputum specimens in frail, older adults may be particularly difficult. Sputum culture may be considered if atypical microorganisms are suspected in a patient who is significantly immunocompromised, a cavitary lesion is noted on chest radiograph, or the patient is not responding to appropriate antibiotic therapy [9]. Though HAP is not covered extensively here, it must be considered in homebound patients recently discharged to home from a hospital, nursing home, or subacute rehabilitation facility and may require different, more broad antibiotic coverage depending on local flora and antibiotic resistance patterns.

10.4.4 Prognosis and Risk Stratification

In general, older adult patients face significant morbidity and mortality from pneumonia, especially when there is attendant frailty and chronic comorbid illnesses. However, with timely diagnosis and treatment, the mortality rate is <10% [15]. Given that timely diagnosis impacts clinical outcomes, clinicians can employ available risk score calculators to help guide decisions like need for hospitalization, intensive care unit (ICU) transfer, and treatment. The two most used risk score calculators are the CURB-65 and PSI.

10.4.4.1 CURB-65

This scale is practical for use in the home setting as it is based largely on clinical criteria easily gathered during the history and physical exam, as well as one relatively routine laboratory test (BUN). The CURB-65 uses a five-point system to predict mortality: (1) presence of confusion, (2) uremia (BUN >19), (3) respiratory rate $\geq$ 30, (4) blood pressure (systolic <90 or diastolic <60), and (5) age greater than 65. Each point on the scale from 0 to 5 confers a greater mortality rate: 0, 0.6%; 1, 2.7%; 2, 6.8%; 3, 14%; and 4 and 5, 28% [13, 16]. Patients with a score of 0–1 should be treated outpatient, and those with score of 4–5 should be admitted if consistent with a patient's goals of care. At the 2–3 range, patients must be closely monitored either in the home or hospital depending on their home support systems and goals of care (see Table 10.3).

10.4.4.2 Pneumonia Severity Index (PSI)

PSI score is used to help determine the need for hospitalization and ICU stay in patients with pneumonia. It is more comprehensive than the CURB-65 (see above) but difficult to implement in the home setting, as it requires multiple laboratory values including arterial pH level, blood urea nitrogen, sodium, and others. As the score increases, the predicted 30-day mortality increases.

Table 10.3 CURB-65 in pneumonia

CURB 65 score	Mortality
One point for each: Presence of confusion	
Uremia (BUN >19)	
Respiratory rate ≥30	
SBP <90 or DBP <60)	
Age greater than 65	
0	<1%
1	3%
2	7%
3	14%
4	28%
5	28%

10.4.5 Pharmacological Therapy

For previously healthy patients with no hospitalizations in the last 90 days, the IDSA/American Thoracic Society (ATS) "Consensus Guidelines on the Management of Community-Acquired Pneumonia in Adults" recommends empiric therapy for patients with CAP who are stable to be managed in the home setting with either a macrolide or doxycycline. However, many homebound older adult patients will not fall into this category due to age, functional impairment, frailty, and multiple comorbidities, including coronary artery disease, chronic lung disease, liver or renal disease, diabetes mellitus, and malignancy. For this group, a fluoroquinolone is the first-line recommended agent; a beta-lactam plus macrolide is an alternative to fluoroquinolone in this situation, specifically an oral fluoroquinolone with respiratory coverage (levofloxacin 750 mg daily, moxifloxacin 400 mg daily, or gemifloxacin 320 mg daily) or a beta-lactam that can treat streptococcal pneumonia (amoxicillin 1 g three times daily, amoxicillin–clavulanic acid 2 g twice daily, or cefpodoxime 20 mg twice daily) *and* macrolide (azithromycin 500 mg × 1 day, 250 mg × 4 days, azithromycin 500 mg daily × 3 days, clarithromycin 500 mg twice daily), or tetracycline such as doxycycline 100 mg twice daily. There is no evidence that treatment for more than 7 days is better than 5–7 days [17] (see Table 10.4).

10.4.6 Aspiration Pneumonia

Use of broad coverage for anaerobes in suspected aspiration pneumonia is controversial, as some guidelines have stated that the likelihood of true anaerobic infection without abscess is low. Most aspiration pneumonias should be treated as community-acquired pneumonias, as the most aspirated organisms are nonresistant mouth flora. It is prudent to treat aggressively in patients presenting with severe symptoms, with

Table 10.4 Antibiotic selections for pneumonia

	First-line antibiotics
Community-acquired pneumonia	Beta-lactam + macrolide (e.g., azithromycin or clarithromycin) -or- Beta-lactam + tetracycline (e.g., doxycycline) -or- Fluoroquinolone (moxifloxacin or levofloxacin)
If anaerobic coverage required for true aspiration	Clindamycin -or- Amoxicillin–clavulanate

obvious abscess on chest radiograph, oral abscesses, witnessed frank aspiration of gastric contents, or those non-resolving with conventional treatment, especially with predisposing factors such as dementia and neurological disease. In these patients, the chance of true anaerobic aspiration pneumonia is higher [9]. If one chooses to treat anaerobic aspiration pneumonia in the home setting, recommended first-line treatment includes clindamycin (450 mg orally 3 times daily) as first-line therapy in addition to usual CAP treatment. Alternative agents include amoxicillin–clavulanic acid (875 mg twice daily) or metronidazole (500 three times daily) *plus* amoxicillin (500 mg three times daily). Another option that is likely effective, but should not be used preferentially, is a 7 day course of a fluoroquinolone as it will cover both CAP and aspiration pneumonia.

10.4.7 Symptom Management

Patients treated for pneumonia at home may need oxygen for a brief period during their acute illness. Many durable medical equipment (DME) companies will supply home oxygen, and it is useful to know how to order it with a local DME supplier before diagnosis. To order oxygen, hypoxia must be documented, thus home-based medical care providers need to add a portable pulse oximeter to their armamentarium and must document the pulse oximeter results from the visit. Hypoxemia must be the primary documented diagnosis as Medicare does not cover oxygen for a pneumonia diagnosis. Medicare will generally cover oxygen if the patient has certain chronic conditions, such as COPD and CHF, exacerbated by pneumonia that now require O_2 support as evidenced by documented hypoxia. Patients who have decided on comfort measures at the end of life and are enrolled in home Hospice may obtain home oxygen through that agency.

10.4.8 Prevention with Vaccinations

(a) Pneumococcal vaccine is recommended for every person aged 65 and older. For patients under 65, pneumococcal vaccine is recommended every 5 years if these patients have chronic illnesses, including HIV, chronic renal disease, immunodeficiency, sickle cell disease, and malignancy [18]. Many younger homebound patients may be immunocompromised due to chronic illness and may fall into this category [18]. Pneumococcal vaccine can be given to patients with pneumonia once they are on treatment with clinical improvement or any time thereafter. There are two types of pneumococcal vaccines now available and recommended for these patients, each encompassing different serotypes: pneumococcal conjugate vaccines (PCV15 and PCV20) and pneumococcal polysaccharide (PPSV23). **Adults** 65 years or older who have not already received a pneumococcal conjugate vaccine should receive either a single dose of PCV15 or a single dose of PCV20. The conjugate and polysaccharide vaccines should not be coadministered. If the conjugate (PCV15) is given, then the 23-valent pneumococcal polysaccharide vaccine (PPV23) is recommended 12 months later. If PCV20 is used, a dose of PPSV23 is *not* indicated [18].
(b) Seasonal influenza vaccination is recommended for all adults yearly. Infection with influenza is associated with the development of pneumonia and higher rates of morbidity/mortality [19].

10.4.9 Nonpharmocologic Therapy

(a) Oxygen: As noted above, patients treated for pneumonia at home may need oxygen for a brief course during or after their acute illness.
(b) Positioning: During the acute illness, standing or sitting upright in a chair or elevating the head of the bed for patients who cannot get out of bed will promote lung expansion and improved air exchange. Aspiration precautions should always be followed, especially for homebound patients with cognitive impairment.
(c) Aspiration precautions: For patients at high risk for aspiration (see section above), all caregivers should be educated and instructed in preventive behavioral measures to avoid aspiration and aspiration pneumonia. These include good daily oral hygiene, keeping the head in a neutral position when swallowing, and keeping patients upright at 90° when feeding and for as long as possible after feeding. If a patient must be fed in bed, the head of the bed should be elevated to at least 30° for at least 1 hour after eating/drinking. Caregivers should feed slowly and allow patients to complete their swallow before feeding continues. If there are aspiration concerns, a speech and language pathologist (SLP) evaluation can be ordered through a community home health agency. SLPs are able to evaluate a patient's swallow function at home and make spe-

cific recommendations about food and liquid consistency to avoid aspiration, as well as provide education and modeling of the precaution behaviors outlined above.

10.5 Cellulitis

Cellulitis is an acute inflammation of the skin mainly involving the deep dermis and surrounding subcutaneous tissues, mostly caused by skin flora that are indigenous to healthy individuals. It is classically characterized by the four cardinal signs of inflammation, *rubor*, *calor*, *tumor*, and *dolor*, or translated from the Latin: redness, warmth, swelling, and pain, respectively [20, 21]. It typically presents as a poorly demarcated area of skin without abscess or purulent discharge. Erysipelas is a superficial cellulitis with mostly lymphatic involvement [21]. This form of cellulitis is often indurated, with a sharp demarcated raised border. It can also cause dimpling of the skin because of localized edema (the "peau d'orange" effect).

10.5.1 Differential Diagnosis and Etiology

Most cellulitis is caused by naturally occurring colonized skin flora, most commonly beta-hemolytic streptococcus (generally group A streptococcus (i.e., Streptococcus pyogenes) and secondarily most common, methicillin sensitive staphylococcus aureus. Methicillin-resistant *Staphylococcus aureus* (MRSA) has also emerged as a frequent cause of skin infections in the community. Patients are most at risk for MRSA if they were recently hospitalized, but there are strains of MRSA causing community-acquired cellulitis independent of recent institutionalization. Identification of possible MRSA infection affects management as described below. Severely immunocompromised individuals may become infected with organisms beyond the usual pathogens, including Gram-negative organisms such as *E. coli* and *Pseudomonas* and with opportunistic organisms such as *Helicobacter cinaedi* and *Cryptococcus* [21]. Diabetic patients' ulcers are also at risk of being infected by Gram-negative organisms (*Enterobacteriaceae* spp., *Pseudomonas aeruginosa*, and *Acinetobacter* spp.).

Risk factors for developing skin infections include any preceding acute or chronic process that results in localized damage to the superficial soft tissues of the body. This includes recent trauma, recent or concurrent dermatitis (either contact or ectopic), venous insufficiency, and chronic edema. Notably, the skin of older adults is especially vulnerable to infection given physiologic aging changes [1]. Any disruption to the lymphatics resulting in chronic or recurrent edema, such as those resulting after mastectomy or lymph node resection, can predispose to cellulitis. Animal or human bites cause cellulitis due to trauma to the skin and transport of mouth flora to the resulting wound. Occasionally, osteomyelitis may evolve outward to cause cellulitis of the overlying skin [21]. Finally, any immunocompromised state such as acquired immunodeficiency disorder syndrome (AIDS) or neutropenia from leukemia, chemotherapy, and organ transplant increases the risk of skin infections, often with unusual organisms [21]. Alternate diagnoses for suspected cellulitis include any process that also causes some or all the signs of skin inflammation, including venous stasis changes, deep vein thrombosis, trauma, vasculitis, as well as other infective processes. Additionally, cellulitis can coexist or be a result of these alternate diagnoses (see Table 10.5).

10.5.2 Investigations at Home

History and physical examination are the mainstay in the diagnosis of skin infections. Appearance of new erythema, swelling, history of pain, and tenderness on palpation are often sufficient to diagnose a skin infection [20–23]. Predisposing risk factors and acuity of symptoms increase the probability of correct diagnosis. However, chronic venous changes and chronic ulcers can make diagnosis on visualization difficult. We do not advise doing skin cultures as these are usually of little to no diagnostic value and will yield skin flora that represents normal colonization [23]. Abscesses and purulent drainage, however, should be cultured according to

Table 10.5 Differential diagnosis of cellulitis

Alternate diagnosis	Comments
Deep vein thrombosis	Determine pretest probability, consider ultrasound if medium/high
Changes of venous insufficiency/stasis dermatitis	Chronic changes, often darker red and hyperpigmented changes, can devolve into secondary infection, especially if venous ulcers develop
Trauma without infection	Ecchymosis, history of trauma, possible hematoma present
Dermatitis (eczema or contact)	Often pruritic, can be chronic
Vasculitis	Systemic signs, lymphadenopathy in certain syndromes, presents diffusely
Insect bite	Local pruritis, very focal symptoms, can develop secondary cellulitis
Drug reaction	Less localized, more diffuse, often presents as hives, can be associated with symptoms of anaphylaxis
Other infections	
Fungal infection (candida or tinea)	Pruritic, scaly, often in intertriginous regions
Osteomyelitis	Acute or chronic, may present with systemic signs and sepsis
Septic bursitis	Localized swelling and redness, presents near a joint
Septic arthritis	Symptoms mostly localized at a joint with some involvement of surrounding skin. Often presents with joint effusion, joint tenderness, and decreased range of motion
Isolated skin abscess	Very focal or minimal to no erythema, purulent discharge present if abscess opened, otherwise fluctuant

Centers for Disease Control (CDC) and IDSA guidelines as the results may change management, especially if infections fail to clear with empiric treatment [22, 23]. Initiation of antibiotic treatment can proceed while awaiting culture results. Blood cultures similarly are of little yield as most skin infections represent local processes [24]. Suspected cellulitis in the lower extremities and sometimes in the upper extremities often present like deep vein thrombosis. At those times, the clinician should consider assessing the probability of deep venous thrombosis (DVT) based on risk factors. The most studied clinical prediction rule is the Wells score [25, 26]. Those with a medium or high pretest probability warrant further evaluation for DVT, such as lower extremity ultrasound dopplers (either in the home if home ultrasonography is available or office-based referral if necessary and within patient's capability). D-dimer may be elevated in both DVT and cellulitis as it is an acute phase reactant. A negative D-dimer may exclude DVT and rule in a cellulitis [26].

10.5.3 Pharmacologic Treatment

The CDC and the IDSA have issued updated guidelines for the antibiotic management of soft tissue infections in response to increasing incidence of MRSA infections in community dwellers. The initial treatment choice depends on whether there is purulence, whereby the skin may be fluctuant, have a yellowish or whitish center, or be draining frank pus. Attempting to aspirate with a needle can also be done to prove purulence if the exam is unclear. An abscess with little to no systemic signs can be incised and drained with curative results and often does not need antibiotics. Additionally, if purulence is suggestive of MRSA infection, appropriate coverage of MRSA is needed. If there is no purulence, then typical coverage of susceptible streptococcus and MSSA is appropriate. However, if the patient fails initial therapy, has severe systemic signs (fever, tachypnea, tachycardia, leukocytosis on labs), and/or is immunocompromised, then MRSA should be covered along with streptococcal species. Of note, MRSA is resistant to all beta-lactam agents (penicillins and cephalosporins), except for one of the newest IV cephalosporins, ceftaroline fosamil. Appropriate oral antibiotic choices for MSSA cellulitis include beta-lactams, mainly penicillins and cephalosporins or clindamycin for those who are allergic to or

Table 10.6 Antibiotic coverage for non-MRSA cellulitis

Antibiotic	Dosing
Penicillins	
Penicillin V	250–500 mg orally every 6 h
Dicloxacillin	500 mg orally every 6 h
Cephalosporins e.g., Cephalexin	500 mg orally 4 times daily
Clindamycin	300–450 mg orally 4 times daily

cannot tolerate beta-lactam-based antibiotics (see Table 10.6). Recommended treatment duration is usually 5 days but may be extended if the patient is not showing signs of improvement [23].

Patients in whom MRSA is suspected are often treated with oral TMP-SMX, a tetracycline, or clindamycin. Rifampin is also an option, although rarely used and should not be used as a single agent. Linezolid is also an option, but the CDC suggests an infectious disease consultation before initiating therapy as linezolid is costly and has potentially severe side effects. Trimethoprim–sulfamethoxazole and doxycycline have unknown or poor coverage for streptococcus, and use of a second agent (such as a beta-lactam) may be recommended to cover both strep and MRSA, especially for initial empiric coverage. Isolated abscesses that require antibiotics can be treated with MRSA coverage alone. Clindamycin covers both streptococcus and MRSA adequately but places patients at significant risk for *C. difficile* colitis. Fluoroquinolones and macrolides are not effective against MRSA due to high rates of resistance (see Table 10.7).

A 2014 evidence-based IDSA guideline considered steroid use (prednisone 40 mg oral daily for 7 days) as an adjuvant treatment for significant symptomatic cellulitis in non-diabetic adult patients. This, however, was based on weak to moderate evidence. Administration of prophylactic antibiotics is appropriate for patients with recurrent cellulitis. These are patients who have 3–4 episodes of cellulitis per year despite failed attempts to control risk factors. Patients can be treated with oral penicillin (250–500 mg orally twice daily) or IM benzathine penicillin (600,000 units for patients who weigh ≤27 kg; 1.2 million units for patients who weigh >27 kg) every 2–4 weeks. Staphylococcal prophylaxis can be tried with clindamycin 150 mg orally once daily for adults. This treatment continues until risk factors are eliminated [23].

Table 10.7 Antibiotic coverage of MRSA cellulitis

Antibiotic	Dosing	Comments
Trimethoprim–sulfamethoxazole (TMP–SMX)	1–2 double-strength tabs twice daily	Only covers MRSA, consider adding beta-lactam for *Streptococcus* coverage (see Table 10.6)
Doxycycline or Minocycline	100 mg twice daily 200 mg orally once then 100 mg twice daily	Only covers MRSA, consider adding beta-lactam for *Streptococcus* coverage (see Table 10.6)
Clindamycin	300–450 mg twice daily	Adequate *Strep* coverage, can use as monotherapy Has increased risk of *Clostridium difficile* colitis
Linezolid	600 mg orally twice daily	Associated with myelosuppression, neuropathy, and lactic acidosis. ID consult recommended
Rifampin	600 mg once daily or 300–450 mg every 12 h	Not routinely used but can be used as adjuvant therapy for persistent Staph infections and/or to eradicate colonization; use only in combination with other agents for *Staph* coverage as resistance with single use is very high

10.5.4 Nonpharmacologic Management

Purulent cellulitis (with subcutaneous abscesses) should be drained, when possible, which will often prove curative if there are not extensive symptoms or systemic signs, such as febrile illness. Simple incision and drainage in most areas of the skin can be accomplished in the home. Abscesses on the face and hands or complex nonhealing wounds often require specialist intervention, either in the office or in the emergency department.

As an adjuvant to pharmacological therapy, elevation of affected extremities and warm compresses can aid in symptomatic control, as both anecdotally promote drainage and thus improve pain and swelling [21, 26]. Finally, nonhealing or worsening cellulitis, despite appropriate diagnosis and appropriate oral antibiotics, may warrant intravenous antibiotics and possibly an infectious disease consult. This complication and/or possible systemic signs with a change in hemodynamics may warrant a higher level of care, such as referral to an emergency department or hospitalization, if such care is within the goals of care of the patient. Signs of deeper tissue infection, including necrotizing infection, also warrant systemic IV antibiotics and hospitalization.

10.6 Summary

Managing *infections in homebound older adults* presents unique challenges that are magnified by frailty, cognitive impairment, functional deficits, and social constraints. Understanding how to navigate and mitigate obstacles in the home is critically important to positive outcomes for older adults. Undoubtedly, infections contribute to significant morbidity and mortality in the homebound population. This was most evident during the COVID-19 pandemic where homebound older adults experienced severe illness and death because of physiologic aging changes in the respiratory, cardiovascular, and immune systems. The COVID-19 pandemic was a stark reminder of the importance of having a multipronged, evidence based, and well-coordinated diagnostic and treatment strategy for this population. In this chapter we have outlined the numerous risk factors for infection in older adults, including frailty, functional impairments, and chronic comorbid illnesses.

References

1. High KP. Infectious diseases. In: Halter JB, Ouslander JG, Studenski S, High KP, Asthana S, Supiano MA, Ritchie CS, Schmader K, editors. Hazzard's geriatric medicine and gerontology. 8th ed. New York: McGraw-Hill; 2022. Chapter 124.
2. Mouton CP, Bazaldua OV. Common infections in older adults. Am Fam Physician. 2001;63:257–68.

3. El Bcheraoui C, Mokdad AH, Dwyer-Lindgren L, Bertozzi-Villa A, Stubbs RW, Morozoff C, Shirude S, Naghavi M, Murray CJL. Trends and Patterns of Differences in Infectious Disease Mortality Among US Counties, 1980-2014. JAMA. 2018;319(12):1248–1260.
4. Gupta K, Hooton T, Naber K, Wullt B, Colgan R, et al. International clinical practice guidelines for the treatment of acute uncomplicated cystitis and pyelonephritis in women: a 2010 update by the infectious diseases society of America and the European society for microbiology and infectious diseases. Clin Infect Dis. 2011;52:e103–20. http://cid.oxfordjournals.org/content/52/5/e103.full. Accessed 22 Sept 2024.
5. Nicolle LE, Gupta K, Bradley SF, Colgan R, DeMuri GP, Drekonja D, Eckert LO, Geerlings SE, Köves B, Hooton TM, Juthani-Mehta M, Knight SL, Saint S, Schaeffer AJ, Trautner B, Wullt B, Siemieniuk R. Clinical practice guideline for the Management of Asymptomatic Bacteriuria: 2019 update by the Infectious Diseases Society of America. Clin Infect Dis. 2019;68(10):e83–e110. https://doi.org/10.1093/cid/ciy1121.
6. Hooton TM, Bradley SF, Cardenas DD, Colgan R, Geerlings SE, Rice JC, et al. Diagnosis, prevention, and treatment of catheter-associated urinary tract infection in adults: 2009 international clinical practice guidelines from the infectious diseases society of America. Clin Infect Dis. 2010;50:625–63. http://www.idsociety.org/uploadedFiles/IDSA/Guidelines-Patient_Care/PDF_Library/Comp%20UTI.pdf. Accessed 22, Sept 2024.
7. McKenzie R, Stewart MT, Bellantoni MF, Finucane TE. Bacteriuria in individuals who become delirious. Am J Med. 2014;127(4):255–7.
8. Bausch K, Stangl FP, Prieto J, Bonkat G, Kranz J. Urinary Infection Management in Frail or Comorbid Older Individuals. Eur Urol Focus. 2024 Aug 30:S2405-4569(24)00164-0.
9. Jackson CD, Burroughs-Ray DC, Summers NA. Clinical Guideline Highlights for the Hospitalist: 2019 American Thoracic Society/Infectious Diseases Society of America Update on Community-Acquired Pneumonia. J Hosp Med. 2020;15(12):743–5.
10. Baillargeon J, Holmes HM, Lin Y, Raji MA, Sharma G, Kuo Y. Concurrent use of warfarin and antibiotics and the risk of bleeding in older adults. Am J Med. 2012;125(2):183–9.
11. Ahmed A, Stephens JC, Kaus CA, Fay WP. Impact of preemptive warfarin dose reduction on anticoagulation after initiation of trimethoprim-sulfamethoxazole or levofloxacin. J Thromb Thrombolysis. 2008;26(1):44–8.
12. Metlay JP, Fine MJ. Testing strategies in the initial management of patients with community-acquired pneumonia. Ann Intern Med. 2003;138(2):109.
13. Wipf JE, Lipsky BA, Hirschmann JV, Boyko EJ, Takasugi J, Peugeot RL, Davis CL. Diagnosing pneumonia by physical examination: relevant or relic? Arch Intern Med. 1999;159(10):1082–7.
14. Maughan BC, Asselin N, Carey JL, Sucov A, Valente JH. False-negative chest radiographs in emergency department diagnosis of pneumonia. R I Med J. 2014;97(8):20–3.
15. CDC/National Center for Health Statistics. Fast facts you Need to Know about Pneumococcal Disease. Centers for Disease Control and Prevention. https://www.cdc.gov/pneumococcal/about/facts.html. Accessed 22 Sept 2024.
16. Lim W, van der Eerden MM, Laing R, Boersma W, Karalus N, Town G, Lewis S, Macfarlane J. Defining community acquired pneumonia severity on presentation to hospital: an international derivation and validation study. Thorax. 2003;58(5):377–82.
17. Dimopoulos G, Matthaiou DK, Karageorgopoulos DE, Grammatikos AP, Athanassa Z, Falagas ME. Short- versus long-course antibacterial therapy for community-acquired pneumonia: a meta-analysis. Drugs. 2008;68(13):1841.
18. Pneumococcal vaccination. https://www.cdc.gov/pneumococcal/vaccines/index.html Accessed 22 Sept 2024.
19. Vaccines by Disease: Flu (Influenza). https://www.cdc.gov/vaccines/vpd/flu/index.html. Accessed 22 Sept 2024.
20. Stevens DL, Bryant AE. Infections of the Skin, Muscles, and Soft Tissues. In: Loscalzo J, Fauci AS, Kasper DL, Hauser SL, Longo D, Jameson J, Editors. Harrison's Principles of Internal Medicine. 21st ed. New York: McGraw- Hill. New York. https://accessmedicine.mhmedical.com/ Accessed 22 Sept 2024.

21. Swartz MN. Clinical practice: cellulitis. N Engl J Med. 2004;350:904–12.
22. Gorwitz RJ, Jernigan DB, Powers JH, Jernigan JA. Strategies for clinical management of MRSA in the community: summary of an experts' meeting convened by the Centers for Disease Control and Prevention. Mar 2006. https://www.cdc.gov/mrsa/pdf/mrsa-strategies-expmtgsummary-2006.pdf. Accessed 22 Sept 2024.
23. Stevens DL, Bisno AL, Chambers HF, Everett ED, Dellinger P, Goldstein EJ, Gorbach SL, Hirschmann JV, Kaplan EL, Montoya JG, Wade JC; Infectious Diseases Society of America. Practice guidelines for the diagnosis and management of skin and soft-tissue infections. Clin Infect Dis. 2005;41(10):1373–406. https://doi.org/10.1086/497143. Epub 2005 Oct 14. Erratum in: Clin Infect Dis. 2005;41(12):1830. Erratum in: Clin Infect Dis. 2006;42(8):1219. Dosage error in article text.
24. Perl B, Gottehrer NP, Raveh D, Schlesinger Y, Rudensky B, Yinnon AM. Cost-effectiveness of blood cultures for adult patients with cellulitis. Clin Infect Dis. 1999;29(6):1483–8.
25. Geersing GJ, Zuithoff NP, Kearon C, Anderson DR, Ten Cate-Hoek AJ, Elf JL, et al. Exclusion of deep vein thrombosis using the Wells rule in clinically important subgroups: individual patient data meta-analysis. BMJ. 2014;348:g1340.
26. Bates SM, Jaeschke R, Stevens SM, et al. Diagnosis of DVT: antithrombotic therapy and prevention of thrombosis, 9th ed. American College of Chest Physicians evidence-based clinical practice guidelines. Chest. 2012;141(2_suppl):e351S–418S.

Chapter 11
Wound Care in Home-Based Settings

Yasmin S. Meah, Fred C. Ko, and David Skovran

11.1 Introduction

Although there are few specific data about the prevalence of wounds in a homebound population [1], wounds are common in persons with similar functional level and comorbidities, such as patients in nursing homes [2]. Chronic wounds, now referred to as hard-to-heal wounds, are a source of frustration to home-based medical providers and more distressingly, negatively impact the quality of life of affected patients and their caregivers. Though challenging and costly to care for, chronic wounds do not routinely require specialty care; however, home-based practitioners need proficiency and experiential knowledge outside their scope of training to care for them successfully. Every provider who takes care of patients in the home setting should be familiar with the major categories of wounds—pressure, venous stasis, lymphatic, arterial, neuropathic, and malignant,—be able to direct the management of these conditions, and develop a working knowledge of general strategies to prevent wounds. Early intervention is the key to successful healing, and the necessity of interdisciplinary collaboration cannot be overemphasized.

Y. S. Meah (✉)
Departments of Medicine, Medical Education, Geriatrics and Palliative Medicine, Icahn School of Medicine at Mount Sinai, New York, NY, USA
e-mail: yasmin.meah@mountsinai.org

F. C. Ko
Departments of Geriatrics and Palliative Medicine and Medicine, Icahn School of Medicine at Mount Sinai, New York, NY, USA
e-mail: fred.ko@mssm.edu

D. Skovran
Department of Medicine and Medical Education, Icahn School of Medicine at Mount Sinai, New York, NY, USA
e-mail: david.skovran@mssm.edu

J. L. Colburn et al. (eds.), *Geriatric Home-Based Medical Care*,
https://doi.org/10.1007/978-3-031-68786-0_11

This chapter will describe the prevalence, pathophysiology, prevention, and treatment options for the wound types listed above. In addition, current documentation and billing codes will be highlighted. Strategies to improve effective collaboration with various disciplines, including certified home health agency (CHHA) nurses, paid and unpaid caregivers, social workers, physical therapists, surgeons, and podiatrists, will be elaborated.

11.2 The Value of Interprofessional Collaboration in the Home-Based Care of Patients with Wounds

Interprofessional collaboration, communication, and partnership are key to wound prevention, palliation, and healing. Alliances between healthcare personnel are built through clear and routine communication, a combined understanding of risk factors unique to each patient, and shared realistic goals of wound healing and pain control. Providers should work in direct collaboration with nurses; joint home visits are occasionally necessary for complex or poorly healing wounds. Nurses who are highly competent in wound care are critical to successful healing; the most effective nurses possess extensive knowledge of dressings, readily counsel caregivers, and report changes in wound state to the primary clinician. Wound care nurses and expert clinicians who offer remote, telemedicine consultation can be helpful in improving wound care outcomes [3, 4]. Physical therapists are also essential to the care team as they can advise on durable medical equipment (such as proper bed surfaces and wheelchair adjustments) and repositioning techniques for caregivers and providers that can significantly improve the course of these ulcers. Additionally, physical therapists may accelerate wound healing using ultrasound and electrical stimulation; they may also conduct lymphatic massage in cases of lymphedema-associated ulcers and direct patients to augment ankle mobility in cases of venous stasis ulcers.

Perhaps most crucial for successful wound treatment in the home are vigilant and dedicated caregivers who maintain skin integrity and adhere to directions on positioning, repositioning, moisture containment, and nutritional augmentation; they also know when to call providers for emerging wounds, non-adherent dressings, new pain, or foul smell. Social workers are often critical in understanding and defining the limitations of caregivers and advocating for the approval of additional hours of paid personnel. Techniques for preventing pressure ulcers are not often intuitive; providers need to dedicate specific and proactive attention to training and counseling caregivers with at-risk patients. Physical therapists can be crucial in this regard, counselling on repositioning and off-loading techniques and guiding critically needed durable medical equipment such as wheelchairs, seat cushions, and bed surfaces. Though ulcers, particularly pressure injuries, may not be entirely avoidable in homebound persons, integrated multidisciplinary teams who are knowledgeable and complementary can increase the likelihood of healing and decrease the risks of infection and uncontrolled pain. In situations in which wound closure is not the goal, palliation is most effective when caregivers, nurses, physical therapists, social workers, and home-based medical clinicians work in concert with aggressive attention to symptoms of distress.

11.3 The Evaluation and Care of Pressure Injuries in the Home

Pressure injuries are among the most common types of wounds in the home-based medical care setting. The description of these wounds as pressure injuries is somewhat constricted as several other physical forces including friction, moisture, and shear stress cause wounds which are largely, but not completely, preventable and treatable. Understanding the physical as well as patient characteristics that lead to these wounds is elemental to implementing effective prevention and therapeutics.

11.3.1 Physics and Anatomy of Wound Development

Correctly characterizing wounds is an essential first step for identifying and justifying preventative strategies and therapies, communicating with fellow providers, documenting and billing, and determining the likelihood of complete healing and/or recurrence.

The staging of pressure injuries is complex, and substantial controversy exists on the validity of accepted scales [5]. The most widely accepted classification system in the USA is the National Pressure Injury Advisory Panel (NPIAP) staging system which categorizes pressure injuries as six stages: Stages I–IV, Unstageable, and Suspected Deep Tissue Injury [6]. In 2016, the NPIAP retitled pressure ulcers as pressure injuries given that tissue injury from pressure does not always manifest as an opening in the skin. Furthermore, two additional categories were added: medical device-related pressure injury which can result from prolonged pressure contact with such equipment as neck braces, BiPAP face masks, catheters, diaper elastics, and bed rails, for instance, and mucosal membrane pressure injury related to prolonged contact with a device to surfaces such as the mouth (i.e., dental appliances) and vagina (i.e., pessaries). In recent iterations of the scale, stages have been co-classified as categories; arguably, categories are more accurate descriptors that counter the common misconception of stages as progressive.

Static prolonged pressure is the primary cause of the development of pressure injuries. It is important to understand that pressure injury stages or categories merely represent the visible degree of tissue injury. The McClemont cone of pressure theory describes the anatomic pressure gradient that develops when bone is pressed upon tissue against a static surface [7]. This concept is crucial to understanding why seemingly more superficial pressure injuries are most commonly the end result of deep pressure. Pressure on tissues causes capillary occlusion, tissue ischemia, and, ultimately, tissue necrosis. Because muscle is closest to bone, it suffers the greatest area of injury; subcutaneous fat is affected in smaller proportion and the skin the least. In addition, muscle and subcutaneous fat suffer far more irreversible damage to sustained periods of pressure than the dermis and epidermis. Thus, "what you see" is often not "what you get"—a phrase often expressed when referring to true pressure wounds of the skin, as the skin damage is just the "tip of the iceberg" when a wound is the result of pressure (Fig. 11.1).

The most susceptible areas are over bony prominences; the most susceptible persons are those with limited or dependent mobility, sarcopenia, nutritional compromise, and arterial and sensory impairment [8]. Although current hospital practice dictates turning the body every 2 h to off-load pressure on high-risk body parts, there is no clear minimum amount of pressure or time necessary to induce cell damage, and this practice is more convention than evidence-based therapy and prevention. In the home, repositioning intervals of every 2 h are next to impossible to implement; a more reasonable set of strategies are interval repositioning of every 3–4 h, ensuring even small movements either by patient cueing or caregiver assistance of particularly vulnerable areas such as the sacrum, hips, ankles, and heels. In patients with peripheral vascular disease in which the lower extremities are particularly vulnerable to capillary compromise under sustained pressure, repositioning intervals may be comfortably extended to 3–4 h by off-loading bony areas with the use of wedge pillows and heel foam protectors.

Shear forces are potent factors in the development of advanced wounds in home-based settings. Shear forces cause stretching and disruption of subcutaneous tissues and capillaries, making them far more vulnerable to damage by pressure [9]. Typical

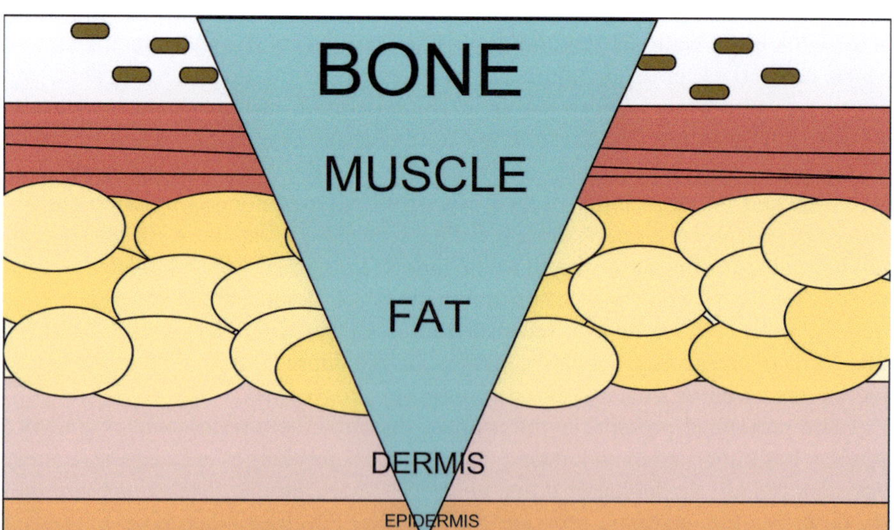

Fig. 11.1 Schematic of McClemont cone of pressure

shear stresses in homebound persons include those generated on the sacrum when a person is shifted upward in bed or glides downward gradually from a partially upright position of 45–90° and on the hip when the person is turned to the side by dragging the body along the greater trochanter. Shear forces accelerate the rate of ulcer manifestation and progression by several orders of magnitude over pressure alone. Older persons with more fragile and inelastic integument due to loss of collagen anchoring proteins and slower rates of tissue repair are more susceptible to injury from shear forces [10]. Minimizing or eliminating shear strain is a crucial primary and secondary prevention strategy, as this force more than pressure alone has been implicated in rapid tissue breakdown and ulceration [11]. The home-based provider should be particularly mindful of certain positions in bed and in wheelchairs and reclining chairs that place patients at high risk of shear injuries; for instance, patients with poor axial tone who sit in wheelchairs without leg supports usually slip forward and down placing a great deal of shear strain on the coccyx and ischial tuberosities. Injuries that result are called "slippage injuries" and characteristically have a tunneling that directs cranially.

11.3.2 Ulcer Stages and Categories

Stage/Category I ulcers emerge without frank denudation or ulceration of the skin and present as red and nonblanchable. In persons with darker skin, these areas are hyperpigmented, and the distinction as a pressure ulcer is often the relative warmth or tenderness to touch compared to surrounding areas. Stage I pressure ulcers are complex wounds to categorize anatomically; though the skin is intact, the degree of damage to deeper tissues may be substantial. If the cause is friction, the damage to deeper tissues may be limited, and thus the true thickness of tissue involvement is limited to the epidermis. The NPIAP cautions against the classification of hyperemia exclusively due to friction a Stage I ulcer; however, many experts agree that distinguishing superficial hyperemia due to friction is difficult in clinical practice and perhaps underestimates the potent role that friction plays in the culmination of decubitus ulcers. Given the high likelihood of substantial deep tissue injury when pressure is the cause, Stage I ulcers should never be taken lightly; they should be seen not simply as at-risk skin involvement but serious deep tissue injury (Figs. 11.2 and 11.3).

Stage/Category II ulcers are partial thickness wounds involving the epidermis and dermis (Fig. 11.4). They usually present as visible denudation of the epidermis and often have depth on the order of millimeters. They may also present as fluid-filled blisters (Fig. 11.5). Although Stage II ulcers may be the result of pressure, they are more frequently the outcome of substantial friction over bony or non-bony areas. They may be promulgated by moisture from urine or feces, heavy exudate, or sweat that separates the bonds between keratinocytes in the stratum corneum, a phenomenon called maceration. Most Stage II ulcers do not progress to Stage III or IV wounds.

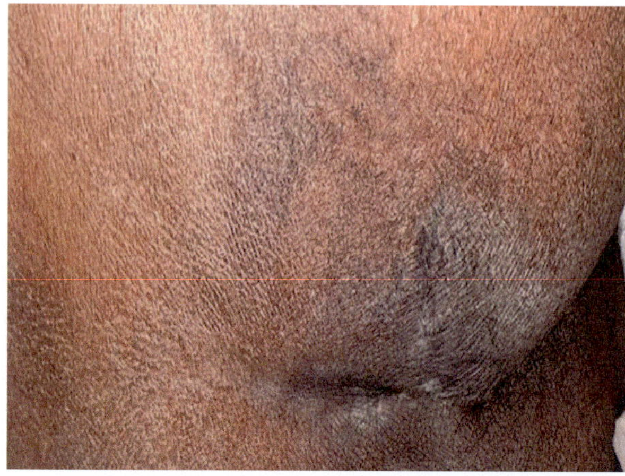

Fig. 11.2 Stage 1 pressure injury of the buttock, dark-skinned

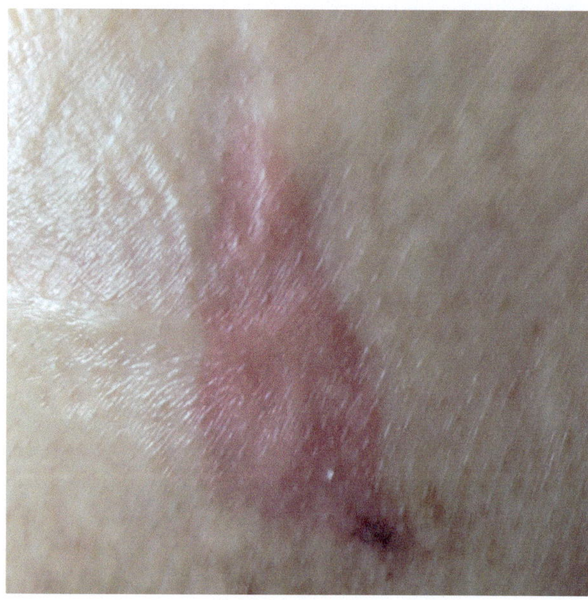

Fig. 11.3 Stage 1 pressure injury of the buttock, light-skinned

Stage/Category III ulcers are shear force or pressure injury wounds. They appear as full-thickness skin loss involving damage or necrosis of subcutaneous fat that may *visibly* extend down to, but not through, underlying fascia, with the ulcer presenting to the naked eye as a deep crater. Classically, these are beefy red craters with depth. Depth, however, can vary based on the anatomic location. In areas in which there is little to no subcutaneous tissue, such as the ankle or scalp, a Stage III ulcer may be quite shallow; in contrast, in areas such as the buttock that have a substantial amount of fat, the depth can be substantial. Stage III ulcers may also extend underneath the dermal and subcutaneous layers of adjacent tissue, a phenomenon known

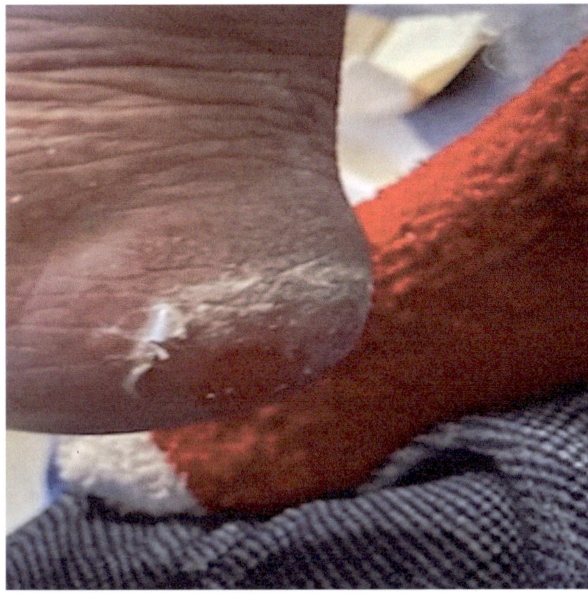

Fig. 11.4 Stage 2 pressure injury of the heel

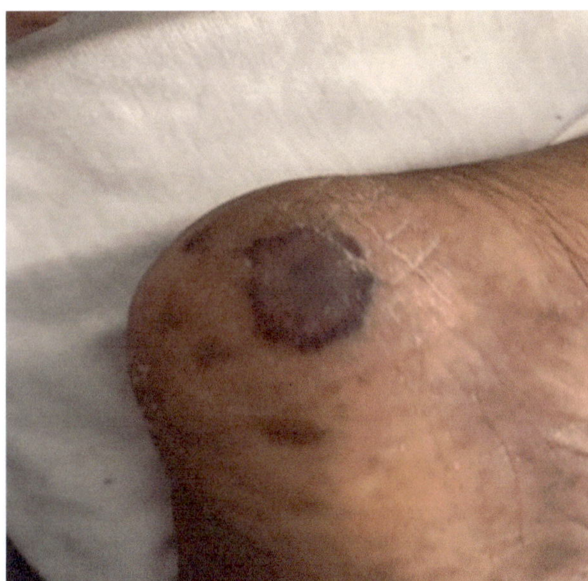

Fig. 11.5 Stage 2 pressure injury of foot, blister

as "undermining" or "tunneling." Deeper tissues such as the muscle, tendon, or bone, although likely affected, are not visible to the naked eye (Fig. 11.6).

Stage/Category IV ulcers are true pressure injury wounds. Like Stage III ulcers, they present with full-thickness tissue loss; in contrast, however, deep tissue layers such as the muscle, tendon, ligaments, or bone are visible. All other characteristics

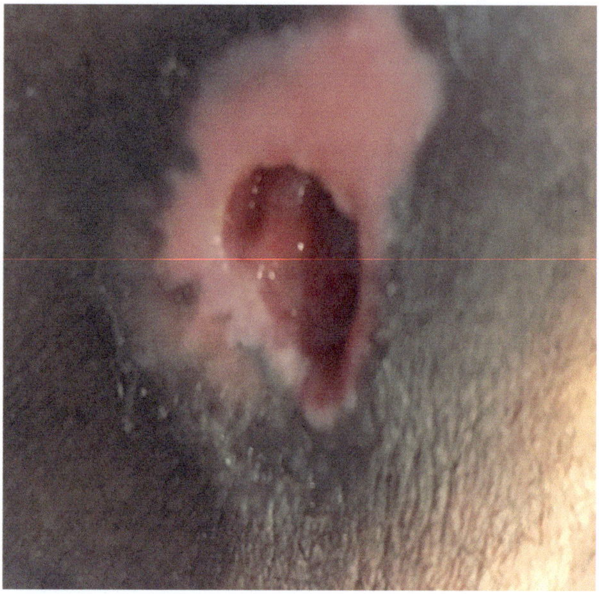

Fig. 11.6 Stage III pressure injury

of Stage III ulcers apply to Stage IV ulcers including widely variable depth depending on anatomic location and transgression to adjacent tissues through undermining and tunneling (Fig. 11.7).

Unstageable ulcers present as full-thickness skin loss, but the true depth of the ulcer is obstructed by necrotic tissue in the form of slough or eschar. Slough is characteristically yellow, tan, gray, green, or brown and may be dense and adherent or soft and viscous. Eschar is tan, brown, or black and can also be dry and adherent or soft and pliable. It is important to recognize that though these necrotic elements may be located on the edge of Stage III and IV wound beds, wounds described as "unstageable" have such a vast degree of such elements which obscure the fullest tissue depth of the wound (Fig. 11.8). Until the slough or eschar is removed from the base of the wound bed, the actual depth of tissue involvement cannot be determined. This practice of removal is generally contraindicated, however, when heel ulcers are the sites of injury. The development of eschar on the heel is considered protective, so dead tissue should not be removed if it is dry (Fig. 11.9).

Deep tissue injury (DTI) characteristically presents as either a blood-filled blister or ecchymosis with purple or maroon-colored intact skin in light-pigmented persons and brawny intact skin in darker-pigmented persons. Affected areas can feel edematous or boggy and are often warmer and tender compared to adjacent skin. DTI pressure ulcers are classically located over bony prominences with highest prevalence at the heel and lesser but still substantial prevalence at the sacrum and buttocks [12] (Fig. 11.10).

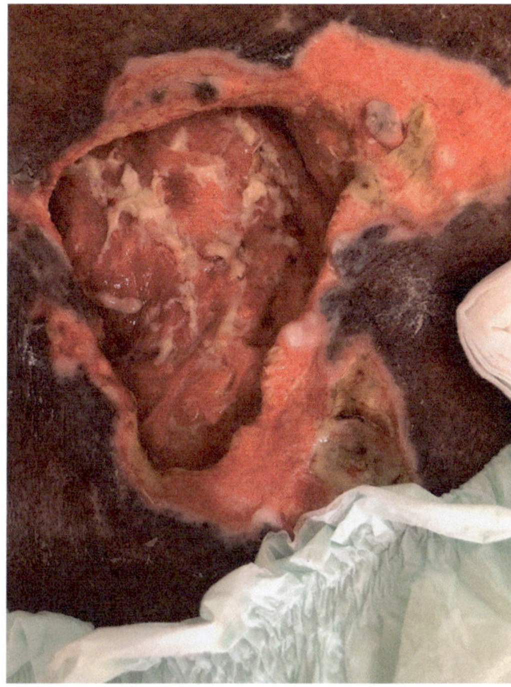

Fig. 11.7 Stage IV pressure injury

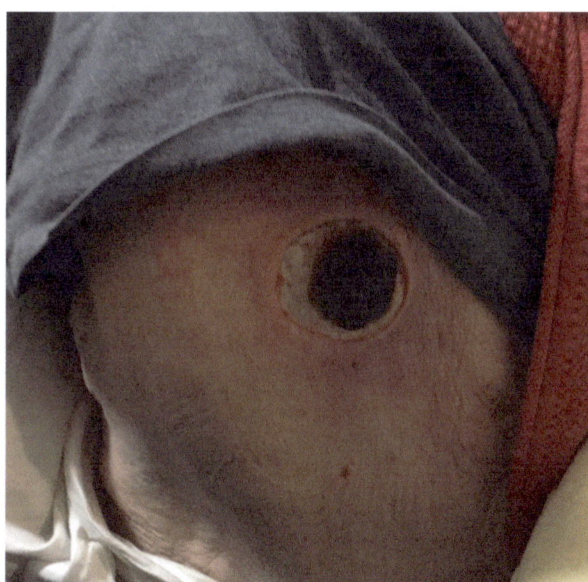

Fig. 11.8 Unstageable pressure injury

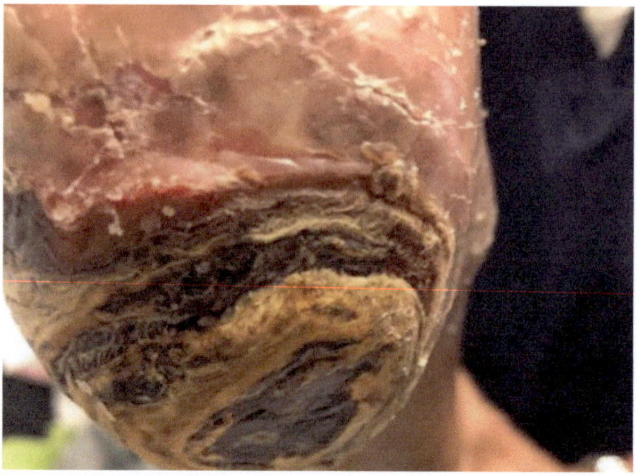

Fig. 11.9 Unstageable pressure injury of the heel

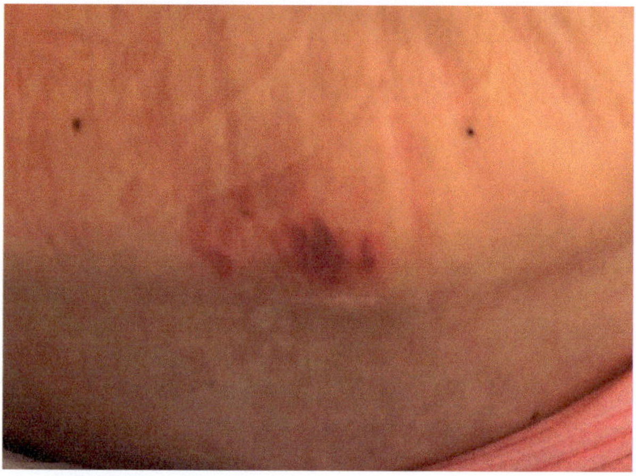

Fig. 11.10 Deep tissue injury

11.3.3 Effective Turning and Repositioning Techniques in the Home-Based Setting

High-risk skin areas in bedbound and chairbound individuals should be inspected thoroughly at every home-based medical care visit. These include, in greatest incidence, the sacrum, ischium, heels and ankles, greater trochanters and scapulae [13], and, in lesser incidence, the back, elbows, ear lobes, and scalp. Areas of vulnerability, however, can vary in persons with paralysis, kyphosis, and other anatomic abnormalities.

Proper repositioning is important for home-based medical care providers to appreciate; providers should instruct caregivers and interdisciplinary personnel on accepted methods for high-risk patients and for those with existing ulcers [14]. Providers should keep in mind, however, that optimal repositioning and repositioning schedules are controversial, and little study has been devoted to the potential significance of small frequent weight shifts that likely prove more practical and potent in home-based settings [15]. Regardless, we recommend the coupling of repositioning and frequent daily skin inspection as integral to preserving skin integrity in immobile and partially mobile patients with the following repositioning and pressure-off-loading techniques whenever possible. The following are suggested methods of positioning and repositioning to minimize friction, pressure, and shear force:

- Use bed linens as a shield and sling to turn and lift immobile persons in bed rather than drag the body directly over surfaces.
- Allow partially mobile persons to move themselves when possible; use assistive devices such as a trapeze to assist patients in mobilizing themselves. Small movements at regular intervals are advised, and caregivers may prompt for regular self-repositioning.
- When recumbent, place persons on their sides at a 30-degree tilt; avoid placing immobile persons directly on their sides to limit pressure on the greater trochanter and lateral malleolus of the ankle [16]. This is an awkward position for most people to maintain so the use of pillows or wedge foam is essential.
- Frequently turn and reposition lying patients every 2–4 h and seated patients every 15–30 min. The repositioning interval can be prolonged up to 4 h for recumbent positions and 1 h for seated persons when using pressure-reducing surfaces.
- Patients in wheelchairs require particular attention to the sacrum, ischial tuberosities, greater trochanters, and heels. Wheelchairs should be properly fitted to ensure pressure on the hips is minimized; patients with limited ability to make even small shifts in weight should have an off-loading, conformable pressure surface such as a gel cushion which helps distribute weight across an expanded surface. Patients who have some degree of upper extremity mobility and axial strength should be reminded to shift side to side in their wheelchair, perform light degree upper arm push-ups, or bend forward until they can slide their hands underneath their buttocks every 15–25 min for 15 s (a strategy called partial unloading). The feet should be properly supported either directly on the floor, through the use of footrests or a foot stool to avoid downward slippage. When escorted in the wheelchair, ensure that the heels are not dragging on the floor.
- With the exception of eating and 30-min postprandial periods, do not leave immobile persons in an upright position more than 30° unless they are on a low air loss mattress. Upright angles greater than 30° have been associated with higher sacral pressures when persons are on standard mattresses.
- Remain cautious about points of pressure and when possible keep bony prominences off-loaded; for instance, do not allow heels to remain static on a supine surface. Rather, elevate with pillows placed just under the calves to keep heels off the bed surface or suspend in foam, sheepskin, or inflatable heel protectors. Pay attention to pressure points on bony surfaces when patients are placed in wheelchairs or transfer slings for prolonged periods.
- Train and monitor caregivers regularly on effective repositioning and off-loading as these techniques are not intuitive.

11.3.4 Ulcer Risk Scales and Utility in Clinical Practice

Several widely accepted scales are used in hospital-based and nursing home settings to define the severity of internal and external risk factors that are most likely to lead to pressure ulcers. Though these scales have not been studied in home-based settings, their scoring breakdown is useful in determining and mitigating risk more holistically.

Decubitus ulcer risk scoring is a key component of the Outcome and Assessment Information Set (OASIS) [17], which is used by Medicare-certified home health agencies (CHHAs) and must be conducted for each patient at defined intervals including on admission. The Braden scale [18], a commonly used tool in the USA, emphasizes risk as a mix of internal (patient specific) and external (environmental and physical) factors.

Because current evidence has shown the use of risk assessment tools is not more effective than clinical judgment alone in preventing ulcers, home-based medical providers rarely use such time-intensive scales [19–21]. Nonetheless, it is important to think of these scales as a framework on which to determine risk and base prevention and therapy, as well as a common language for the interdisciplinary care team. We summarize the essentials here as a general inventory of risk factors. In addition, we have supplemented risk factors with practical considerations beyond what is captured in accepted scales.

11.3.4.1 Patient Characteristics Influencing Pressure Ulcer Development

- *Physiologic age*: Advancing age with increased comorbid conditions that enhance the likelihood of incontinence, skin breakdown, and reduced capability of repair all contribute substantially to intrinsic risk.
- *Comorbid conditions*: Diseases such as cardiopulmonary disease, atherosclerotic disease, or diabetes, which impair tissue oxygenation, increase the risk of tissue ischemia and thus pressure ulcer formation. Diseases such as dementia promulgate other risk factors such as immobility, sensory impairment, nutrition, and incontinence; dementia of all types poses the greatest risk for pressure ulcers.
- *Degree of immobility*: Poor or limited ability to make small adjustments in movement necessary to offset pressure related ischemia is critical to the development of wounds. Highly immobile patients such as those with paraplegia, severe degenerative joint disease, or advanced dementia make them far more likely to experience high shear forces when mobilized and develop pressure wounds if not repositioned frequently, particularly if they are unable to make the small bodily adjustments that are critical to avoiding nocturnal ischemia in mobile persons.
- *Cognition*: Persons who suffer from impaired cognition or communication may lack the ability to move or direct their caregivers on turning and repositioning, particularly when in discomfort from prolonged periods of pressure. Furthermore, such persons may be incontinent and thus may be prone to urinary or fecal dermatitis.

- *Sensory impairment*: Those with impaired sensation such as those with spinal cord injuries, peripheral vascular disease, or scarred integument from previous deep tissue ulcers are unable to feel the painful stimuli from pressure-related ischemia and therefore unlikely to spontaneously move to relieve pressure.
- *Nutritional state*: A compromised nutritional state which often accompanies advancing age, frailty, and multiple comorbid conditions, especially dementia, is a clear risk factor for pressure ulcer formation and stalled healing. For one, as the patient loses weight, contact points of bony prominences are more pronounced and susceptible to pressure and friction injury. Additionally, the reduction in protein due to reduced intake or increased catabolism, as well as other nutrients such as vitamin A, C, and zinc, causes tissues to lose reparative capability [22]. The roles of macronutrients such as protein, carbohydrates, fats and fluid, and micronutrients such as amino acids (notably, arginine, and glutamine), vitamins (A, C, and D), and minerals (zinc, selenium, and iron) are substantial in wound healing; however, the benefits of individual supplementation are controversial.

11.3.4.2 External Risk Factors for Pressure Ulcer Development

- *Friction and shear forces*: Prolonged upright positioning and repositioning of the body without surface barriers such as a sheet can subject the body to both persistent and dynamic shear forces. Removing bed linens or diapers with the body pressed on the surface can cause significant friction and shear force injury. Pressure-relieving devices including foam or pillow off-loaders and static and dynamic bed surfaces coupled with proper positioning and repositioning schedules can reduce risk.
- *Microclimate*: The heat, moisture, and pH climates around bony prominences are significant cofactors in developing and propagating pressure injuries. The microclimate is usually the consequence of several phenomena: (a) moisture from urinary incontinence, fecal incontinence, sweat, or heavily exuding wounds can cause maceration and dermatitis and increase the likelihood of dynamic friction and shear forces to induce tissue injury, and (b) heat generated by friction that changes the architecture and load-bearing integrity of collagen and elastin degrades natural skin emollients that protect and lubricate the skin and causes capillary dilatation and thermal injury. The use of absorptive surfaces which are used to capture urine and stool may compound this phenomenon; diapers and woven incontinence pads, for instance, are usually not breathable and can augment local heat and pH [23]. In addition, the use of wipes which may be alkaline in pH can change the natural acidic barrier of the skin and increase bacterial load, destroy local collagen, inhibit macrophage and fibroblast activity, and accelerate the development and propagation of pressure injuries at susceptible sites. Careful attention to hygiene with the use of pH balanced cleansers, frequent incontinence care, the application of barrier creams and emollients, and the prudent use of nonlayered incontinence pads are important complements to interval off-loading and repositioning.

11.3.5 Direct Care of Pressure Injuries in the Home

The key to successful wound care is a comprehensive and collaborative approach; multiple interventions need to be implemented to maximize success and likelihood of wound closure and the prevention of wound recurrence. Collaboration with interdisciplinary personnel, consultants, and caregivers is essential to optimal wound healing. Adequate pain palliation is also essential; pain control allows for direct wound care, and palliative care goals are intrinsic to good home-based medical care.

The comprehensive care of wounds can be separated into several direct and indirect tasks. Direct wound care is the most relevant to the home-based medical provider and perhaps the most daunting because of poor training and misconception of such care as germane only to surgeons, podiatrists, or wound care nurses.

The following summary of wound care is most relevant to the care of pressure injuries. Most principles, however, can be extrapolated to the care of venous stasis ulcers, arterial ulcers, neuropathic wounds, and diabetic foot ulcers. The care of each of these wound types has particular nuances discussed in detail in the following sections.

11.3.5.1 Pressure Wound Assessment

Accurate classification and measurements are important for effective communication with interdisciplinary providers, monitoring for progress and identifying appropriate therapy. The therapy can be complex and involve an array of topical treatments, debridement modalities, support surfaces, and mechanical closure devices. Classifying wounds not simply by stage but also by percentage slough, necrosis, characteristics of the surrounding tissue ("periwound"), and degree of tunneling and undermining is a critical skill for home-based providers.

Beyond staging, the following assessments should be performed for each wound:

1. Size of the wound in length, width, and depth. It is best to use paper tape to measure. The asymmetry of many wounds means that the length and width are often not simple. We, nonetheless, recommend the following approach:
   (a) Use the clockface as the reference for communication and documentation. Use the head and feet as reference points for 12 o'clock and 6 o'clock, respectively.
   (b) Measure caudal-cranial width across the longest part of the wound.
   (c) Measure lateral width across the longest part of the wound.
   (d) Measure depth of the wound with a cotton swab or the finger gently placed to the base of the wound bed. Note the degree to which deeper tissues such as tendon and bone can be visualized.
   (e) Use the cotton swab to measure the depth of undermining and note the extent along the clock face. In addition, use the cotton swab to measure the depth of tunneling. Be as descriptive as possible; for example, "Undermining

from 2 o'clock to 6 o'clock with maximum depth of 3 cm at 4 o'clock and minimum of 0.5 cm at 2 and 6 o'clock."

2. Determine the percentage of slough and necrosis. Necrosis, or eschar, should be noted as wet or dry and adherent or friable.
3. Note the degree of exudate as mild, moderate, or heavy and the quality as serous, purulent, or bloody.
4. Document the quality and extent of the peripheral wound bed or periwound. The degree and extent of maceration, visible as bleached and edematous tissue, should be noted. In addition, any erythema or hyperpigmentation (especially in dark-skinned persons), bruising, tenderness, or crepitus should be noted. Finally, scar tissue, which is vulnerable to additional breakdown, should also be recorded.
5. Wounds should be classified as the most advanced stage by depth and should not be reclassified as they heal. For example, as a Stage III pressure ulcer becomes more shallow, it should be described as a "healing Stage III ulcer," not reclassified as a Stage I or II ulcer.

11.3.5.2 Wound Bed Preparation: Cleansing, Initial and Maintenance Debridement, and Primary and Secondary Dressings

The general principles of direct wound care are summarized as follows:

1. Remove senescent or dead tissue with chemical, mechanical, autolytic, or sharp debridement.
2. Cleanse with the goal of removing biofilm—even though you cannot see it, it is there.
3. Keep wounds with craters moist but not excessively so; the goal is to keep the wound bed mitotically active, self-sanitizing between dressing changes, and at a relatively acidic pH.
4. Cover pressure injuries that have intact skin with either a dressing or an absorptive emollient to prevent opening. Only intact skin with clear underlying pus or crepitus should be intentionally opened.
5. Fill dead space with packing materials tailored to the degree of exudate; choose packing materials with antimicrobial activity in areas with a high risk of infection.
6. Occlude all wounds with padding necessary to absorb excess exudate and adhesives that restrict entry of urine, stool, or sweat and maintain the internal environment at an acidic pH.
7. Protect the perimeter of the ulcer from maceration with the use of barrier creams or wipes before applying adhesives. Barrier wipes will also allow for greater adhesion and reduce skin trauma on removal of adhesives.

Wound Cleansing: Preservative-free normal saline or hypochlorous acid (i.e., Vashe™) should be used to cleanse most hard-to-heal wounds [24]. In general, povidone-iodine solution, hydrogen peroxide, isopropyl alcohol, and sodium hypochlorite (a bleach solution that is commercially available as Dakin's Solution™) should be avoided or used only in limited circumstances given their high destruction of viable tissue and consequential delay in wound healing.

Povidone-iodine solution has a role in keeping dry gangrene desiccated; it should be applied liberally over the eschar and up to 2.5 cm of the periwound and allowed to dry; the area may subsequently be covered with a nonocclusive dressing such as gauze.

Dakin's Solution™ is advised as a time-limited application of 1/2 to 1/4 strength solution to foul-smelling wounds just long enough to control the smell and reduce visible biofilm. It can be caustic and painful; it should be avoided for long-term use, and should pain be significant, discontinued entirely. In home-based settings, Dakin's Solution™ is used to reduce extensive areas of dense senescent tissue (slough) or biofilm. This is particularly useful for densely adherent slough with substantial surface involvement. Prior to application of higher strength solutions, adequate analgesia may be necessary with subcutaneous or subsurface lidocaine 2% administered via injection.

Hypochlorous acid (Vashe™) is an alternative wound cleanser that has shown significant bacteriostatic and bacteriocidal activities compared with Dakin's Solution. It is not cytotoxic, offers a pH of 5.5 that approximates healthy tissue, and significantly reduces colony counts of *Staphylococcus* and *Pseudomonas* when applied to a wound bed for several minutes. In home-based settings, we often use hypochlorous acid as a maintenance wound wash for wounds with a mild to moderate degree of slough or to reduce bioburden in between dressing changes for wounds that tend to reaccumulate visible biofilm quickly.

Initial and Maintenance Debridement: Debridement, or the removal of visible and invisible nonviable tissue, is essential to reducing infection and promoting and speeding closure. Known as wound bed preparation (WBP), debridement is a two-phase process that may or may not follow sequentially. Initial debridement consists of the primary removal of visible nonviable tissue such as fibrin slough and necrotic eschar. Maintenance debridement involves the ongoing removal of cellular components such as nondividing or senescent fibroblasts and keratinocytes and proteins of the extracellular matrix that can impede an advancing tissue edge and the cellular turnover necessary for tissue healing [25]. Debridement should be a continual process until complete wound closure.

Mechanical debridement is the most nonspecific type of debridement, with effects on both viable and nonviable tissue; its greatest utility is in the removal of biofilm. Three common methods of mechanical debridement are described below:

- Wet-to-dry dressing debridement: Saline-saturated gauze dressings are placed in a wound bed, long enough to allow the gauze to dry; the gauze is then pulled out with force.
- Gauze debridement: Woven gauze moistened with saline is used to forcefully rub areas of slough, bacterial biofilm, or necrosis.
- High-pressure saline debridement: Saline administered to a wound under high pressure removes bacterial biofilm and cellular debris. In home-based wound care, we often create a highly effective device by attaching a 30–60 cc syringe to

a 16-, 18-, or 20-gauge peripheral venous cannula (with the needle removed) or the tubing of a winged infusion set (butterfly) and clipping the tubing to approximately 5–10 cm (Fig. 11.11).

Autolytic debridement involves the use of dressings that promote the body's natural enzymes to continually remove cellular debris from the wound. All moist, occlusive dressings promote autolytic debridement; as an exclusive means to care for the wound, autolytic debridement is most effective in treating shallow ulcers with a low amount of drainage.

Chemical debridement involves the application of agents that degrade or digest extracellular proteins sustaining necrotic or nonviable tissue in wound beds. It is usually selective for senescent or dead tissue although penetration and effectiveness can be variable depending on the depth, density, and moisture of the devitalized tissue. Dakin's Solution™, or sodium hypochlorite (bleach), is a caustic chemical that achieves significant debridement of necrotic eschar or slough particularly if dense. It is often used at 1/4 strength to limit toxicity to surrounding tissue. On occasion, with wounds requiring more rapid debridement and in which sharp debridement is difficult to perform because of the location or high density of necrotic tissue, we use full strength or 1/2 strength Dakin's Solution™ as a one-time application to loosen the nonviable tissue. Before soaking the area with Dakin's saturated gauze, we anesthetize the tissue with lidocaine to minimize the severe pain that can be associated with this application.

Enzymatic debridement (collagenase): Because collagen in healthy tissue is shielded by mucopolysaccharides, only exposed collagen in devitalized tissue is susceptible to degradation by metalloproteinases contained in collagenase [26]. For

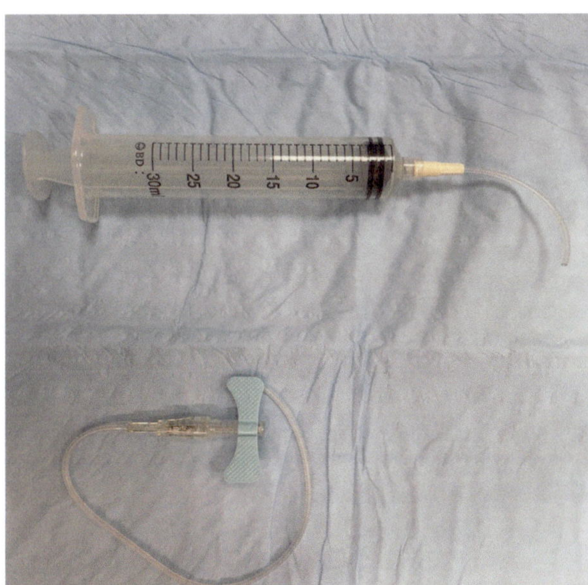

Fig. 11.11 Syringe attached to clipped butterfly tubing for wound irrigation

maximal success, dense slough or eschar should be crosshatched with a #10 blade before application to achieve penetration and uplifting of the collagen fibers which anchor the base of the eschar to the wound bed. In settings where sharp cross-hatching is not possible, however, application of collagenase can still promote substantial degradation of collagen.

Sharp debridement is indicated when chemical debridement has been unsuccessful, when more rapid tissue closure is desired, or when preparing the wound bed for negative-pressure wound therapy (NPWT). It is usually accomplished with a rounded scalpel (#10 or #15 blade), a dermal curette, or scissors using counterpressure from a hemostat or forceps to ensure an accurate tissue plane between viable and nonviable tissue. Sharp debridement accelerates rates of wound closure on the order of days to weeks over chemical or autolytic debridement alone.

Home-based primary care clinicians should undergo appropriate training before executing this bedside skill. Some suggestions for resources include online training modules with videos (e.g., https://www.woundsource.com/), hands-on wound care courses with a sharp debridement skills laboratory, or spending several sessions side by side with a clinician expert, such as a vascular surgeon, podiatrist, experienced primary care physician, or nurse practitioner with ample experience in debridement.

11.3.5.3 When Surgical Debridement, Amputation, and/or Closure Are Necessary

It is occasionally necessary to consult a surgeon for operative debridement or amputation. In cases of extensive necrosis or infection or in the case of expansion of a wound despite aggressive home-based measures, surgical debridement and closure may be necessary, if such intervention is consistent with the patient's overall status and goals of care. In our practice, most patients request in-home care alone, so external consultation is often difficult. On occasion, surgical consultants can make joint home visits or virtual consultations to advise on necessary next steps. For foot and ankle wounds, home-based podiatrists can be important resources for more extensive debridement.

11.3.5.4 Bacterial Colonization, Critical Colonization, and Local Wound Infection

Reducing bacterial burden in the wound bed involves three main strategies including regular cleansing and irrigation, removing devitalized tissue, packing with antimicrobial dressings, and/or creating an acidic wound environment that inhibits bacterial proliferation [27]. Contamination and colonization of ulcers are common; several factors including bacterial burden, host immunity, and degree of devitalized tissue can cause colonization to progress to critical colonization (otherwise known as local wound infection marked by foul smell, local purulence, or retarded wound healing but not generally requiring antibiotic therapy), invasive tissue infection with penetration of the surrounding healthy tissue (i.e., cellulitis or abscess), and, ultimately, systemic infection. The most common organisms invading devitalized tissue are *Staphylococcus aureus*, *Streptococcus pyogenes*, and *Pseudomonas aeruginosa* [28]; less common species include *Proteus* sp. and *Escherichia coli* [29].

In the event of surrounding tissue penetration or systemic infection, oral, intravenous, or intramuscular antibiotic therapy may be necessary and should be tailored to the most likely organisms in the area affected. For instance, sacral wounds may require enhanced coverage of gram-negative species. Although not routinely recommended, if a wound bed is suspected to have a high bacterial burden given persistently foul smell, slow wound healing, persistent exudate on the order of days to weeks, or frank pus, sampling for culture can guide antibacterial therapy and uncover highly resistant species. Providers should use the *Levine* quantitative swab technique when culturing a wound to ensure that colonizing bacteria are selected out from invasive species: The wound bed is first cleansed with normal saline and patted dry; a sterile culture swab is spun and pressed for 5 s over a 1 cm^2 area of the healthiest appearing tissue that is free of exudate, pus, or necrosis. This technique helps to ensure the bacteria that is collected is that which is infecting the area rather than contaminant.

11.4 Primary Dressings, Secondary Dressings, and Adhesives in Home-Based Wound Care

In general, the choice of wound care dressings should be tailored to the appearance of the wound bed, the size, depth, and degree of tunneling and undermining, the degree and quality of exudate, the degree and quality of devitalized tissue, and the appearance of the perimeter of the wound (known as the periwound). When ordering and documenting dressings, it is best to characterize layers as primary (i.e., directly on top of the wound), secondary (the layer directly adjacent to the primary layer), and tertiary (anchoring or adhesive) dressings.

The following tables summarize some of the common dressings and adhesives used in home-based settings with indications for each. This table is not meant to be restrictive or exhaustive; rather it should give the clinician a general repertoire and vocabulary for various dressing types. Home-based medical care providers should note that limitations in formulary are often be imposed by the nursing agency; some nursing agencies favor certain brands over others. Because the care is often like that of other wounds, we have used pressure injuries as the standard indication and have noted when certain dressings are also indicated for other wounds (Tables 11.1 and 11.2).

Some guiding principles for wound dressings are as follows:

1. *Stage I and Suspected Deep Tissue Injury ulcers may be left uncovered or covered.* In areas subject to moisture or irritation from urine or feces, an emollient moisture barrier such as vitamin A/D cream or zinc oxide may be used. In addi-

Table 11.1 Primary dressings in home-based wound care

Primary dressing	Primary forms	How it works	Optimal uses	Other indications and contraindications
Hydrogels	Manufactured as amorphous gel or gel sheets	Lubricates and softens tissue Promotes autolytic debridement	Shallow wounds (depth less than 1 cm) with minimal exudate Deeper wounds (depth greater than 1 cm) with significant granulation tissue and without dense necrotic tissue or slough Wounds with thin layers of necrosis or slough in preparation for sharp debridement Painful wounds in which a cooling effect is desired	Not recommended for moderately to heavily exudative wounds or venous stasis ulcers Can be mixed with 2% lidocaine gel or morphine liquid for additional analgesia Ideal for palliative care settings as frequency of dressing changes can be up to 1 week; users are advised to refer to manufacturer insert of each product for details
Hydrocolloids	Manufactured as sheet, powders, and pastes, the latter with more absorptive capacity	Hydrophilic colloid particles bound to polyurethane which absorbs fluid from the wound and creates a gel-like covering Over dry wounds acts as an impermeable barrier to moisture and a cushion against friction	Well-granulating wounds with mild exudate Shallow wounds with thin necrosis or slough in preparation for sharp debridement Over bony prominences subject to repeated trauma from friction or shear stress such as the sacrum	Not recommended for use in deep wounds, infected wounds, or venous stasis ulcers Often used as secondary dressing for stage II or shallow stage III ulcers Advised in palliative care settings as frequency of dressing changes can be up to a week

Primary dressing	Primary forms	How it works	Optimal uses	Other indications and contraindications
Alginates	Manufactured as pads and ribbons. Pads can also be cut into ribbons	The absorption of wound fluid causes the seaweed-derived fibers to form a gel that promotes a moist wound environment	Given their high absorptive capacity, alginates are ideal for heavily exuding wounds Ideal for filling large craters, tunnels, and undermining Excellent primary dressing for venous stasis ulcers Can be used with antimicrobial gels in infected wound beds When impregnated with silver offers additional barrier to bacterial growth	Not recommended for use in wounds with low drainage as the dressing can dry out the wound or impregnate into the wound causing difficulty in removing residual fibers Dressing frequency can be every other day For wounds with minor bleeding, alginates can induce hemostasis
Hydrofibers (aka hydrocolloid fiber)	Manufactured as pads and ropes; many come impregnated with silver	Like an alginate, the absorption of wound fluid causes this synthetic carboxymethylcellulose (CMC) fiber to create a gel (similar to a hydrocolloid dressing) with enhanced absorption over alginates [66]	Same as alginates	Non-recommended uses are the same as alginates Benefit over alginates is that the frequency of wound care dressings can be several days longer [67]

(continued)

Table 11.1 (continued)

Primary dressing	Primary forms	How it works	Optimal uses	Other indications and contraindications
Foams and hydropolymer derivatives	Manufactured as sheets (conformable or shaped to body part), sheets with peripheral adhesives or ropes; may be impregnated with silver or other antibacterial products that inhibit colonization	Foam dressings are composed of a polymer or urethane foam with craters that trap the exudate. The polyurethane coating enhances the creation of a moist wound environment, thus promoting autolytic debridement or chemical debridement when coupled with an enzymatic ointment. Hydropolymers offer enhanced absorption with a backing layer that has breathability allowing for significant evaporation of wound exudate [68]. Differing antibacterial properties of impregnated and manufactured types are useful for limiting the bacterial burden of wounds in high-risk areas, wounds with foul odor, or wounds that are chronically colonized	A primary dressing for any sized cavity with moderate to heavy exudate A secondary dressing for heavily exudative wounds; may be placed on top of the primary dressing; the latter can include alginates or hydrofibers A secondary dressing for non-exudative wounds to limit shear force during the healing process Primary or secondary dressing for venous stasis ulcers Primary or secondary dressing for friable or painful neuropathic foot wounds	Polyurethane foam dressings with high moisture vapor transmission rates (MVTR) may allow for more days between dressing changes for highly exudative wounds Foams are not indicated as primary dressings for dry wounds or wounds with minimal exudate as they may stick to the wound bed and removal may cause trauma or pain

Primary dressing	Primary forms	How it works	Optimal uses	Other indications and contraindications
Gauze	Dry gauze sheets or bandages, petroleum-impregnated gauze, iodine-impregnated gauze strips, elastic gauze bandage	Gauze sheets trap moisture through the lattice; layering multiple sheets maximizes absorption	Petroleum impregnation offers a nonstick and less painful variation that can promote a moist wound bed with varying occlusive properties Iodine-impregnated gauze strips offer wicking properties for small infected or moderately exudative wound spaces Elastic gauze bandages, when wrapped with tension, can compress venous stasis or bleeding wounds As a secondary dressing, gauze can provide adequate off-loading of pressure	Dry gauze is only used as a secondary dressing over dressings with more potential to keep wound beds moist With rare exception, dry gauze should not be applied as a primary dressing to any wound Moist gauze as a wet-to-wet dressing is effective as a primary dressing for diabetic foot wounds Wet-to-dry gauze, in which moist gauze is allowed to dry before removal, is contraindicated in palliative care settings due to excess trauma and pain

Table 11.2 Secondary and tertiary dressings/adhesives

Dressing	Common uses and considerations in home-based wound care
Transparent film	Waterproof yet permeable to oxygen, these are mostly used as secondary and tertiary adhesive dressings in home-based care. Used to anchor the primary dressing, transparent films provide occlusion so that moisture is trapped within the wound, and maceration of the periwound is minimized. Adherence to the periwound is aided by the use of adhesive skin preparations. Transparent dressings can also be used as a primary dressing for shallow wounds, first-degree and second-degree burns, and blisters
Gauze	Dry gauze is used as an inexpensive common secondary dressing for heavily exudative wounds whether under a foam dressing or without; gauze bandages are also used to anchor primary and secondary dressings and to create substantial off-loading particularly for foot wounds
Foam	Often used as a secondary dressing for heavily exudative wounds particularly sacral ulcers in which there is the added benefit of reducing friction and pressure as well as venous stasis ulcers. For venous stasis wounds, we do not advise foam dressings with adhesive as the latter can denude the surrounding tissue during removal
Woven abdominal pads	Like foam, woven abdominal pads can offer substantial absorption, albeit at slightly less effective capacity but also at far less expense. Particularly for wounds requiring frequent wound changes and less bulk, woven abdominal pads are cost-effective alternatives to foam with higher absorptive strength than gauze
Paper tape	The closing ability of paper tape is adequate for wounds in which the edges are closely approximated and the area is free of moisture [69]. Its place in decubitus wound closure, however, is fairly limited to very small wounds (i.e., a centimeter or less in diameter and depth) as a secondary dressing. Paper tape offers the advantages of low cost and low allergenic potential. The primary disadvantage is that it poorly seals in areas with significant moisture or high shear stress. When placed exclusively over the dressing without contact with the skin, it can provide adequate adhesion
Cloth tape	Stretchable perforated cloth tape is a mainstay of home-based wound care. Unlike silk or rubber tape, stretchable cloth tape offers breathability, high adhesion particularly when coupled with adhesive skin preparations, and conformability to allow ease of movement. These qualities reduce moisture of the periwound and offer high occlusion to sweat, urine, and feces and reduced blister rates over traditional cloth tapes [70]. The cost of stretchable tape, however, is significantly greater than standard silk or rubber-based tape

tion, a thin adhesive barrier such as a transparent dressing, a hydrocolloid, or a foam dressing is advised to limit friction.

2. *Stage II ulcers require different therapies based on the appearance and type.*
   - Blisters can be *left uncovered or covered* with an emollient such as vitamin A and D cream or zinc oxide or a primary dressing such as a thin transparent adhesive (Tegaderm™), a hydrocolloid, or a foam dressing. All barriers are optional but can facilitate the goal of reducing friction and limiting moisture.
   - Superficial ulcers should *always be covered and require filling* if there is substantial depth, i.e., more than 0.5 cm, with dressings that are more hydrating

if the exudate will barely moisten the primary dressing and more absorptive if the exudate is substantial and likely to saturate the primary dressing. Primary dressings such as hydrocolloids can be used for the majority of Stage II wounds with some degree of drainage. Hydrogels, which are hydrating and can come as a true gel or a solid matrix, keep the wound bed moist and cool. They are usually reserved for very shallow wounds without substantial devitalized tissue and with nominal exudate [14]. They may promote debridement of devitalized tissue albeit at a slower rate than the application of collagenase [32]. Packing with more absorptive dressings such as calcium alginate or carboxymethylcellulose (CMC)-based hydrofibers is necessary when the exudate is substantial and the depth is significant (i.e., greater than 0.5 cm). Occasionally, for highly exudative wounds, a foam dressing, secondary layers of gauze, or woven abdominal pads are indicated. Barrier creams and skin preparations that promote waterproof seals between the skin and the adhesive dressing should be used to limit the maceration of the periwound.

3. *Stage III and IV ulcers are treated similarly.* The goal is to fill the crater bed with the right material to promote absorption while maintaining a moist, bacteria-free wound environment. We often use collagenase at the base of the wound if there is visible slough or eschar or hydrogel if there is a high degree of granulation tissue and mild drainage. Although hydrogel can be used in the wound base if there is dry eschar or dense slough, we advise its use solely to soften the eschar or slough in preparation for further sharp debridement within a week. Collagenase, though superior to hydrogel in this regard, is used similarly; cross-hatching with a #10 blade any dense areas of slough or eschar before application allows for increased penetration to the anchoring layers of the base; this step, however, is not necessary [30]. When drainage is moderate to severe, common dressings to fill such cavities include alginate, CMC-based hydrofibers, and foam dressings. Heavily exudative wounds often require significant layering with secondary dressings such as foam, excess gauze, or woven abdominal pads. The sacrum is particularly susceptible to substantial moisture from feces and urine; we invariably use several layers of secondary dressings for such wounds as well as a tight adhesive with conformability such as perforated cloth tape or a transparent adhesive dressing to maximize occlusion.
4. *Heel wounds*: These wounds deserve special attention as the management of Stage III, IV, and Unstageable ulcers of this area differs considerably from the care of wounds elsewhere in the body. In general, heel wounds with eschar should be kept dry with daily painting of betadine [31]. Dry eschar is protective of the underlying tissue and if removed can lead to poor wound healing and limb loss. If the area is moist, use of the strategies for general Stage III and IV wounds can be applied.

11.4.1 Support Surfaces and Cushions in the Treatment of Pressure Wounds

As part of the armamentarium of pressure wound care, pressure-reducing and pressure-relieving support surfaces are integral. Although data are conflicting on ideal support surfaces for the prevention and healing of pressure wounds, there is consensus that higher-specification foam mattresses as well as air, gel, and water-based surfaces and/or mattresses are superior to standard hospital bed mattresses [32, 33].

Pressure redistribution surfaces and cushions (wheelchair and heel, for instance) are classified as static or dynamic depending on whether or not they vary the pressure beneath the patient at timed intervals. The Centers for Medicaid and Medicare Services (CMS) has further classified bed surfaces into Group 1, 2, or 3 classifications based on their degree of pressure reduction or redistribution. In general, Group 1 surfaces provide the least amount of pressure reduction or redistribution and Group 3 the greatest [34].

Static bed overlays or mattresses, also known as constant low-pressure devices, distribute weight over large contact areas thus reducing pressure to a single body prominence. These surfaces are largely considered preventive Group 1 support surfaces if composed of gels, foam, water, or air; therapeutic Group 2 if composed of a powered low air loss mechanism; or therapeutic Group 3 support surfaces if composed of fluidized air and particulates such as silicone beads [35]). Dynamic overlays, on the other hand, are largely considered therapeutic, Group 2 surfaces, though evidence also supports their use as preventative redistribution surfaces. Dynamic support surfaces such as alternating pressure cushions, mattress overlays, or mattresses contain air pockets that variably inflate and deflate to adjustable high- or low-pressure states. Kinetic or tilting beds allow for pressure redistribution through total body mobilization. The following table summarizes the qualifications for Group 1, 2, and 3 support surfaces as determined by CMS (Table 11.3).

Other foam and sheepskin pressure redistribution modalities are available which are particularly useful for bony prominences and other areas subject to high rates of shear stress even when a patient is on a bed support surface. For prevention and therapy of heel ulcers, in particular, sheepskin and foam boots are more effective than mattress support surfaces alone in redistributing pressure to the calves, which are far less vulnerable to pressure and shear force related injury [42]. It is recommended that all immobile persons who are maintained on any group surface either wear sheepskin or foam boots or have their heels suspended in the air through the use of low-cost cushions or rolled towels placed under the calves [36].

Table 11.3 Pressure-relieving support surfaces in home-based medical care

Pressure-relieving surface group	Group 1	Group 2	Group 3
Examples of support surfaces used in home care	• Gel mattress overlay • Alternating pressure pads • Static air or gel mattresses	• Powered alternating pressure mattress • Powered pressure-reducing low air loss mattress	Air-fluidized silicone bead beds
Criteria for Medicare coverage	All patients who are completely immobile qualify Partially mobile patients and patients with any stage pressure ulcer on the body qualify if they have at least one of the following risk factors: • Incontinence (fecal, urinary or both) • Poor nutritional state • Circulatory compromise • Sensory impairment	Patients must have either • Multiple stage II pressure ulcers on the trunk or pelvis that have been under comprehensive treatment for the past 30 days. Treatment must have included the use of a group 1 support surface and clear documentation that the wounds have nonetheless worsened or not improved • Large or multiple stage 3 or 4 ulcers on the trunk or pelvis • rece$nt (i.e., within 60 days) skin graft or flap for a stage 3 or 4 pressure ulcer	Immobile patients with stage 3 or stage 4 pressure ulcers who • Would require institutionalization if the device was not provided • Have previously failed therapy with a group 2 device
Conditions for discontinuation or downgrading to a lower group	–	–Ulcer(s) healed –Beyond 60 days of flap or graft skin closure	Ulcer(s) healed

(continued)

Table 11.3 (continued)

Pressure-relieving surface group	Group 1	Group 2	Group 3
Additional considerations	Advised for all bedbound individuals (14,50)	Clinicians should be diligent about documenting the comprehensive care of the wound which should include modification of risk factors such as incontinence, nutritional state, and immobility by frequent and proper repositioning	Monthly, detailed documentation must be submitted to US Medicare to acquire and retain group 3 support surfaces in the home –Must adequately document that wound care is comprehensive and includes direct wound care management with qualified staff, limitation of incontinence associated moisture, and nutritional support –Must also document dedicated caregivers who assist with the comprehensive wound care plan and can respond quickly to a malfunctioning group 3 bed which has lost power or is leaking air. Nonfunctioning group 3 bed systems, which become rock-hard when air is lost or noncirculating, can cause expansion of a wound in hours

11.5 Venous Leg Ulcers

Chronic leg ulcers caused by chronic venous insufficiency (CVI) are the second most common wound-type treated in home-based medical care settings (Figs. 11.12 and 11.13). Varicose veins are the most common cause of CVI [37]. In studies of community-dwelling persons 60 and older, however, other comorbid vascular conditions such as peripheral arterial disease, diabetes mellitus, hypertension, and congestive heart failure have also shown potent links to venous ulceration [38]. Venous stasis skin changes can present as skin hyperpigmentation, eczema, or hard thickened areas with unusual friability of the overlying skin when edematous. Superficial trauma and pressure may accelerate venous ulcer development.

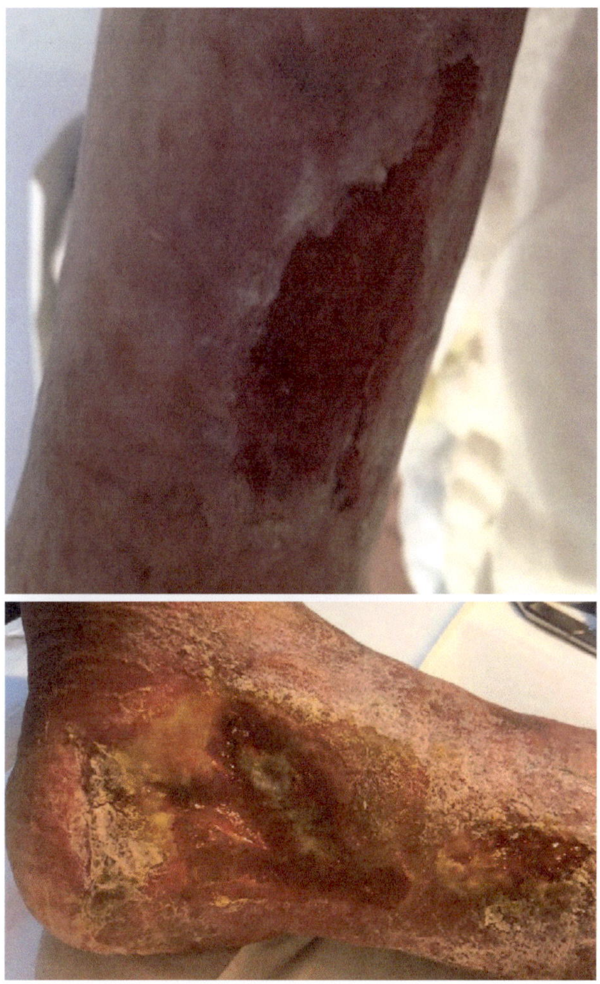

Figs. 11.12 and 11.13 Venous stasis ulcers

Coexisting lymphedema marked by impairments in the lymphatics can dramatically reduce the chances of venous stasis ulcer (VSU) healing. Limbs affected by lymphedema show a classic cauliflower-like change in the skin and edema that fails to reduce even with elevation; patients who are affected often suffer from obesity or have a history of local irradiation, lymph node dissection, neoplastic penetration, or a family history of lymphedema (Fig. 11.14).

Venous leg ulcerations occur between the knee and the ankle. They are classically but not exclusively located over the medial and lateral malleolus of the ankle (also known as the gaiter area). These wounds often begin as small shallow ulcerations with serous exudate that can rapidly expand over the course of days to weeks. The odor can be profound and cause significant distress. When ulcers erupt, the periwound is often very edematous, with substantial erythema, scaling, and weeping. The pain of such wounds is not usually severe unless there is an active infection; such discomfort must be distinguished from the frequently described "achiness" of CVI. Wounds, when infected, present with a burning pain. Unlike decubitus and arterial ulcers, there is usually no eschar. The wound bed often contains nearly homogenous granulation tissue; occasionally they can also be shrouded with superficial fibrinous necrosis or slough [39] (Fig. 11.10). Traumatic wounds that occur on the limbs affected by venous insufficiency are common; they often arise from a

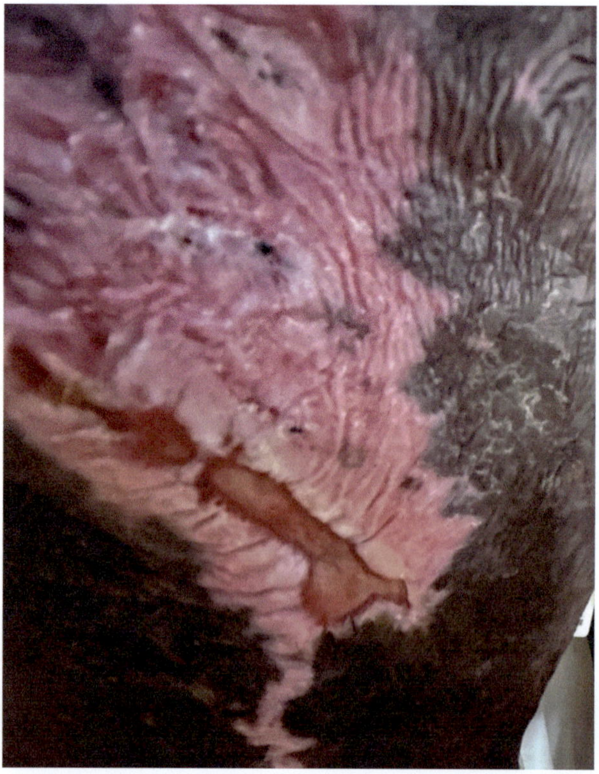

Fig. 11.14 Lymphedema ulcer

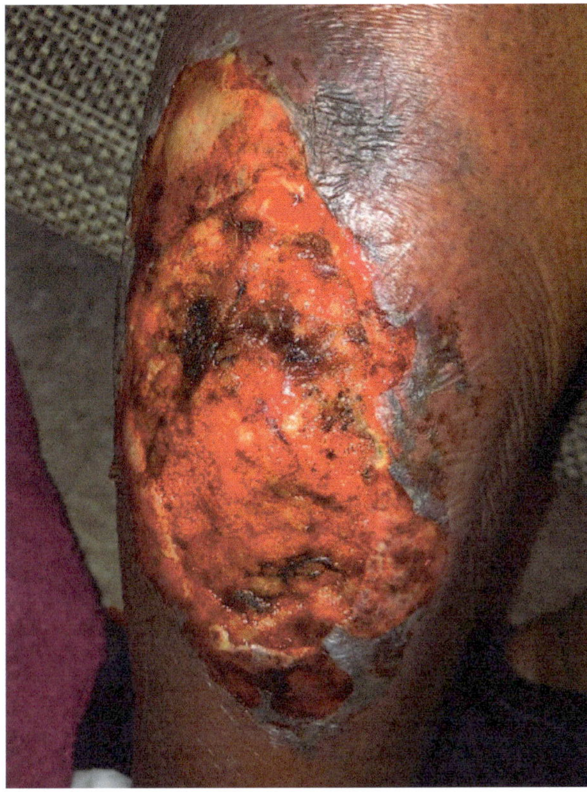

Fig. 11.15 Traumatic wound in leg affected by venous insufficiency

minor injury such as a scrape against the bolts or leg supports of a wheelchair. They can have the temperament of a venous ulcer, often oozing and failing to close with local wound dressings (Fig. 11.15).

Prior to developing a treatment plan for venous ulcers, it is critically important to differentiate the wound from an arterial ulcer, as the more substantial compressive therapies can be detrimental to persons with arterial compromise. Combination arterial-venous wounds are common. Some symptoms that distinguish arterial ulcers are substantial pain of the extremity at rest with worse pain during elevation or activity. Arterial wounds usually have a pale, gray, or yellow bed, have nominal to no exudate, and are often covered with eschar. Venous wounds, however, are rubrous and exudate heavy; the surrounding skin is often brawny.

If a venous stasis ulcer is suspected and compression therapy is being considered, then the site should be evaluated for adequate blood flow via a palpable dorsalis pedis pulse or a bedside Doppler ultrasound. The resting ankle-brachial systolic pressure index (ABI) is a simple test that can be performed with a stethoscope and a sphygmomanometer at the bedside and is used to determine the quality of blood flow [40]. The person should be placed in the supine position for at least 10 min before performing the test; if the person smokes, the test should be performed no less than 2 h after the last cigarette. The systolic pressure is first taken over both brachial arteries with a sphygmomanometer; subsequently a systolic pressure is obtained at the dorsalis pedis and posterior tibialis arteries, while an appropriately sized cuff is placed over the leg between the ankle malleoli and the calf. The higher systolic pressure of the two inferior arteries is divided by the higher systolic pressure of the arms to obtain the ABI. In cases in which the home-based medical provider has access to a portable Doppler probe, the measurements will be more accurate. An ABI between 0.91 and 1.3 is considered normal, and the wound should be treated as a venous stasis ulcer. An ABI should not be completed on a person if they have excruciating pain in the lower legs or a suspected deep vein thrombosis. In such cases, we advise referral to a mobile vascular laboratory or a home-based podiatrist for assessment of arterial flow by Doppler.

Compression is the mainstay of effective venous stasis ulcer care. When a venous stasis ulcer develops, a compression dressing should be applied over a primary dressing; this is true even in cases of traumatic wounds that occur in limbs affected by venous insufficiency. There are two main options for compression: an Unna boot (compression dressing) and the four-layered bandage dressing. The Unna boot consists of a paste bandage that is impregnated with zinc oxide, glycerin, and gelatin. It is applied without tension in a circular fashion from the foot just distal to the metatarsals to below the knee. An elastic wrap or tubular support bandage is applied as a final layer and forms a cast after drying. The four-layered bandage involves the application of compressive elastic dressings at mid-stretch and with overlap to allow creating an even distribution of tension across the limb. Excessive tension by the bandager is both unnecessary and potentially deleterious; clinicians should practice with the use of videos before applying [41, 42]. The first layer is an absorbent padding. It should be wrapped in a spiral fashion with a 50% overlap. The second layer is a light conforming wrap that is also wrapped in a spiral fashion with 50% overlap. The third layer is a compression layer. It should be applied in a Fig. 11.8 fashion with a 50% overlap and 50% stretch. This will apply about 17 mmHg pressure. The fourth layer is also compression. It is wrapped in a spiral fashion with 50% overlap and 50% stretch, which results in 20 mmHg pressure. Several studies comparing the Unna boot with the four-layer compression dressing have showed no differences in the effectiveness of healing venous stasis ulcers [43]. For ease of application and removal, we opt for the four-layer compression dressing in the home.

Evidence supports the greater effectiveness and faster healing times of a four-layer compression dressing over single component dressings, such as elastic gauze. For home-based persons for whom we cannot obtain an adequate arterial evaluation, we will use a two-layer compressive wrap composed of a primary absorptive layer and a single compressive layer; although the healing time is slower, it can be effective particularly in persons who are recumbent.

Cleansing prior to coverage with a compression dressing should be performed with care to minimize trauma to the surrounding skin. We recommend gently patting the wound with saline or sterile water-doused gauze [44]. Additional dry gauze can be used to pat the wound dry. Primary dressings with high absorption are usually preferred such as alginates, CMC-based hydrofibers, or foam. Hydrocolloids offer a soothing overlay but are less absorptive; they can be used over venous stasis ulcers with mild drainage. Finally, nonstick gauze or petrolatum-impregnated gauze may be used though their absorption capability is extremely low. They do offer the benefits of low cost and less painful removal.

Factors predicting a high likelihood of healing within 1 year of compression therapy include an ulcer width of less than 20 cm, eruption less than a year, significant reduction of lower extremity edema during the first 2 months of therapy, and granulation tissue accounting for more than 10% of the wound bed [45]. Conversely, risk factors that predict a lower likelihood of wound resolution within a year include larger wound sizes, wounds present for over a year, substantial necrotic slough within the wound bed, obesity, immobility, particularly at the ankle joint, and substantial lower extremity edema that persists beyond the early months of therapy. As venous stasis wounds are often difficult to heal and recurrent, such risk factors are useful in helping providers determine realistic chances of wound closure.

11.6 Arterial Ulcers

11.6.1 Etiology, Risk Factors, and Signs and Symptoms of Arterial Ulcers

Peripheral arterial occlusive disease (PAOD) is common and associated with significant morbidities including arterial ulceration of the lower extremities. All patients presenting with lower extremity ulcers should be considered for the concurrent presence of arterial insufficiency. Only those patients who will benefit from invasive management or whose therapeutics may change based on the presence or absence of arterial disease, however, should undergo further testing in a vascular laboratory [46, 47].

Arterial ulcers frequently occur in areas of the lower extremities subjected to pressure or repetitive trauma and can share significant overlap in appearance and etiology with pressure injuries (Fig. 11.16) [55]. Commonly affected areas include the metatarsal and phalangeal heads, web spaces between the toes, lateral malleolus, heels, tibia, and bony prominences of the foot frequently exposed to pressure from a shoe or brace or the pressure of a bed surface. Though heels are sites highly susceptible to pressure injury, the density of soft tissue that cushions the bone means that when ulcers do evolve, they are often the product of coexisting peripheral arterial disease (Fig. 11.17).

Arterial ulcers often have well-demarcated margins with a round, "punched out" appearance; the wound bed is often yellow, tan, or black in color and has minimal exudate. These wounds can look indistinguishable from Stage 3, 4, or deep pressure injuries. The clue is often in the location—areas such as the lower leg or thigh where pressure injuries do not typically develop, for instance. The surrounding skin can

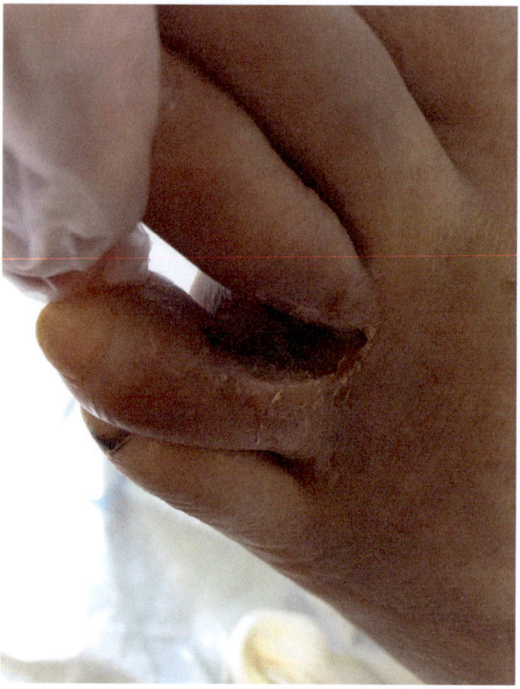

Fig. 11.16 Arterial ulcer of the digital webspace

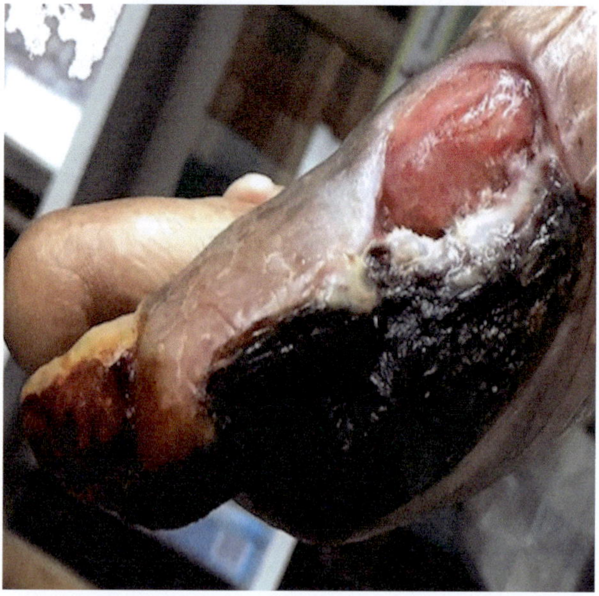

Fig. 11.17 Arterial heel ulcer

offer additional clues—the absence of hair, a shiny quality to the skin, a cool temperature, or the lack of palpable pulses.

A more accurate assessment of arterial blood flow in the extremities can be achieved by measuring the ankle brachial index (ABI) described above using a stethoscope or Doppler ultrasound. In home-based settings, the latter is often difficult to perform without a portable Doppler ultrasound machine. The ABI provides a ratio of ankle to brachial artery systolic blood pressure, which predicts the effectiveness of peripheral circulation and severity of PAOD. The screening value for PAOD is defined by a resting ABI of ≤0.90 [48]. More specifically, an ABI that ranges from 0.91 to 1.30 indicates an absence of significant arterial disease, and wounds, if present, are healable. An ABI that ranges from 0.41 to 0.90 indicates mild to severe arterial insufficiency with varying degrees of wound healing potential. An ABI ≤0.40 indicates critical lower extremity ischemia and low probability of wound healing. The availability of ABI data can help clinicians gauge the potential for arterial ulcer healing in homebound patients.

11.6.2 Arterial Wound Management

The restoration of peripheral blood flow by revascularization is the intervention that will most likely promote healing of arterial ulcers but is often not practical or desirable in homebound patients with limited life expectancy. Therapeutics thus focus on the optimization of modifiable risk factors (smoking, diabetes, hyperlipidemia, etc.), the avoidance of constrictive garments and pressure dressings, pressure modulation through offloading techniques previously described, and the elevation of the head of bed (4–6 in. but no more than 30°) to maintain the lower extremity position below the level of the heart to help improve arterial flow.

The management of arterial ulcers distinctly differs from the care of other types of wounds in the following ways: maintaining a dry wound bed, avoiding the unroofing of eschar (unless moist and/or with evidence of eschar lift from pus or underlying exudate), and mitigating the high risks of wound infection, pain, and malodor. Like pressure ulcers, arterial ulcers benefit from substantial mitigation of pressure and friction through multilayered dressings such as gauze wraps applied without tension. To keep the wound bed dry, both healable and non-healable dry ulcers should be cleansed with povidone-iodine or chlorhexidine and then patted dry to remove any excess solution; subsequently, a protective dry wound dressing such as gauze can be applied.

In cases of non-arterial wounds, the removal of eschar by debridement promotes cell turnover and leads to faster wound healing. However, in the setting of arterial insufficiency, debridement and unroofing of eschar may cause the premature exposure and desiccation of poorly vascularized subcutaneous fat and augment chances of local infection. Consider the eschar as a protective covering which may allow for subdermal closure and thus should not be disrupted unless it shows signs of lift. In cases in which the reversion of vascular supply is not possible, skilled clinicians need to use their judgment and exercise frequent visits to ensure that the decision to remove dry necrotic tissue has a favorable consequence.

In contrast to dry arterial wounds, when treating a moist arterial ulcer with or without slough or wet necrosis, the use of autolytic, soft mechanical (via saline-doused gauze rubbed across the wound bed), or chemical debridement (via the application of 1/4 strength Dakin's or Vashe wound solution to the wound bed for 5 min every other day) is appropriate to reduce biofilm, promote wound bed stability, and enhance conditions that may promote closure even when the vascular supply is unlikely to improve. Arterial wounds with a high degree of biofilm have the potential to close if the biofilm is continually reduced and debrided. Dressings with analgesic cooling properties such as a hydrogel applied under a non-pressured dressing such as a gauze wrap or an adhesive hydrocolloid that maintains a moist wound environment can be applied after debridement to optimize cell migration and matrix formation. Cadexomer iodine and iodine-impregnated foam dressings may reduce interim biofilm accumulation and are often used in lieu or in addition to the above mechanisms of biofilm disruption.

Arterial ulcers are especially prone to infection. The signs and symptoms of a wound-related infection may include (a) increased bacterial burden as suggested by a nonhealing wound, new necrotic slough, friable or dark red hypergranulation tissue, absence of granulation tissue, increased exudate, and malodor; (b) localized infection as indicated by new or worsening pain, increased periwound induration, erythema, or warmth, and increased wound size; or (c) systemic infection as determined by the presence of lethargy, fevers, delirium, and sepsis [48]. The restoration of arterial blood flow via bypass or atherectomy, which is often considered palliative, is central to controlling wound-related infection. In patients who are not candidates for revascularization surgery, however, systemic antibiotic therapy coupled with methodical and frequent biofilm removal remains the treatment of choice for infected arterial ulcers.

Wound odor typically results from tissue necrosis or bacterial colonization; it may not be solely indicative of wound infection. While wound odor is not directly harmful to the patient, it may indicate the degree of bacterial burden and pose psychological stress on the patient and caregivers. Effective strategies to reduce the development of malodor include methodical biofilm removal, frequent dressing changes, and timely changing of bed linens soiled by exudate. Daily to three times weekly application of topical metronidazole (1% solution, 0.75% or 0.8% gel, or topical powder from crushed metronidazole tablets) is particularly effective in treating wounds with high anaerobic bacteria burden [49]. In addition, odor-controlling dressings that contain activated charcoal or cadexomer iodine that remove excess drainage and inhibit bacterial growth are helpful [50].

Peripheral arterial disease and arterial ulcers are painful. The pain can be constant or intermittent and present only with wound dressing changes. Positioning the lower extremities below the level of the heart may alleviate limb pain due to arterial insufficiency. This can be accomplished by hanging the affected leg over the side of the bed to improve flow. If dressing changes prove to be painful, oral or topical analgesic administration (in the form of topical lidocaine 4% or 5% gel or EMLA™

cream) 30–60 min prior to wound manipulation is indicated. Because systemic analgesia is superior to topical therapies in achieving pain control, the administration of a nonopioid or opioid analgesic at sufficient doses is frequently required to achieve optimal pain management. Moreover, the use of non-adherent dressings such as nonstick gauze, hydrogel-impregnated dressings, or foam can minimize disruption of arterial ulcers and is less likely to cause pain on removal; dressings that have desiccated and are adherent should be moistened with room-temperature saline before removal.

11.7 Treatment of Neuropathic Ulcers and Diabetic Foot and Ankle Ulcers

Although neuropathic ulcers can arise in multiple conditions that affect the peripheral nerves, diabetes accounts for the large majority encountered in community-based settings. In our practice, diabetic ulcers are frequently encountered as part of a constellation of poorly controlled diabetes, debility, and arterial disease (Figs. 11.18, 11.19 and 11.20). Pressure injury due to the insensate limb is a particular risk for both the ambulatory and nonambulatory patient. Wheelchairs, for instance, if not properly fitted and equipped with the proper inflated cushion and padded leg lifts, may pose a significant risk for the patient with an insensate limb.

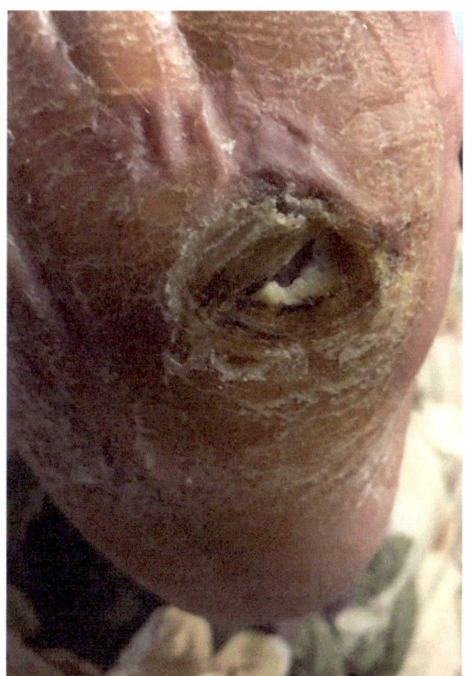

Fig. 11.18 Diabetic foot ulcer, first metatarsal phalangeal joint, plantar surface

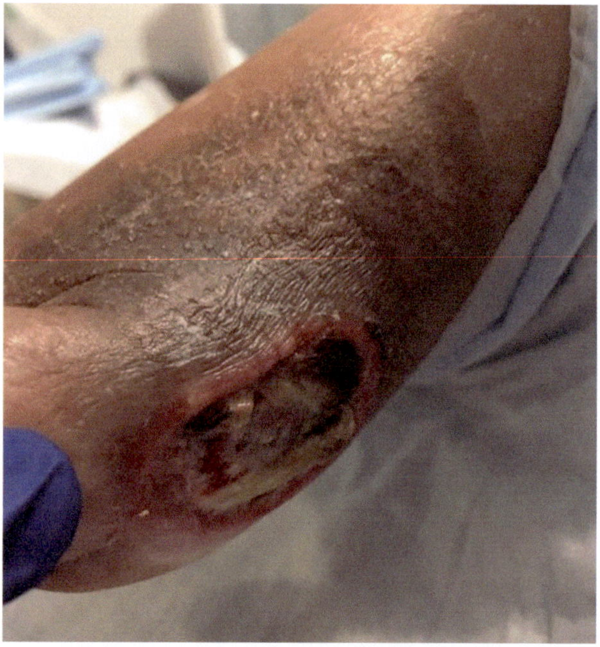

Fig. 11.19 Diabetic foot ulcer, first metatarsal phalangeal joint, medial surface

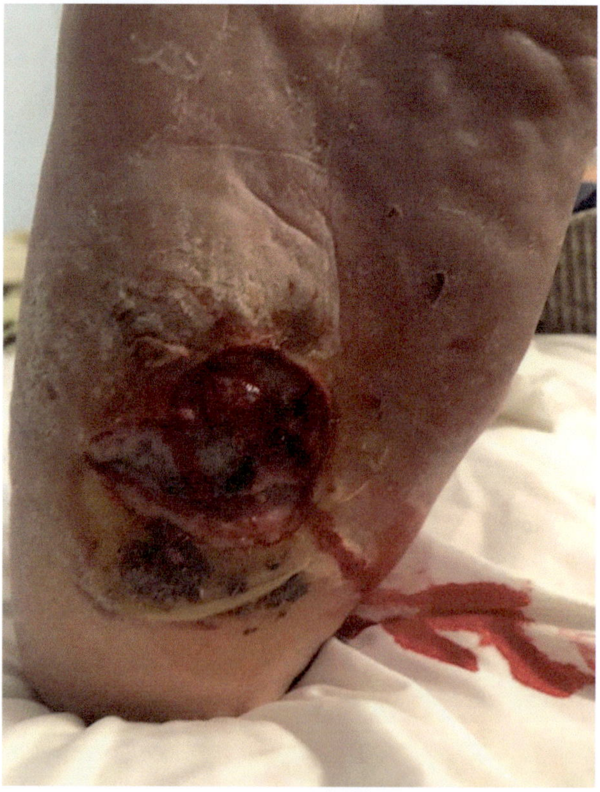

Fig. 11.20 Diabetic foot ulcer, midfoot

In general, the care of these wounds is similar to the care of pressure ulcers and arterial ulcers [51]. Diabetic foot and ankle ulcers may often be associated with arterial insufficiency, and ABIs are essential to determining if large versus small vessel disease is involved. The former may require revascularization to enhance the likelihood of wound closure. Small vessel disease, however, requires glucose control coupled with pressure off-loading through the use of specialized boots if ambulatory, sheepskin or foam heel protectors if bedbound, or immobile [52] and specially fitted shoes if ambulatory.

Direct care of diabetic neuropathic wounds of the foot often involves dressings that control a high bacterial burden. Cadexomer iodine preparations, which come as an ointment, gel, or paste, can be used to fill cavities, absorb excess exudate, enhance autolytic debridement, and reduce bacterial burden and have been shown to offer a lower-cost alternative to more expensive antibiotic preparations and to twice-daily saline soaked gauze dressings or moist-to-moist dressings [53, 54]. Though daily moist-to-moist dressings are an acceptable standard of care for diabetic neuropathic foot ulcers, it is labor-intensive and in home-based settings, not routinely possible.

Neuropathic wounds in persons without diabetes are treated with the same modalities used for pressure ulcers, as the etiologies are often quite similar. The absence of localized pain may be associated with substantial wound size and depth before noticed. Patient and caregiver vigilance in monitoring skin over bony or friction-prone surfaces is essential to prevention.

11.8 Home-Based Treatment of Malignant Wounds

Malignant wounds in the homebound are particularly challenging to manage because such wounds have a high morbidity and almost always occur when prognosis is grim and life expectancy is short. Malignant wounds occur when there is direct infiltration of tumor into the skin and subcutaneous tissues, leading to vessel erosion or occlusion and subsequent tissue death. The necrosis of superficial tissues in turn leads to sloughing, drainage, foul smell, and localized bacterial colonization. Such wounds can then become ulcerating or fungating. Skin metastases can occur in as many as one in ten patients with metastatic cancer [55]. The most common cancers associated with cutaneous spread leading to wounds are breast, head and neck, and skin cancers [56].

One of the most distressing symptoms of malignant wounds is odor, resulting from the necrosis of tissue and products of anaerobic bacteria that colonize the wounds. Topical metronidazole (cream preferred over gel which contains alcohol that may sting on application), medicinal honey, and oral chlorophyll [57] have been shown to reduce odors from malignant wounds. Silver or other antimicrobial-impregnated formulations can also reduce odor.

Drainage can be copious. Using absorptive dressings, like alginates, hydrofibers, hydrocolloids, or topical sucralfate cream is indispensable in the care of malignant wounds.

Alginates and hydrofibers also offer immediate hemostatic properties, but their removal can be traumatic and lead to more bleeding; homecare providers are urged to use caution with such dressings and to consider saturating the dressing with saline just prior to removal. A provider may need to balance the goal of managing drainage with minimizing the frequency of painful dressing changes. If the drainage is not manageable with highly absorptive dressings, an ostomy bag may be used.

Malignant wounds tend to bleed. Erosion of the wound or tumor into a superficial vessel can lead to frank hemorrhage. Minor oozing and spotting can be minimized with nonstick dressings such as a hydrogel wafer, petroleum-impregnated gauze, nonstick gauze or foam dressing, and reduced frequency of dressing changes. Topical adrenergic agents like oxymetazoline (usually available as a nasal decongestant), topical or systemic tranexamic acid, or systemic aminocaproic acid have also been effective in managing bleeding wounds.

Pain from malignant wounds can be targeted with several local therapies, like topical lidocaine or morphine suspended in topical sucralfate or hydrogel, or with a systemic approach if warranted by the severity or persistence of the pain. The quantities advised are approximately 1 mg of morphine to 1 g of hydrogel to achieve a 0.08–0.1% mixture; a compounding pharmacy is often necessary to create this. Such agents can also be used to treat painful pressure and venous stasis wounds.

11.9 Indications for Negative-Pressure Wound Therapy

Accelerated wound closure with the use of negative-pressure wound therapy (NPWT) is becoming more mainstream in home-based wound care. NPWT involves the attachment of a semiocclusive foam or gauze dressing to a vacuum device and a collection reservoir through plastic tubing (Figs. 11.21 and 11.22). A solid seal that inhibits passage of air is critical to promoting a moist wound environment and preventing overdrying [58]. NPWT works through several theorized mechanisms:

- Macrodeformation, or the physical approximation of the wound surface.
- Microdeformation, or the promotion of cellular proliferation at the wound surface.
- Creation of a moist wound environment with low oxidative exposure.
- Positive alterations in blood flow in the deeper wound bed despite reductions on the surface [59].

For poorly healing Stage 3 and 4 pressure ulcers, venous ulcers, and neuropathic wounds with minimal closure or expansion despite standard wound therapies over the course of 3 months, NPWT can greatly augment wound closure rates provided certain personnel are available [60]. Increasingly NPWT is being exercised as a first-line therapy for the above conditions, but the lack of capable or confident caregivers to help manage the device limits practical use. One absolute requirement is the ready availability of caregivers, such as family, to care for the device when troubleshooting. Caregivers paid through public insurance are often prohibited from

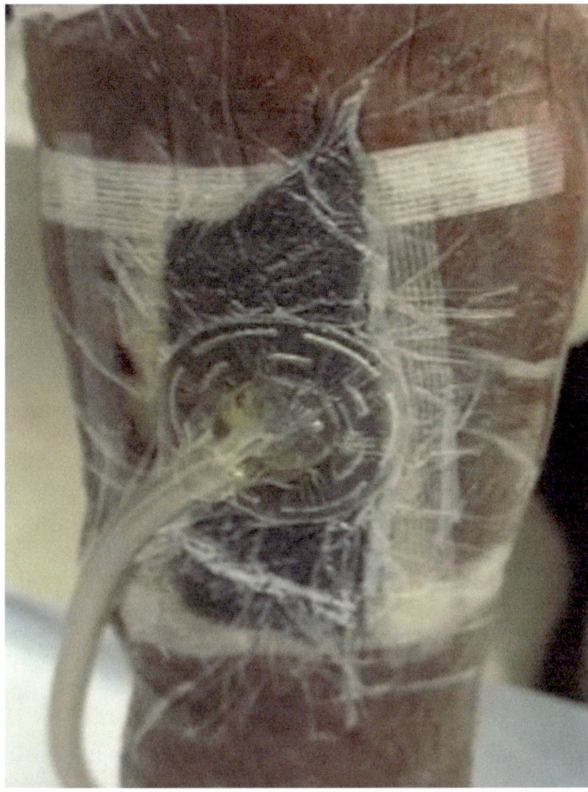

Fig. 11.21 Negative-pressure wound therapy applied to a traumatic wound of leg affected by chronic venous insufficiency

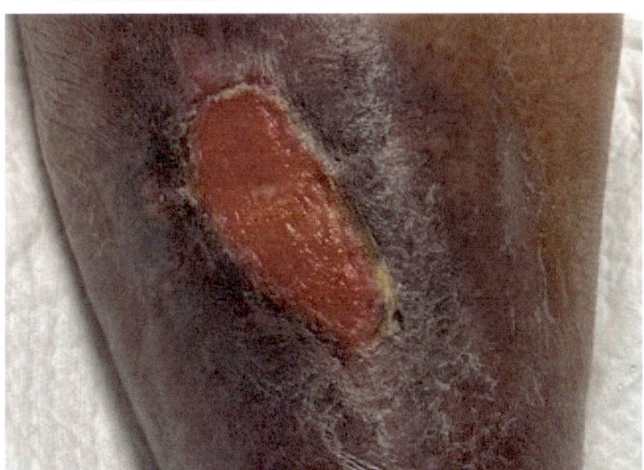

Fig. 11.22 Healing traumatic wound treated by negative-pressure wound therapy

operating or adjusting the device. A second absolute requirement is nursing staff that are well-trained to operate the device and its attachments correctly. Familiarity with the device, possible adverse consequences, and troubleshooting capabilities are essential. Though many companies offer help on demand, this is not a reliable means to provide the daily care necessary for effective NPWT. In our experience, the home-based medical provider's role is to ascertain the ability of caregivers to operate, troubleshoot, and call the providers when the device malfunctions or power is lost. Faulty equipment or dressing attachment can cause delays in wound healing and, more distressingly, can cause infection, pain, or additional wounds to arise from maceration. Home-based medical providers should optimize the wound bed before application; this will mean adequate debridement to remove the majority of eschar or slough and treatment of underlying infection. Consultation with the NPWT on-staff nurse is helpful to providers less experienced with NPWT. Complications of these devices include bleeding and infection, the latter often due to retained dressings or infrequent dressing changes [61]. Regular assessment of the wound with accurate and rigorous documentation is the responsibility of the primary provider for insurance coverage of the device; use up to 3 months without significant closure is a criterion for termination of the device.

11.10 Nutritional Counselling and Supplementation

The roles of adequate nutrition and glycemic control are particularly crucial to the healing of pressure ulcers, venous ulcers, and diabetic foot ulcers. Catabolic states cause an increased susceptibility to pressure ulcers. The rate of healing of venous and pressure ulcers indirectly correlates with albumin levels (commonly used as a marker of protein malnutrition) [62]. Similarly, the rate of healing of diabetic foot ulcers inversely correlates with hemoglobin A1c levels [63].

When possible, the advice of a dietitian is beneficial in treating patients with wounds who also suffer from nutritional deficiency; typically, we use albumin levels of less than 3.5 g/dL, an elevated C-reactive protein, hemoglobin levels less than 8, and hemoglobin A1c levels greater than 8 as markers of a compromised state that is likely to substantially prolong the time to healing.

In our practice, we typically liberalize caloric intake for patients with pressure ulcers to 30–35 kcal/kg per day through dietary changes or oral nutritional supplements (ONS) when necessary; we also advise augmenting protein intake to 1.25–1.5 g/kg per day. Practically this often means offering more calorie dense foods (i.e., ice cream shakes) with protein fortification (i.e., adding nut butters or protein powder). Several small randomized and non-randomized controlled trials suggest that arginine and vitamin C-enriched nutritional supplementation may reduce the time to healing for hard-to-heal wounds [64]. Unfortunately, the cost of arginine-based marketed powders is currently not reimbursable by private or public insurance and can be prohibitive.

11.11 Billing for the Assessment of Wounds and Wound Care

Careful and complete documentation is an important first step to accurate billing for wound care. Documentation should involve attention to intrinsic and extrinsic risk factors and discussions with caregivers and healthcare personnel on the mitigation of each. In addition to accurate documentation of the wound stage and size, wound bed preparation and methods of debridement must be clearly documented. In general, Current Procedural Terminology (CPT) codes are used in home-based wound care *only* if an active debridement modality such as mechanical, enzymatic, chemical, or sharp debridement is conducted on the day of the visit [65]. In other words, if the wound was measured and the dressing applied and no debridement was performed, the codes for active wound care cannot be reported.

- Debridement of biofilm performed on the skin, epidermis, or dermis is reported with the active wound care management CPT codes 97,597 and 97,598. This code series can also be used when the tissues debrided are at the base of deeper wounds when no specific tissue layer (i.e., fascia, muscle, or bone) is identified. This code series includes high-pressure irrigation of the wounds and the application of chemical debriding agents. Any one of these methods qualifies as an active wound management modality.
- Debridement of nonviable tissue (eschar, slough) whether by mechanical, chemical, enzymatic, or sharp modalities is coded as is coded with CPT code 97602.
- In cases when debridement of nonviable tissue is performed in preparation for negative-pressure wound therapy, and the goal is for closure of the wound by primary intention, CPT codes are of the 15,002–15,005 series.

Wounds cannot be billed by individual lesion; rather aggregate size of all of the wounds by square centimeter is what determines the appropriate CPT code and whether additional CPT codes are necessary. For instance, code 97597 is billed for debridement of nonviable tissue for the first 20 cm^2 of aggregate wound size, and debridement of any additional square centimeter is billed with the addition of code 97598.

11.12 Summary

Wound care and prevention are critically important skills for home-based practitioners to master. Pressure injuries are frequently encountered in home care; their causes are multifactorial and not wholly avoidable. The care of such wounds, whether a superficial Stage I or deep Stage IV, is multidimensional and requires careful and regular attention, proper documentation, tailored dressings, comprehensive treatment regimens, and interdisciplinary partnership with shared goals of closure and palliation of pain and psychological distress. Primary and secondary prevention of pressure injuries require root cause analyses of instigating, propagating, and perpetuating factors. Venous stasis and lymphedema ulcers, arterial ulcers, neuropathic wounds, and malignant wounds are encountered less frequently, but their management, though complex, can be extrapolated from the care of pressure injuries.

References

1. McDermott-Scales L, Cowman S, Gethin G. Prevalence of wounds in a community care setting in Ireland. J Wound Care. 2009;18(10):405–17.
2. Park-Lee E, Caffrey C. Pressure ulcers among nursing home residents: United States, 2004. NCHS Data Brief. 2009;14:1–8.
3. Vowden K, Vowden P. A pilot study on the potential of remote support to enhance wound care for nursing-home patients. J Wound Care. 2013;22(9):481–8.
4. Etingen B, Wirth M, Patrianakos J, Kartje R, Baharestani M, Weaver F. Outcomes of telehealth for wound care: a scoping review. Adv Skin Wound Care. 2022;35:1–15.
5. Kottner J, Balzer K, Dassen T, Heinze S. Pressure ulcers: a critical review of definitions and classifications. Ostomy Wound Manage. 2009;55(9):22–9.
6. Edsberg LE, Black JM, Goldberg M, Mcnichol L, Moore L, Siegreen M. Revised National Pressure Ulcer Advisory Panel Pressure Injury Staging System: revised pressure injury staging system. J Wound Ostomy Cont Nurs. 2016;43(6):585–97.
7. McClemont EJ. Pressure sores. No pressure—no sore. Nursing (Lond). 1984;2(21):1–3.
8. Cushing CA, Phillips LG. Evidence-based medicine: pressure sores. Plast Reconstr Surg. 2013;132(6):1720–32.
9. Gefen A, Farid KJ, Shaywitz I. A review of deep tissue injury development, detection, and prevention: shear savvy. Ostomy Wound Manage. 2013;59(2):26–35.
10. Ganceviciene R, Liakou AI, Theodoridis A, Makrantonaki E, Zouboulis CC. Skin anti-aging strategies. Dermatoendocrinology. 2012;4(3):308–19.
11. Bennett L, Kavner D, Lee BY. Shear vs. pressure as causative factors in skin blood flow occlusion. Arch Phys Med Rehabil. 1969;60:309–14.
12. VanGilder C, MacFarlane GD, Harrison P, Lachenbruch C, Meyer S. The demographics of suspected deep tissue injury in the United States: an analysis of the international pressure ulcer prevalence survey 2006-2009. Adv Skin Wound Care. 2010;23(6):254–61.
13. Barczak CA, Barnett RI, Childs EJ, Bosley LM. Fourth national pressure ulcer prevalence survey. Adv Wound Care. 1997;10(4):18–26.
14. Seiler WO. Decubitus ulcers: treatment through five therapeutic principles. Geriatrics. 1965;40:30–44.
15. Krapfl LA, Gray M. Does regular repositioning prevent pressure ulcers? J Wound Ostomy Cont Nurs. 2008;35(6):571–7.
16. Moore Z, Cowman S. Using the 30° tilt to reduce pressure ulcers. Nurs Times. 2012;108(4):22–4.
17. Centers for Medicaid and Medicare services. Home Health Quality Initiative [Internet]. 2015. http://www.cms.gov/Medicare/Quality-Initiatives-Patient-Assessment-Instruments/HomeHealthQualityInits/index.html.
18. Braden B, Bergstrom N. Braden Scale [Internet]. 1988. http://www.bradenscale.com/images/bradenscale.pdf.
19. Anthony D, Papanikolaou P, Parboteeah S, Saleh M. Do risk assessment scales for pressure ulcers work? J Tissue Viability. 2010;19(4):132–6.
20. Kottner J, Balzer K. Do pressure ulcer risk assessment scales improve clinical practice? J Multidiscip Healthc. 2010;3:103–11.
21. Pancorbo-Hidalgo PL, Garcia-Fernandez FP, Lopez-Medina IM, Alvarez-Nieto CJ. Risk assessment scales for pressure ulcer prevention: a systematic review. Adv Nurs. 2006;54(1):94–110.

22. Dorner B, Posthauer ME, Thomas D. The role of nutrition in pressure ulcer prevention and treatment: National Pressure Ulcer Advisory Panel White Paper [internet]. 2009. http://www.npuap.org/wp-content/uploads/2012/03/Nutrition-White-Paper-Website-Version.pdf.
23. Zeevi T, Levy A, Brauner N, Gefen A. Effects of ambient conditions on the risk of pressure injuries in bedridden patients—multi-physics modelling of microclimate. Int Wound J. 2018;15:402–16.
24. Niezgoda JA, Sordi P, Hermans MH. Evaluation of Vashe wound therapy in the clinical management of patients with chronic wounds. Adv Skin Wound Care. 2010;23(8):352–7.
25. Panuncialman J, Falanga V. The science of wound bed preparation. Clin Plast Surg. 2007;34(4):621–32.
26. Shi L, Carson D. Collagenase Santyl ointment: a selective agent for wound debridement. J Wound Ostomy Cont Nurs. 2009;37(6 Suppl):S12–6.
27. Basterzi Y, Ersoz G, Sarac G, Sari A, Demrikan F. In-vitro comparison of antimicrobial efficacy of various wound dressing materials. Wounds. 2010;22(7):165–70.
28. Ebright JR. Microbiology of chronic leg and pressure ulcers: clinical significance and implications for treatment. Nurs Clin North Am. 2005;40:207–16.
29. Bessa LJ, Fazii P, Di Giulio M, Cellini L. Bacterial isolates from infected wounds and their antibiotic susceptibility pattern: some remarks about wound infection. Int Wound J. 2015;12(1):47–52.
30. Smith and Nephew Inc. Measurement and Application Process for Collagenase SANTYL® Ointment [Internet]. 2014. http://www.santyl.com/hcp/application.
31. Shannon MM. A retrospective descriptive study of nursing home residents with heel eschar or blisters. Ostomy Wound Manage. 2013;59(1):20–7.
32. Legood R, McInnes E. Pressure ulcers: guideline development and economic modelling. J Adv Nurs. 2005;50(3):307–14.
33. McInnes E, Asmara JB, Bell-Syer S, Dumville J, Cullum N. Preventing pressure ulcers—are pressure-redistributing support surfaces effective? A Cochrane systematic review and meta-analysis. Int J Nurs Stud. 2012;49(3):345–59.
34. National Pressure Ulcer Advisory Panel Terms and Definitions Related to Support Surfaces [Internet]. 2007. http://www.npuap.org/wp-content/uploads/2012/03/NPUAP_S3I_TD.pdf.
35. Center for Medicaid and Medicare Services. Medicare Policy Regarding Pressure Reducing Support Surfaces—JA1014 [Internet]. 2010. http://www.cms.gov/Medicare/Medicare-Contracting/ContractorLearningResources/downloads/JA1014.pdf.
36. Junkin J, Gray M. Are pressure redistribution surfaces or heel protection devices effective for preventing heel pressure ulcers? J Wound Ostomy Cont Nurs. 2009;36(6):602–8.
37. Eberhardt RT, Raffetto JD. Chronic venous insufficiency. Circulation. 2014;130:333–46.
38. Greer N, Foman NA, MacDonald R, Dorrian J, Fitzgerald P, Rutks I, Wilt TJ. Advanced wound care therapies for nonhealing diabetic, venous, and arterial ulcers. Ann Intern Med. 2013;159(8):532–42.
39. Lazarides MK, Giannoukas AD. The role of hemodynamic measurements in the management of venous and ischemic ulcers. Int J Low Extrem Wounds. 2007;6(4):254–61.
40. Aboyans V, Criqui MH, Abraham P, Allison MA, Creager MA, Diehm C, Fowkes FGR, Hiatt WR, Jonsson B, Lacroix P, Marin B, McDermott MM, Norgren L, Pande RL, Preux P-M, Stoffers HE, Treat-Jacobson D. Measurement and interpretation of the ankle-brachial index: a scientific statement from the American Heart Association. Circulation. 2012;126:1–20.
41. Moffatt C. Four-layer bandaging: from concept to practice. Part 2: Application of the four-layer system. 2005. http://www.worldwidewounds.com/2005/march/Moffatt/Four-Layer-Bandage-System-Part2.html#ref17.
42. Introduction to Profore. [Internet] Date unknown. http://www.smith-nephew.com/professional/products/advanced-wound-management/profore.
43. Polignano R, Bonadeo P, Gasbarro S, Allegra C. A randomised controlled study of four-layer compression versus Unna's boot for venous ulcers. J Wound Care. 2004;13(1):21–4.

44. Kelechi T, Johnson JJ. Guideline for the management of wounds in patients with lower-extremity venous disease. J Wound Ostomy Cont Nurs. 2012;39(6):598–606.
45. Milic DJ, Zivic SS, Bogdanovic DC, Karanovic ND, Golubovic ZV. Risk factors related to the failure of venous leg ulcers to heal with compression treatment. J Vasc Surg. 2009;49(5):1242–7.
46. Hirsch AT, Criqui MH, Treat-Jacobson D, Regensteiner JG, Creager MA, Olin JW, Krook SH, Hunninghake DB, Comerota AJ, Walsh ME, McDermott MM, Hiatt WR. Peripheral arterial disease detection, awareness, and treatment in the primary care. JAMA. 2001;286(11):1317–24.
47. Hopf HW, Ueno C, Aslam R, Burnand K, Fife C, Grant L, Holloway A, Iafrati MD, Mani R, Misare B, Rosen N, Shapshak D, Benjamin Slade J Jr, West J, Barbul A. Guidelines for the treatment of arterial insufficiency ulcers. Wound Repair Regen. 2006;14(6):693–710.
48. Wound infection in clinical practice. An international consensus. Int Wound J. 2008;5(Suppl 3):3–11.
49. O'Brien C. Malignant wounds: managing odour. Can Fam Physician. 2012;58(3):272–4.
50. Fleck CA. Fighting odor in wounds. Adv Skin Wound Care. 2006;19(5):242–4.
51. Andrews KL, Houdek MT, Kiemele LJ. Wound management of chronic diabetic foot ulcers: from the basics to regenerative medicine. Prosthet Orthot Int. 2015;39(1):29–39.
52. Rai NK, Suryabhan AM, Kumar M, Shukla VK, Tripathi K. Effect of glycaemic control on apoptosis in diabetic wounds. J Wound Care. 2005;14(6):277–81.
53. Chow I, Lemos EV, Einarson TR. Management and prevention of diabetic foot ulcers and infections: a health economic review. Pharmacoeconomics. 2008;26(12):1019–35.
54. Apelqvist J, Ragnarson TG. Cavity foot ulcers in diabetic patients: a comparative study of cadexomer iodine ointment and standard treatment. An economic analysis alongside a clinical trial. Acta Derm Venereol. 1996;76(3):231–5.
55. Lookingbill DP, Spangler N, Helm KF. Cutaneous metastases in patients with metastatic carcinoma: a retrospective study of 4020 patients. J Am Acad Dermatol. 1993;29:228–36.
56. Recka K, Montagnini M, Vitale C. Management of bleeding associated with malignant wounds. J Palliat Med. 2012;15(8):952–4.
57. Merz T, Klein C, Uebach B. Fungating wounds—multidimensional challenge in palliative care. Breast Care. 2011;6(1):21–4.
58. Orgill D, Bayer L. Update on negative pressure wound therapy. Plast Recon Surg. 2011;127(Suppl 1S):105S–15S.
59. Malmsjo M, Ingemansson R, Martin R, Huddleston E. Wound edge microvascular blood flow: effects of negative pressure wound therapy using gauze or polyurethane foam. Ann Plast Surg. 2009;63(6):676–81.
60. Orgill D, Bayer L. Negative pressure wound therapy: past, present and future. Int Wound J. 2013;10(Suppl 1):15–9.
61. Update on serious complications associated with negative pressure wound therapy systems: FDA Safety Communication. [Internet]. 2011. http://www.fda.gov/MedicalDevices/Safety/AlertsandNotices/ucm244211.htm.
62. Legendre C, Debure C, Meaume S, Lok C, Golmard JL, Senet P. Impact of protein deficiency on venous ulcer healing. J Vasc Surg. 2008;48:688–93.
63. Christman AL, Selvin E, Margolis DJ, Lazarus GS, Garza LA. Hemoglobin A1c predicts healing rate in diabetic wounds. J Invest Dermatol. 2011;131(10):2121–7.
64. Neyens JCL, Cereda E, Meijer E, Cereda EP, Meijer C, Lindholm C, Schols JMGA. Arginine-enriched oral nutritional supplementation in the treatment of pressure ulcers: a literature review. Wound Med. 2017;16:46–51.
65. Billing and Coding Guidelines for Wound Care (Revised 2/10/2022). https://www.cms.gov/medicare-coverage-database/view/article.aspx?articleId=55818&ver=17.
66. Barnea Y, Weiss J, Gur E. A review of the applications of the hydrofiber dressing with silver (Aquacel ag®) in wound care. Ther Clin Risk Manag. 2010;6:21–7.
67. Harding KG, Price P, Thomas S, Hofman D. Cost and dressing evaluation of hydrofiber and alginate dressings in the management of community-based patients with chronic leg ulceration. Wounds. 2001;13(6):229–36.

68. Carter K. Hydropolymer dressings in the management of wound exudate. Br J Community Nurs. 2003;8(9 Suppl):S10.
69. Chao TC, Tsaez FY. Paper tape in the closure of abdominal wounds. Surg Gynecol Obstet. 1990;171(1):65–7.
70. Koval KJ, Egol KA, Polatsch DB, Baskies MA, Homman JP, Hiebert RNJ. Tape blisters following hip surgery. A prospective, randomized study of two types of tape. Bone Joint Surg Am. 2003;85(10):1884–7.

Chapter 12
Social and Ethical Issues in Home-Based Medical Care

Thomas E. Finucane and Thomas K. M. Cudjoe

12.1 Brief Summary

Ethical and social issues permeate the care of homebound patients who depend on others. Patients who can speak up for themselves often face very difficult choices. Patients who lack the capacity to speak for themselves may present even more complex decision-making problems. The determination of capacity generally cannot be done with simple or objective tests except in the most clear-cut cases. This determination is critical with respect to both the definition and management of potential elder abuse and to the use of advance directives.

12.2 Key Points

1. The determination of capacity requires an understanding of the task at hand.
2. This determination often requires judgment beyond the medicolegal.
3. Elder abuse is one extreme of a continuum of caregiver or companion behaviors that ranges from the heroic to the criminal.

T. E. Finucane (✉)
Johns Hopkins Bayview Medical Center, Baltimore, MD, USA
e-mail: tfinucan@jhmi.edu

T. K. M. Cudjoe
Division of Geriatric Medicine and Gerontology, Center on Aging and Health, Johns Hopkins University School of Medicine, Baltimore, MD, USA
e-mail: tcudjoe2@jhmi.edu

J. L. Colburn et al. (eds.), *Geriatric Home-Based Medical Care*,
https://doi.org/10.1007/978-3-031-68786-0_12

4. In end-of-life decision-making, designated substitute decision-makers, sometimes called "healthcare agents," are likely to be more useful than living wills in most jurisdictions.
5. Clinicians who make home visits are uniquely positioned to judge capacity, identify abuse, and help with advance care planning.

12.3 Introduction

In the poem "He Makes a House Call," Dr. John Stone wrote that "Health is whatever works, and for as long" [1]. He located this definition of health within the context of a house call and could well have been talking about a homebound patient with disabling conditions and the fabric of caregivers on whom such a dependent patient depends. Many homebound patients who are quite ill nonetheless lead full and authentic lives and are quite happy to do so. After making home visits for just over a year, a clinician once observed that as a result "I have radically redefined what I mean when I say that a patient is really sick."

Office visits and home visits differ in important ways that are relevant to the perspective of a home-based medical provider. First, in the more standard clinic-based encounter, a patient arrives at a clinician's place. The initiative for the visit has originated with the patient or companions, which may require a substantial commitment from both, and they frequently have an agenda. Clinicians are often, in a certain way, responding. In home visits, in contrast, the context and the contract are quite different; clinicians take the initiative to go to the patient. If the patient/companion initiative is not required, engagement with a home-based clinician may be weaker. More often, when a patient recognizes the home-based clinician's commitment to the patient's health and the willingness to do what it takes to provide needed care, a high level of trust will develop, and patient engagement is augmented. The difference between clinic visits and home visits in clinician-patient relationship can be seen indirectly. If a patient stops coming to the clinic, his clinician might or might not track him down. An unanswered knock on the front door of a homebound patient, in contrast, may create a distinctly different sense of obligation.

Second, clinicians visiting a home may incidentally obtain additional dimensions of information almost completely unavailable in the clinic. The distinction between medical and social needs, always a challenging matter in care of vulnerable adults, may be far more direct and dramatic to a clinician in the living room. Meeting the medical and social needs of a homebound patient can present tragic challenges and trade-offs.

A third difference between clinic visits and home visits can be called the "locus of control." In the clinic, patients are usually outnumbered strangers in strange lands. The power dynamic strongly favors the healthcare system. During a house call, patients are at home: "Here, you are in charge - of figs, beans, tomatoes, life" [1].

A lengthy array of ethical and social issues arise in the care (often long term) of a homebound patient who is often frail, dependent, chronically ill, cognitively impaired, living in poverty, or some combination of these characteristics. In this chapter, we will focus on two important issues: (1) mistreatment of vulnerable adults and (2) advance planning for life-threatening illness. Because the constructs of "vulnerable adult" and of "advance directives" both depend heavily on whether a patient has the capacity to make decisions, we begin with a discussion on capacity.

12.4 Autonomy, Capacity, and Respect for Persons

12.4.1 Adult Protective Services

In general, referral to Adult Protective Services for review of relationships and living situation is reserved for persons who lack the physical or cognitive capacity to provide for their daily needs or to defend themselves in an abusive or neglectful situation. In general, advance directives take effect when the individual no longer has the capacity to make complex decisions about life-sustaining medical treatment but has previously left guidance about such decisions. In these models, capacity is often considered as a binary value; patients either have it or lack it.

12.4.2 Decisional Capacity Is Not a Yes-Or-No Characteristic

In general, people are assumed to have the ability to speak for themselves; the possibility that they lack this ability is not routinely considered. Questions about capacity usually arise in patients with neurologic or psychiatric symptomatology. Competence is considered more to be a legal term, determined by a judge, and "capacity" to be a clinical term, determined by treating physicians.

For practical purposes, it would be most useful to classify a patient as either having or lacking capacity. Several problems arise in this endeavor, however. First, cognitive capacity may wax and wane due to disease, medications, illness, and other patient-related factors. A common characteristic of Lewy body dementia and of severe infection is variability in sensorium. Second, decisions may change depending on circumstances. A competent, determined bedtime decision to get up at 6 a.m. and work in the garden may be replaced by an equally competent and determined decision at 6 a.m. to stay in bed. Third, judgments about capacity depend on the task at hand. Competence at playing bridge does not imply competence at playing shortstop. Similarly, a person may be capable of accepting the risk of a fall and consequent prolonged interval on the floor but not capable of deciding about major surgery or toxic chemotherapy. "Judgments of incompetence are therefore impossible to understand unless a task is assumed or specified" [2]. Fourth, and perhaps

Table 12.1 Suggested abilities to look for when determining capacity

Accurately understand the choices
Manipulate relevant information and weigh risks and benefits
Communicate a decision
Be consistent

the most important, is the generally subjective nature of competency determinations. The essence of this problem was well summarized many years ago: "The search for a single test of competence is a search for the Holy Grail. Unless it is realized that there is no magical definition of competency to make decisions about treatment, the search for an acceptable test will never end … judgments (about competence) reflect social considerations and societal biases as much as they reflect matters of law and medicine" [3].

The general elements that suggest a patient has capacity are shown in Table 12.1, although this is necessarily a simplification. In addition, the ability to make a reasonable decision has been proposed as a criterion and discussed at length, without clear resolution. Here most clearly, decisions about what is reasonable may not be a matter for objective determination.

12.4.3 Threshold for Evaluation and Certification of Incapacity

Even when a person can satisfy these criteria, social considerations and societal biases will influence many determinations. The capacity to make decisions is most often sought when the outcomes are high stakes and the patient's wishes do not conform to the clinician's recommendations. Stated differently, patients may be perceived to have capacity to say "yes" to a clinician but perceived to lack capacity to say "no." Tools have been developed to assist clinicians in assessing capacity, particularly in critical or high stakes decision-making [4].

In one view, great weight should be given to stated preferences even if the patient has marginal or limited capacity unless there is avoidable suffering or a clear risk of severe and avoidable harm; in these circumstances, coercive activity is more easily acceptable. Defining what level of risk is unacceptable may remain a cause of argument.

In another view, a patient's dignity (and the social contract) may require action if the patient's situation surpasses some level of offensiveness even if no physical harm results [5]. Extreme squalor, indifference to personal hygiene, and very odd social behaviors or relationships may provoke some clinicians to diagnose abuse or self-neglect and alert the authorities. Ignoring a cognitively impaired or mentally ill person who is being exploited or simply can no longer care for herself is unconscionable. But certifying that someone is incapacitated and then depriving him/her of his/her freedom simply to enforce a socially acceptable lifestyle are also wrong. Personal as well as societal biases will influence many determinations.

12.4.4 Practical Matters

The idea of capacity is closely linked to philosophical ideas about free will and personal responsibility; this is one reason the determination of capacity will remain controversial and difficult. The practical importance of this observation is that for any person who is conversational, the only valid way to judge capacity is to have a conversation with that person. Documentation of capacity is best done by a careful record of that conversation. Scores on popular cognitive tests have little additional value. The ability to describe the consequences of the proposed options and to explain why a particular option is being chosen is enough to satisfy most clinicians.

A sample note is given in Box 12.1. For patients whose communication abilities are limited, the determination of capacity will be more difficult. A simple language description of the patient's understanding of and reasoning about treatment options is generally the best way to document how the clinician judged the patient to have or lack decisional capacity about the specific management plan in question.

Box 12.1 Sample Informed Consent Discussion

Today Ms. Jones and I discussed her recent hospitalization, especially the fall, fracture, rhabdomyolysis, renal failure, and brief maintenance on dialysis. She describes this as the worst 4 weeks of her life and realizes that her life was in danger during that hospitalization. She clearly states, however, that she would rather go through the entire experience a second time, including the risk of death, than leave her home. She can name several important danger points, including the bathroom, the front steps, and especially the basement steps on the way back up with clean laundry. She feels she has made all home modifications that are reasonable and affordable and sees no other good options. She is not willing to consider any alternative housing, including her daughter's home. Was interested in an assisted living facility but is unwilling to spend that amount of money for room and board. She remains estranged from her husband and son, whom she does not wish us to contact. Her mini-mental state examination (MMSE) today is 21/30, stable. I believe she understands the risks of her decision to stay home and is willing to undertake them, especially given her lack of reasonable/acceptable alternatives.

12.5 Elder Abuse and Self-Neglect

Tolstoy begins Anna Karenina, "All happy families are alike. But every unhappy family is unhappy in its own way." Most care at home is provided with dedication and generosity and much of it in highly constrained circumstances. Some degree of caregiver impatience, burnout, and anger is common. Patient, caregiver, and circumstantial factors may increase the risk of decompensation. When the patient is somehow too vulnerable and the interactions are too cruel, a patient may be said to suffer abuse. As with the concept of capacity, some cases are clear-cut and beyond dispute. In many situations, however, there is no bright line but rather a continuous gradation from niceness to criminal behavior occurring in the context of a family with its history and a cultural understanding that may differ from the clinician's.

In this section, we will consider homebound, vulnerable adults of any age. When considering older adults, the term "elder abuse" is commonly used.

Definitions of elder abuse are variable, primarily focused on risk, harm, and safety and often discussed in the language of rights and victims. Table 12.2 shows a common schema for subtyping abuse and neglect.

Table 12.3 lists a variety of definitions [6–9]. Purported signs of abuse and neglect include pressure sores, weight loss, and medication nonadherence. The first two of these are common among chronically ill patients who are receiving absolutely good care. The third is highly prevalent in all care settings and patient groups. Here are three situations which might be classified differently according to the different definitions:

1. An older couple has a long tradition of bitter arguments. Hurtful remarks by each other are common and repetitive.
2. One partner asks for the tenth time in 2 hours whether they have had lunch yet today. The other responds sharply with the intention of discouraging further repetition of that question.
3. A bedbound patient with urinary frequency wears a diaper. The caregiver allows a certain interval of time to pass between diaper changes.

Each of these three interactions meets at least one of the definitions of elder abuse. How long a person may be left wet in a diaper, if there are no adverse medical consequences, before a finding of neglect should be made is a very complex question indeed.

Table 12.2 Common subtyping of abuse and neglect

Physical abuse
Social or mental abuse
Sexual abuse
Financial exploitation
Neglect
Self-neglect

Table 12.3 Some definitions related to elder abuse and additional resources

World Health Organization [6]: A single, or repeated act, or lack of appropriate action, occurring within any relationship where there is an expectation of trust which causes harm or distress to an older person
Administration for Community Living [7]: Any knowing, intentional, or negligent act by a caregiver or any other person that causes harm or a serious risk of harm to a vulnerable adult
Centers for Disease Control and Prevention [8]: An intentional act or failure to act that causes or creates a risk of harm to an older adult
National Research Council [9]: "Elder mistreatment" refers to (a) intentional actions that cause harm or create a serious risk of harm (whether or not harm is intended) to a vulnerable elder by a caregiver or other person who stands in a trust relationship to the elder or (b) failure by a caregiver to satisfy the elder's basic needs or to protect the elder from harm
American Bar Association [10]: A state-by-state summary of relevant definitions of abuse from the American Bar Association and state-by-state adult protective services reporting laws

Despite the lack of a serious definition, "elder abuse" is described as common, important, underdiagnosed, and underreported. A variety of laws have been passed, centers established, and guidelines promulgated—without consistent definition. Further, in 2018 the US Preventive Services Task Force "conclude(d) that the current evidence is insufficient to assess the balance of benefits and harms of screening for abuse and neglect in all older or vulnerable adults" [11]. They do not recommend screening.

Our failure to understand, diagnose, and prevent elder abuse is often attributed to a lack of research. An even more fundamental lack is a consensus definition on which to base the research. Homebound patients, often with high-level physical or mental disability or both, may require a great deal of long-term care in very difficult circumstances.

Questions of referral to Adult Protective Services Protective Services (APS) or consideration of guardianship are often more legal, tactical, medicolegal, and economic than they are medical, social, or ethical. Most states have mandatory reporting requirements for suspected abuse.

Because there are no data to suggest that referral to APS is more likely to help than to harm, clinicians in states with mandatory reporting of elder abuse are in an extremely difficult position. Involving the legal system in the care of a patient is difficult for many physicians, who are primarily interested in finding the optimal situation, both medical and social, for their patients. In addition, the clinician's duty to protect the patient's confidentiality is in direct conflict with this duty to report, unless the patient requests that the information be conveyed.

In addition to the social situation and historical clues, evidence of physical harm must be evaluated carefully. Home visits will usually provide a much richer picture of the situation. Adjustments in the home environment may suggest themselves on-site. Possible alternative sources or sites of care may be realistically considered while in the home. Questions such as "are you afraid you may be hurt at home?" or "is there anyone who is hurting you?" might be preferred to a question such as "do you feel safe at home?" since some people may interpret the use of the word "safe"

Table 12.4 Characteristics of patient, caregiver, or both associated with risk of elder abuse

High level of impairment and dependency with many care needs
Psychiatric illness and/or substance abuse
History of abusive relationships
Limited financial and/or social resources
Social isolation

to be a question about grab bars in the bathroom and smoke alarms in the kitchen. Table 12.4 shows characteristics of patients and caregivers that have been associated with elder abuse.

Neglect, sometimes included as a form of elder abuse and sometimes considered separately, is also difficult to define. Many caregivers, such as adult children, have no direct legal duty to the person for whom they care. If such caregivers, making the best of a bad situation, provide inadequate care by some test and are referred to APS, they may interpret the referral as a provocation and may then worsen the situation. If well done, in contrast, APS referral may work as a form of coaching, providing a new perspective and suggestions for improvement in a very cloistered situation.

However well intentioned, referral of a patient to APS is generally equivalent to an accusation. This allegation of abuse or neglect is often being made against the person who is providing the bulk of the patient's care. This may lead to discontinuation of the clinician-patient and perhaps the caregiver-patient relationship, thus leading ultimately to harm. Ideally, such referrals would be made with the patient's permission and the consent of the caregiver. It would be seen as a step toward improving situations which are overwhelming to the caregiver.

12.6 Advance Directives

For home-based medical care patients who have capacity, decisions about potentially life-sustaining treatment can be very difficult. Three things are generally true about most patients: They do not wish to suffer, they do not wish to die, and they do not wish to talk openly about the trade-offs. Each of these wishes becomes more apparent to patients as death comes nearer. In a questionnaire study, subjects without cancer were more likely to decline noncurative, toxic chemotherapy for an advanced cancer than subjects who had advanced cancer [12]. Fair evidence shows that clinicians and caregivers may underestimate a patient's quality of life and desire to accept aggressive treatment.

In a separate study, the majority of patients with metastatic colon or lung cancer taking chemotherapy did not understand that this therapy was very unlikely to be curative. Patients who rated their physician most favorably had the highest rate of misunderstanding. "Physicians may be able to improve patients' understanding, but this may come at the cost of patients' satisfaction with them" [13].

Seeing patients at home, clinicians may be more able to understand how a chronically ill patient is living and what the benefits and burdens of treatment might be. Because of the relationship's nature, they may be able to improve a patient's understanding without undermining the relationship. A study done in a home-based primary care program, however, showed that homebound patients with poor prognosis remain reluctant to participate in advance care planning, except when death is near and certain [14].

The right of a patient with capacity to decline treatment, even if it would be lifesaving, is reasonably well established in most cases. A far more complex, and legally less well-defined, question arises when a patient can no longer decline, or accept, such treatment. In an attempt to preserve autonomy when capacity is no longer present, two legal instruments have been devised. These intend to allow a competent patient to leave advice about how medical decisions should be made if the patient were to become incapacitated. In a living will, the patient leaves specific guidance about certain medical treatments that may be considered in the uncertain future. With a healthcare agent, the patient designates substitute decision-makers who are then authorized to make decisions on behalf of the patient.

The nomenclature can be confusing. In some states, "advance directives" are synonymous with "living wills," and "healthcare agents" are treated separately. In other states, "advance directive" is the umbrella term that includes both "living wills" and "healthcare agents." We will use the latter schema. A substitute decision-maker may be acting because the patient, previously competent, has designated his/her for this task. Some terms used by states to refer to the designated decision-maker include healthcare agent, healthcare proxy, healthcare representative, attorney in fact, healthcare surrogate, and patient advocate [15]. If no substitute decision-maker is designated, then a default decision-maker may be identified. Terms used to refer to this person are also quite variable and may overlap or directly contradict the terms used in other states [15].

To make matters worse, there is a great deal of variability among the states in the degree of authority that is granted to default substitutes compared to designated substitutes. In Virginia and Washington, DC, the default substitute has nearly as much authority as the designated substitute. Maryland tends to be much more restrictive in the authority of the default substitute. State-by-state advance directive forms are available online [16]. Because of their wide variability, clinicians should know the relevant specifics if they are engaging patients in these discussions.

12.6.1 Living Wills

In general, the discussion of the living will is a complex matter for a patient. The patient must keep these two hypothetical circumstances in mind. The clinician asks the patient to imagine both that the patient has become sick enough that decisions about life-sustaining treatments are needed and that they have become unable to make those decisions. The patient then makes a binding, but revocable, decision about which treatments they would decline or accept. One way to phrase this to the patient, very carefully, is to ask if there are conditions where the patient would rather be dead than accept treatment to try to prolong life.

Many clinicians can recall patients who have left advance directives to limit treatment (e.g., "I never want to be intubated again") but then change their minds and do not reject treatment when it would avert death.

A paper entitled "The End of History Illusion" raises further serious questions about the concept of advance directives. Based on measurements made on over 19,000 adults from age 18 to 68 years, the authors conclude that "Young people, middle-aged people, and older people all believed they had changed a lot in the past but would change relatively little in the future. People, it seems, regard the present as a watershed moment at which they have finally become the person they will be for the rest of their lives" [17]. If these subjects were reinterviewed 10 years later, they would presumably again report that they had changed greatly in the interim but would not change much in the future. Decisions about what would be worse than death might seem immutable at the time they are made and be highly inaccurate after some time has passed.

Perhaps because decisions like these may be so changeable, many states have strictly limited the situations in which living wills are valid. In several states, they refer only to treatment limitation in the event of terminal illness. In several, they are valid only if the patient is terminally ill or in a persistent vegetative state. Each state's designated categories should be carefully understood before completing a living will with a patient.

Advance care planning (ACP) about future events, as opposed to real-time medical decision-making, has been assumed to be essential for high-quality care when death is near. In contrast a series of good trials "could not identify meaningful differences in health care use, patient quality of life, or goal-concordant care between those randomly assigned to receive either ACP or usual care" [18].

12.6.2 Designated Substitute Decision-Maker

As noted above, the name for a substitute decision-maker who is designated by the patient varies greatly among jurisdictions (agent, representative, proxy, and surrogate, among others). Once again varying among jurisdictions, a substitute who has been designated is usually given a great deal of authority to make medical decisions on behalf of a patient who is no longer able to make their own decisions. In Maryland, the healthcare agent can make virtually any decision that the patient could make if the patient were still capable unless the signer has added restrictions to the document. An important exception is involuntary psychiatric treatment, which cannot be given on the basis of an agent's authorization. Other states place some restrictions on the authority of the agent to decline life-sustaining treatment. Finally, many states allow a patient to designate the substitute and grant decisional authority to that agent at the time the document is signed.

Designating a substitute decision-maker is generally a far simpler task cognitively than deciding about hypothetical treatment decisions during hypothetical future life-threatening illnesses in the context of a hypothetical incapacitating cognitive impairment, decisions which are often very difficult for a competent patient. In addition, the discussion about designating an agent probably has less emotional impact than the discussion required to complete a living will (imagine you have both advanced cancer and Alzheimer's disease). We suggest a discussion about healthcare agents, built around this question. "You know that if we need to make any decisions about treatment, we'll ask you how you would like things to be done. But let's say that something happened to you. Let's say you hit your head on the windshield and we couldn't talk to you. Who is it that we should talk to about your care?"

The formalities for recording advance directives vary from state to state. Some but not all require notarization. In many states, lawyers are not required. Repositories in which to store advance directives are available online, or a copy may be scanned into the electronic medical record. There is little published experience about their utility. We advise patients to give copies of the documents to their physician, the person(s) named as agent, and one or two other close friends.

12.7 Social Isolation and Loneliness

Approximately one in four community-dwelling older adults in the United States experiences social isolation [19], "the objective lack of (or limited) social contact with others" [20]. Estimates vary with varying definitions, but the "diagnosis" connotes that the individual is endangered or harmed by limited social connections. Being homebound increases the risk of being socially isolated, and socially isolated older adults are more likely to become homebound [21].

Social isolation is distinct from loneliness, "the perception of social isolation or "distress that results from discrepancies between ideal and perceived social relationships" [20], although definitions of "loneliness" also vary widely. Homebased primary care practitioners may be the major source, perhaps the only source, of connection for some of these older adults.

Isolation and loneliness are associated with a wide variety of illnesses and adverse outcomes [22], but confounding is likely. For example, the strong association between dementia and isolation may be due to reduced ability or desire to socialize or both. The association between dementia and isolation is strong, but this is not proof of causation, and strong evidence to identify interventions that improve real outcomes in this group of people is lacking. People who become isolated due to circumstances beyond their control will likely differ from those who seem to willfully isolate themselves, who may value medical intervention less than we would hope.

12.7.1 Assessing Social Isolation and Loneliness

Home-based medical care providers are well situated to identify individuals experiencing social isolation and loneliness. Several validated scales aim to quantify the presence of or risk for social isolation [23]. None of these scales has been validated in a population of homebound older adults with high morbidity burden and high prevalence of cognitive and functional impairment. The three-item UCLA Loneliness Scale was developed for use in telephone surveys as a shortened version of the Revised UCLA Loneliness Scale, a 20-item scale. The three-item scale is widely used in research and clinical settings [20].

Box 12.2 Three-Item UCLA Loneliness Scale [24]

Lead-in and questions are read to respondent.

The next questions are about how you feel about different aspects of your life. For each one, tell me how often you feel that way.

1. First, how often do you feel that you lack companionship: Hardly ever (1), some of the time (2), or often (3)?
2. How often do you feel left out: Hardly ever (1), some of the time (2), or often (3)?
3. How often do you feel isolated from others: Hardly ever (1), some of the time (2), or often (3)?

Scoring: Sum the total of all items. Higher scores indicate greater degrees of loneliness.

These scales can introduce a conversation about an individual's connectedness. Such conversations may help clinicians to understand an individual's emotional and instrumental supports and to design practical assistance, for example, organizing a plan about how to manage an emergency.

12.7.2 Approaches to Social Isolation and Loneliness in Home-Based Care

Realistic care plans to address social isolation and loneliness among recipients of home-based care depend on understanding an individual's circumstances. Socially isolated individuals are less likely to participate in advance care planning, and substitute decision-makers may be unavailable [25].

Because discussions about social isolation are often very personal, individuals who prize their privacy may feel questions about family and friends are intrusive and irrelevant to medical care. Presentation of the risks associated with social isolation should be factual and as nonthreatening as possible, and the focus should be on patient autonomy and shared problem-solving. Developing goals that are feasible and sustainable, practitioners benefit from a practical, working knowledge of local resources. Providing care to a socially isolated and homebound older adult poses a unique set of challenges. Without social connections to offer emotional, instrumental, and informational support, many of these needs may fall to the home-based primary care team.

A number of strategies and interventions have been studied to try to address social isolation and loneliness in older adults and have been analyzed in multiple systematic reviews, none of which have focused on homebound older adults [26–29]. The quality of studies in this area and evidence for efficacy is limited, given the complexity and individual nature of the problem; however, it is worth considering if any of these options might be things a patient or care partner could try.

Strategies include finding options outside the home for older adults who are willing, such as by attending day programs, senior centers, community groups, or religious services to interact with others. For older adults who cannot or are not willing to leave the home, other options can be considered. For instance, for those who have access to tablets or computers, technology can be used to connect older adults to others, such as through one-on-one connections, online social groups, support groups, or exercise classes [30]. Other interventions that have been studied include psychological therapies, animal therapy, befriending programs (one-on-one volunteer visits or telephone support) [31], and leisure or skill development [32]. Exploring potential connections to neighbors, people from religious organizations or shared cultural groups, or volunteers through programs such as hospice are other options. For older adults who need food assistance, studies suggest that Meals on Wheels provides social, as well as nutritional benefit from receiving meals [29]. Although the evidence base for these interventions is murky, interventions such as befriending programs and online support groups might be best suited for home-based care practices to consider developing.

Further study is needed to explore interventions for underserviced and marginalized groups of older adults, such as older adults identifying as LGBTQ+, indigenous seniors, non-English speakers, and new immigrants [32].

12.8 Conclusion

In an important essay, Broyard points out that "To most physicians my illness is a routine incident in their rounds, whilst for me it is the crisis of my life." In home-based medical care, the illness is neither routine nor an incident. The clinician has a far richer understanding of the patient's (and the caregiver's) situation. Decisions made in this context can more fully honor and respect the patient as a person [33].

References

1. Stone J. He makes a house call (internet). 2014. https://utmedhumanities.wordpress.com/2014/03/16/he-makes-a-house-call-john-stone/. Accessed 23 May 2023.
2. Faden RR, Beauchamp TL. A history and theory of informed consent. New York: Oxford University Press; 1986. Chapter 8.
3. Roth LH, Meisel A, Lidz CW. Tests of competency to consent to treatment. Am J Psychiatry. 1977;134(3):279–84.
4. Chow GV, Czarny MJ, Hughes MT, Carrese JA. CURVES: a mnemonic for determining medical decision-making capacity and providing emergency treatment in the acute setting. Chest. 2010;137(2):421–7. https://doi.org/10.1378/chest.09-1133.
5. Foster C. Putting dignity to work. Lancet. 2012;379(9831):2044–5.
6. Elder abuse: the health sector role in prevention and response (Internet). Geneva: World Health Organization; 2016. https://cdn.who.int/media/docs/default-source/ageing/ea-infographic-en-jun-18-web.pdf?sfvrsn=6dc7f167_2. Accessed 20 Jun 2023.
7. What is elder abuse? (Internet). Administration for Community Living. 2019. https://acl.gov/programs/elder-justice/what-elder-abuse. Accessed 20 Jun 2023.
8. Fast facts: preventing elder abuse (Internet). CDC. 2021. https://www.cdc.gov/violenceprevention/elderabuse/fastfact.html. Accessed 20 June 2023.
9. National Research Council (US). Panel to review risk and prevalence of elder abuse and neglect. In: Bonnie RJ, Wallace RB, editors. Elder mistreatment: abuse, neglect, and exploitation in an aging America. Washington, DC: National Academies Press (US); 2003.
10. American Bar Association Commission on Law and Aging. 2021. https://www.americanbar.org/content/dam/aba/administrative/law_aging/2020-abuse-definitions.pdf. Accessed 20 Jun 2023.
11. US Preventive Services Task Force, Curry SJ, Krist AH, Owens DK, Barry MJ, Caughey AB, Davidson KW, Doubeni CA, Epling JW Jr, Grossman DC, Kemper AR, Kubik M, Kurth A, Landefeld CS, Mangione CM, Silverstein M, Simon MA, Tseng CW, Wong JB. Screening for intimate partner violence, elder abuse, and abuse of vulnerable adults: US Preventive Services Task Force final recommendation statement. JAMA. 2018;320(16):1678–87.
12. Slevin ML, Stubbs L, Plant HJ, et al. Attitudes to chemotherapy: comparing views of patients with cancer with those of doctors, nurses, and general public. BMJ. 1990;300:1458–60.
13. Weeks JC, Catalano PJ, Cronin A, et al. Patients' expectations about effects of chemotherapy for advanced cancer. N Engl J Med. 2012;367(17):1616–25.
14. Carrese JA, Mullaney JL, Faden R, et al. Planning for death but not serious future illness: qualitative study of housebound elderly patients. BMJ. 2002;325(7356):125.
15. Mathew S, Gershengorn HB, Hua M. Terminology for surrogate decision making varies widely by state. J Palliat Med. 2018;21(8):1060–1.
16. CaringInfo. A program of the National Hospice and Palliative Care Organization. https://www.caringinfo.org/planning/advance-directives/by-state/. Accessed 20 Jun 2023.
17. Quoidbach J, Gilbert DT, Wilson TD. The end of history illusion. Science. 2013;339(6115):96–8.
18. Morrison RS, Meier DE, Arnold RM. What's wrong with advance care planning? JAMA. 2021;326(16):1575–6. https://doi.org/10.1001/jama.2021.16430. PMID: 34623373; PMCID: PMC9373875.
19. Cudjoe TK, Roth DL, Szanton SL, Wolff JL, Boyd CM, Thorpe RJ Jr. The epidemiology of social isolation: national health and aging trends study. J Gerontol Ser B. 2020;75(1):107–13.
20. National Academies of Sciences, Engineering, and Medicine. Social isolation and loneliness in older adults: opportunities for the health care system. Washington, DC: National Academies Press; 2020.
21. Cudjoe TK, Prichett L, Szanton SL, Roberts Lavigne LC, Thorpe RJ Jr. Social isolation, homebound status, and race among older adults: findings from the National Health and aging trends study (2011–2019). J Am Geriatr Soc. 2022;70:2093.

22. Jawaid A. Protecting older adults during social distancing. Science. 2020;368(6487):145. https://doi.org/10.1126/science.abb7885.
23. Donovan NJ, Blazer D. Social isolation and loneliness in older adults: review and commentary of a National Academies Report. Am J Geriatr Psychiatry. 2020;28(12):1233–44.
24. Hughes ME, Waite LJ, Hawkley LC, Cacioppo JT. A short scale for measuring loneliness in large surveys: results from two population-based studies. Res Aging. 2004;26(6):655–72.
25. Cudjoe TKM, et al. Advance care planning: social isolation matters. J Am Geriatr Soc. 2020;68(4):841–6.
26. Galvez-Hernandez P, González-de Paz L, Muntaner C. Primary care-based interventions addressing social isolation and loneliness in older people: a scoping review. BMJ Open. 2022;12(2):e057729.
27. Fakoya OA, McCorry NK, Donnelly M. Loneliness and social isolation interventions for older adults: a scoping review of reviews. BMC Public Health. 2020;20(1):129.
28. Courtin E, Knapp M. Social isolation, loneliness and health in old age: a scoping review. Health Soc Care Community. 2017;25(3):799–812.
29. Thomas KS, Gadbois EA, Shield RR, Akobundu U, Morris AM, Dosa DM. "It's not just a simple meal. It's so much more": interactions between meals on wheels clients and drivers. J Appl Gerontol. 2020;39(2):151–8.
30. Gadbois EA, Jimenez F, Brazier JF, Davoodi NM, Nunn AS, Mills WL, Dosa D, Thomas KS. Findings from talking tech: a technology training pilot intervention to reduce loneliness and social isolation among homebound older adults. Innov Aging. 2022;6(5):igac040.
31. Fakoya OA, McCorry NK, Donnelly M. How do befriending interventions alleviate loneliness and social isolation among older people? A realist evaluation study. PLoS One. 2021;16(9):e0256900.
32. Freedman A, Nicolle J. Social isolation and loneliness: the new geriatric giants: approach for primary care. Can Fam Physician. 2020;66(3):176–82.
33. Broyard A. Doctor talk to me. New York Times. Accessed 26 Aug 1990.

Chapter 13
Palliative Care

Christine S. Ritchie and Martha L. Twaddle

13.1 Emerging Models of Home-Based Palliative Care

With an increasing recognition that many individuals with serious illness will experience high illness burden and functional challenges for years and not just months, home-based palliative care (HBPalC) is emerging as an important component of home-based medical care that presages and complements services provided by hospice and can serve as a useful adjunct to home-based primary care [1]. A number of HBPalC models are filling the landscape of community-based care. The most common models fall into the following categories: HBPalC programs that are part of the continuum with hospital-based palliative care programs, HBPalC programs as a subset of home-based primary care programs, stand-alone consultative HBPalC programs, payer-based combined primary/palliative care, or palliative care programs provided by hospices and functioning outside of the traditional hospice benefit.

There is significant overlap between home-based primary care and HBPalC (see Fig. 13.1). Practically speaking, because of the relatively poor prognosis and high symptom burden of many patients seen in home-based primary care, all home-based primary care practices must be practicing *primary palliative care* (see Table 13.1). However, for patients with particularly refractory pain or other symptoms; complex depression, anxiety, or grief; existential distress; or needs for assistance with

C. S. Ritchie (✉)
Division of Palliative Care and Geriatric Medicine, Department of Medicine, Harvard Medical School, Massachusetts General Hospital, Boston, MA, USA
e-mail: csritchie@mgh.harvard.edu

M. L. Twaddle
Palliative Medicine, Northwestern University Feinberg School of Medicine, Chicago, IL, USA
e-mail: martha.twaddle@northwestern.edu

J. L. Colburn et al. (eds.), *Geriatric Home-Based Medical Care*,
https://doi.org/10.1007/978-3-031-68786-0_13

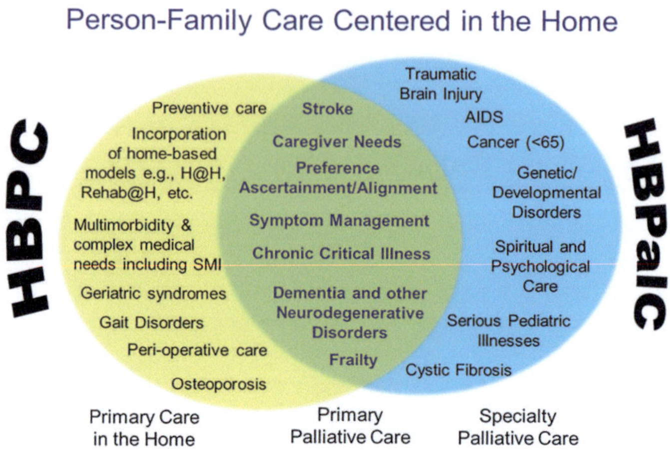

Fig. 13.1 Homecare medicine and palliative care: skills and settings

Table 13.1 Primary palliative care

Key components of primary palliative care
Pain/symptom assessment and management
Social/spiritual assessment
Understanding of and communication around illness/prognosis
Identification of patient-centered goals of care

conflict resolution around goals or methods of treatment, the provision of specialty palliative care in the home is essential to provide quality care.

Specialty palliative care involves healthcare professionals certified in hospice and palliative care. By definition, palliative care promotes an interprofessional approach that requires the active collaboration of medicine, nursing, and social work along with a combination of other disciplines such as mental health, pharmacy, and spiritual care as indicated [2, 3]. Specialist palliative care providers work in two ways: first, by providing direct care to patients and their families, and second, by providing consultative support to primary care or other specialty providers (as a consultant in the home or clinic) and enhancing and supporting their care of the patient and family. The critical competencies for HBPalC include the ability to manage complex and refractory symptoms, prognosticate, recognize the signs and symptoms of approaching death, address and help coordinate the associated care and support needs of patients and their families before and after the death, and support bereavement.

Palliative care does not lend itself well to fee-for-service payment models. The nature of the care provided is often time-intensive and involves team members who traditionally have no or limited direct insurance reimbursement mechanisms for their time and expertise (such as social work and chaplaincy). It is most effective (and has been best adopted) in integrated healthcare systems where care is value driven. In this payment model, optimizing care in the home for individuals with serious illness can demonstrate improved patient and caregiver-centered outcomes while at the same time reduce the unnecessary suffering and added cost of care incurred in more expensive hospital or institutional settings.

13.2 Home-Based Palliative Care Outcomes

By and large, studies of HBPalC demonstrate reduction in acute care use and overall costs [4]. A randomized study of outpatient palliative care in lung cancer patients demonstrated better quality of life, improved survival of almost 3 months, and reduction of utilization across the entire course of illness [5]. An RCT of a HBPalC also demonstrated improved satisfaction, fewer hospital and emergency department visits, and lower costs [6]. A study in Canada of HBPalC demonstrated reduced hospitalizations and more days at home [7]. A propensity-matched study of home vs. hospital-based palliative care also suggested longer survival rates for those receiving HBPalC with a recognition that residual confounding may have explained some of these differences [8]. While fewer studies have demonstrated individual level benefits in symptoms and quality of life, mixed-methods analyses suggest value in these domains as well [9].

13.3 Key Processes of Care in HBPalC

13.3.1 Elucidation of Goals of Care and Treatment Preferences

Key elements of person-centered care include eliciting care goals and treatment preferences. This exploration naturally leads to the development of a care plan that aligns with patient and family values. Care goals are dynamic in nature and deeply contextualized by patients' personal definition of what constitutes meaning and significance, their cultural and social framework, their experience of illness, and the priority they place on certain health outcomes. Providers must become adept at eliciting and understanding patient and caregiver values and goals, recognizing that these goals will shift over time as their illnesses progress and/or what is important to them reprioritizes. A number of tools are available to elicit patient and caregiver values and goals. The questions in Table 13.2 offer examples of questions that can be used to better understand patients' values and goals.

Table 13.2 Useful questions to elicit patients' values and goals for care

What are the most important things in your life now?
What do you hope for?
What are your fears? Are there things about your current situation that worry you?
What do you understand about your condition and your overall health?
How much information about your condition do you find helpful? How much detail do you like or do you prefer to have me speak to your (daughter, son, husband, wife, or friend) about these issues?
If you become sicker, how much are you willing to go through for the possibility of gaining more time?
How much does your family understand about what is important to you and your wishes for your treatment?

13.3.2 Prognostication

Along with communication skills, the ability to prognosticate is one of the most important skills of those involved in the care of the very ill and one of the critical competencies in generalist and specialty level palliative care [10, 11]. Providing a time frame and, when necessary, conveying a sense of urgency considering limited life expectancy allow patients and families to make informed decisions as to how their time will be spent and the opportunity to prioritize activities and treatment plans. The skill of prognostication requires knowledge of the typical trajectories of illness and insight as to the implications of physical signs and symptoms of illness as they manifest alongside and are impacted by the psychosocial and spiritual dynamics of the individual and their family. The provider must be familiar with the evidence from the literature and be able to gather complete information in a patient assessment including exploring the psychosocial and spiritual aspects of the individual and family. The complex thinking and decision-making skills involved in prognostication also rely heavily on the wisdom honed from clinical experience. Most importantly, the ability to communicate prognosis to a patient and family is a critical skill to know, because of culture, religion, or patient/family preferences what to convey, how, and to whom. Table 13.3 provides a few considerations when engaging in conversations around prognosis.

13.4 Physical Aspects of Care Including Symptom and Safety Issues

13.4.1 Common Symptoms in the Home

Patients for whom home is the optimal setting for care delivery most often have advanced or complex illnesses coupled with significant functional impairment or disability. These individuals often experience a significant symptom burden as a

Table 13.3 Considerations when providing prognostic information

Find out what the patient/caregiver understands about the illness and their general sense about how things are going, e.g., "What is your understanding of your current health situation?"
Find out what kind of information the patient/caregiver desires, e.g., "How much do you want to know?" "Are you the kind of person that likes to hear numbers and facts or do you prefer more general information?"
Provide information while acknowledging limitations of prognostic estimations, e.g., "Every person is different. What usually happens to someone in your situation is..."
Avoid specific numbers and use time ranges, instead use time frames, e.g., "days to weeks," "weeks to months," etc.
Check for understanding, e.g., "What is your understanding of what we have discussed?"
Acknowledge and support the expression of emotion, e.g., "It sounds like you are upset/concerned/sad…"

result of their underlying diagnoses and comorbidities. Managing symptoms in the home setting presents unique challenges, particularly if symptoms are dynamic, rapidly escalate, or require intravenous medications for effective relief. In a study of 318 adults followed by a home-based medical care program, 43% reported severe burden from one or more symptoms. The symptoms with the highest level of severity were depression, pain, appetite, and shortness of breath [12]. We briefly discuss management of these four most prevalent symptoms.

13.4.2 Depression

Depressive symptoms are prevalent in patients with advanced, life-threatening illnesses with up to 42% experiencing depression at the end of life. Depression may be an indication of inadequately managed symptoms; therefore, addressing pain, dyspnea, and other symptoms as part of the overall treatment strategy is a key first step to addressing depressive symptoms.

Very few pharmacologic studies have been conducted that address depression in advanced illness; consequently, therapeutic recommendations do not differ greatly between palliative and non-palliative patients. For patients with advanced illness, three factors influence choice of antidepressants (see Table 13.4): (1) the time frame for treatment, (2) concurrent medical conditions, and (3) pharmacologic properties of the drug.

With respect to time frame for treatment, patients with a life expectancy of several months may benefit from a selective serotonin reuptake inhibitor (SSRI) or tricyclic antidepressants (TCA) as long as the need for immediate onset of action is not present. The European Association for Palliative Care recommends mirtazapine, sertraline, and citalopram as reasonable considerations for first-line therapy. For those who are weeks to a few short months from death, psychostimulants such as methylphenidate and modafinil offer more immediate onset within 24–48 h of initiation of therapy [13]. Concurrent medical conditions also guide therapy. For those

Table 13.4 Considerations for pharmacologic treatment for depression in advanced illness

Antidepressant type	Time frame for treatment	Concurrent medical conditions	Comments
Tricyclic antidepressants, e.g., nortriptyline	≥2 weeks	May be useful in setting of peripheral neuropathy	Greater risk for overdose Can prolong the QTc interval Can contribute to orthostatic hypotension
Selective serotonin reuptake inhibitor, e.g., sertraline	4–6 weeks[a]	Different agents may have more activating or sedating effect; tailor to patient symptoms	Can cause serotonin syndrome; use care when using in combination with trazodone or other agents affecting serotonin metabolism
Tetracyclic antidepressant, e.g., mirtazapine	1–2 weeks	Reasonable in heart failure and diabetes May increase anticoagulant effect of warfarin	May increase appetite May reduce nausea Sedative effect may be beneficial for some Caution for serotonin syndrome in older adults
Psychostimulants, e.g., methylphenidate	24–48 h		Caution in heart disease or cognitive disturbances (e.g., delirium)

[a]One-third of the overall effect of selective serotonin reuptake inhibitors (SSRIs) after 6 weeks of treatment is seen in the first week [15]

with a history of seizure disorder, bupropion should be avoided. For those with chronic pain, antidepressants that also have a positive impact on pain (such as venlafaxine and duloxetine) should be considered. Relevant pharmacologic properties of antidepressants include availability of liquid formulation and side effects of the medication. Antidepressants that are available in liquid formulation (for when swallowing pills becomes more difficult) include fluoxetine, sertraline, paroxetine, citalopram, escitalopram, doxepin, and nortriptyline. Side effects such as orthostatic hypotension, dizziness, constipation, and prolonged corrected QT (QTc) interval tend to be most pronounced with TCA. Weight gain can be a potentially positive side effect of SSRI and mirtazapine and is, at times, a desired outcome. Sedation is also common with mirtazapine and trazodone and may be beneficial to patients with insomnia and depression, whereas agents with more activating properties (psychostimulants, SSRI) may be a side effect that is more beneficial to those with fatigue or psychomotor slowing [14].

Nonpharmacologic therapy includes supportive psychotherapy and existential therapy.

Supportive psychotherapy involves supporting adaptive coping mechanisms and minimizing emotional reactions such as shame and self-loathing that contribute to distress. Existential therapy often focuses on self-worth and self-determination in the context of increasing loss of control. Common forms of existential therapy include dignity therapy, therapeutic life review, and meaning-centered psychotherapy. Dignity therapy, a brief individualized psychotherapeutic intervention targeted at psychosocial and existential distress, has been shown to increase dignity, purpose, and meaning and reduce depressive symptoms [16, 17]. Dignity therapy can be provided by a social worker or trained volunteer. The questions commonly used in dignity therapy to elicit better understanding of patient/caregiver needs can be easily adapted to the home setting [18]. A useful overview question is "What do I need to know about you as a person to give you the best care possible?" Other related questions include many listed in Table 13.2 and questions to elicit other appropriate avenues for social and spiritual support: "Who else should we get involved to help you through this difficult/challenging time?"

13.4.3 Pain

Pain is a common symptom experienced by individuals with serious or life-limiting illness, regardless of the underlying etiology. Pain is multidimensional in nature and can be exacerbated by depression, existential distress, and psychosocial circumstances. Because of the complex nature of pain, careful assessment is needed to optimally characterize pain, determine, if possible, the cause of each type of pain being experienced, and base management on the nature of the pain. Key elements of pain that ideally should be elucidated include character, location, frequency, relieving and aggravating factors of the pain, response to previous medication and treatment, and severity.

Pharmacologic pain management includes opioids, nonopioid analgesics (including acetaminophen), and nonsteroidal anti-inflammatory drugs (Table 13.5). Nonpharmacologic management may include guided imagery, transcutaneous electrical nerve stimulation (often facilitated through home physical therapy), therapeutic exercise, and treatments often considered alternative or complementary, such as acupuncture, massage, and other mind-body approaches.

13.4.4 Loss of Appetite

Appetite is affected by illness, drugs, dementia, and mood disorders. In a study of older adults from assisted living facilities or senior centers, decreased emotional well-being was most closely associated with poor appetite, highlighting the need to assess for and address depression [19]. Often, loss of appetite for patients with life-limiting illnesses such as metastatic cancer or end-stage heart failure is a prognostic indication that the patient's condition is advanced. In these instances, helping caregivers be comfortable with the patient's reduced interest in eating and offering ways the caregiver can demonstrate love and affirmation other than through food are the most straightforward approach to manage loss of appetite.

Table 13.5 Considerations for pharmacologic treatment of pain in advanced illness

Analgesic type	Concurrent medical conditions	Common adverse effects	Comments	Starting dose	Usual effective dose (maximal daily dose)
Acetaminophen	Caution in liver disease and in advanced age	Can cause nausea Most side effects relate to impact on liver: itching, loss of appetite, dark urine, clay-colored stools	Narrow dosing window Caution in accounting for presence of acetaminophen in many OTC meds	650 mg q4h to 500 mg q6h	2–3 g/d (4 g)
Nonsteroidal anti-inflammatory agents	Caution in heart failure, kidney disease, hypertension, history of GI bleed, and advanced age	Gastrointestinal bleeding Renal impairment and acute renal failure Salt and water retention Bronchial spasm/asthma Cardiovascular risk	Misoprostol or proton pump inhibitors reduce risk for GI bleeding; consider topical over systemic formulations	Ibuprofen OTC: 200 mg q8h Rx: 400 mg q6–8h Naproxen Sodium: OTC:220 mg q12h Rx: 250 mg q6–8h	Ibuprofen: 400–800 mg q6–8h (3200 mg) Naproxen Sodium: OTC: 440–660 mg q12h Rx: 250–500 mg q8–12 (1000 mg)

(continued)

Table 13.5 (continued)

Analgesic type	Concurrent medical conditions	Common adverse effects	Comments	Starting dose	Usual effective dose (maximal daily dose)
Tramadol	Dose reductions necessary in older adults, renal impairment, and end-stage liver failure	Nausea and constipation common lightheadedness, dizziness, drowsiness, or headache	Lowers seizure threshold Can cause hypoglycemia Risk for serotonin syndrome if provided concomitantly with serotonergic medications	12.5–25 mg q4–6h	Variable (variable)
Opioids	Avoid morphine in renal insufficiency (note that in persons of advanced age, creatinine may overestimate glomerular filtration rate)	Sedation, nausea, and itching are common and often resolve Constipation does not resolve with time and requires prophylactic bowel stimulants or osmotic agents	Once total daily dose established from short-acting agents, long-acting agent can be considered. Transdermal patch formulations should not be offered as first-line treatment until opioid dosing needs are known	Oxycodone immediate release: 2.5–5 mg q4–6h	Oxycodone immediate release: 5–10 mg q4–6h

For those who are not in the final stages of life, simple approaches to treat loss of appetite include removing dietary restrictions, supplementing intake by increasing the protein and calorie density of food, and considering nutritional supplements. Protein intake can be supplemented by adding milk powder, whey protein, dried peanut butter powder, egg whites, or tofu to food. Caloric density can be enhanced by adding olive or grape seed oil to sauces, fresh or cooked vegetables, and grains or pasta. Multiple small meals are often preferred over fewer large meals. The value of nutritional supplements in frail older adults remains controversial, but they appear most beneficial in older adults with evidence of undernutrition and are reasonable to consider as a time-limited trial. The three most common appetite stimulants used for anorexia include megestrol acetate, dronabinol, and mirtazapine. Megestrol acetate has been demonstrated to increase quality of life in patients with cancer and in nursing home residents. However, weight gain is not sustained, and megestrol acetate can worsen heart failure, impair function of the corticoadrenal axis, and increase incidence of deep venous thrombosis and as such should be used cautiously [20]. Dronabinol has been shown to improve appetite in patients with AIDS, and one small study has shown benefit in advanced dementia; however, it has significant CNS side effects and therefore has not been widely used in older adults [21]. As noted above, mirtazapine is more likely than other antidepressants to stimulate appetite and lead to weight gain and therefore is often considered in the setting of anorexia. Studies in nursing homes and in cancer patients with anorexia, however, have not shown conclusive benefit [22, 23].

Decisions regarding enteral nutrition at the end of life should be consistent with treatment goals and patient preference. With the exception of head and neck cancer and esophageal cancer, no studies have demonstrated improved survival in cancer or advanced dementia with enteral support. In advanced dementia, careful spoon-feeding, allowing adequate time for feeding, avoiding distractions, and using verbal cueing are optimal.

13.4.5 Dyspnea

Dyspnea is common in the setting of advanced illness. Like with pain, characteristics of dyspnea and potential causes should be part of the initial and ongoing assessment. Common modalities that also can be effective include the use of a fan, breathing techniques, mindfulness and relaxation, anxiety management, and energy conservation. Breathing techniques that can reduce the sensation of dyspnea include pursed lip breathing, prolonged exhalation, and posture modification. Evidence from randomized controlled trials suggests that a simple fan can reduce feelings of breathlessness and improve physical activity in patients with advanced illness [24]. In addition to mindfulness and relaxation, guided imagery and distraction strategies (e.g., music, TV, reading by self or caregiver) can be beneficial. Morphine and other opioids can mitigate the sensation of breathlessness and often reduce dyspnea at much lower doses than are required to address pain.

13.4.6 Medication Safety

The practice of safe prescribing and administration differs in the home compared to the institutional setting. For example, in the home it is the patient themselves or a non-healthcare professional who is most often assessing the symptom burden in real time and dispensing the medication prescribed for relief. Education and the regular review of the safety issues involved in the storage and utilization of medications in the home are an important area of focus for visiting healthcare professionals. Each home visit ideally includes a review of the medications and a check as to where they are stored, how the safe disposal of used and unused, topical medications or needles is handled, and whether any family members, especially children, could be at risk because of the medications. Unfortunately, it is not unusual to have issues with the misuse of medications in the home setting, including diversion by the patient themselves or other people in the household or outsiders having access to the medications. These issues may range from misuse such as the patient taking medications for reasons other than for which it was prescribed (such as medicating anxiety with pain medication) to family members taking the medications or patient/family selling the prescribed medications. Home-based medical providers must assess the risk before prescribing, as well as pay careful attention to utilization and refill patterns. For patients receiving medications such as opioids or benzodiazepines, a medication "contract" with the patient is ideally a routine part of practice. This would include only one clinician prescribing the medication at anticipated intervals with no refills/reissues after hours and on weekends and ideally one pharmacy dispensing. When misuse becomes evident, the medication, amount dispensed, or delivery route may need to be altered to enhance compliance and safety without sacrificing symptom control. Unfortunately, in cases where diversion is discovered, the patient/family must be notified that the physician or practitioner is no longer able to prescribe unless the issue can be securely corrected [25].

13.4.7 General Safety Issues in Advanced Illness

In addition to the safety issues related to medication, general safety in the home is always of concern. Given the correlation of functional impairment with advanced complex illness, the home-based medical provider should routinely assess for general patient safety with each visit. Issues may include the safe use of oxygen with patients who continue to smoke, the risk of falls with the presence of oxygen tubing, electrical cords, throw rugs, and uneven or poorly lit surfaces. Safety in the bathroom includes assessing for presence for or need for assistance devices such as handrails, bath benches, and perhaps an elevated toilet seat with sidebars. Reviewing how the patient navigates their home, how they exit and enter, and whether they are still driving despite advanced illness and impairment is vitally important. Here the interdisciplinary team of palliative care is particularly helpful as team members are available to help secure such resources as additional help in the home, assistance devices, food delivery, and transportation.

13.5 Psychosocial Aspects of Care in the Home

A number of psychosocial factors influence quality of life for patients with serious illness along with their caregivers. Environmental and social resources and constraints include the patient's home and the ability of the patient's home to accommodate his/her physical needs, the patient's neighborhood, and built environment. Perceived or real discrimination, negative life events, high illness burden, and multiple comorbidities can be major sources of difficulty, while religious involvement and social support are often protective. Involving social work and pastoral care early can reduce both patient and caregiver distress.

13.6 Hospice Care

Over 1500 years ago, hospices emerged as places of "hospitality" for travelers on pilgrimage throughout the Middle East. These places of safety evolved into the early hospitals of Europe, most often operated and staffed by religious orders. Dame Cicely Saunders of Great Britain, trained as a nurse, social worker, and then as a physician, is recognized as the creator of the modern concept of hospice care. She pioneered the application of the scientific approach to the care of the dying, establishing many of the current best practices of palliative medicine including the control of pain via around-the-clock administration of analgesic therapy. Hospice entered the United States in 1974 under the guidance of Florence Wald, PhD, Dean of the Graduate School of Nursing at Yale University. Working in consultation with Dame Saunders, Dean Wald opened the Connecticut Hospice in New Haven 1974. This introduction of hospice care model into the United States was a significant shift from the British model as it emphasized care in the home, a model that is most common within the United States to this day [26].

13.6.1 Hospice as a Part of Healthcare

Hospice is a highly developed form of palliative care within the continuum and has been supported for over 30 years by defined insurance benefits, beginning with the United States Congress authorizing the Medicare Hospice Benefit (MHB) in 1986. The MHB, through the *Conditions of Participation* [27], addresses the types of services provided within hospice care, the persons eligible to elect the benefit, and the payment system that supports the care. Hospice programs secure Medicare certification by demonstrating compliance with these federal regulations and may thus receive reimbursement for patient care from Medicare. Medicaid and commercial insurance programs generally mimic the MHB, with some variability in the levels of hospice care provided. To elect hospice care and receive reimbursement under the MHB, a patient must be deemed "terminally ill" or having a prognosis of 6 months or less if the illness follows a typical course. This initial certification of the terminal illness is the responsibility of the hospice medical director (HMD) along with patient's attending physician, if they have one.

13.6.2 The Medicare Hospice Benefit

The Hospice Medicare Benefit is divided into benefit periods, initially two 90-day periods followed by an unlimited number of 60-day increments. Each benefit period requires the hospice medical director to recertify and document in narrative form the patient's eligibility as to prognosis and goals of care. The MHB requires and covers four levels of care: routine home care (RHC), general inpatient (GIP), respite, and continuous care, which is also referred to as crisis care. More than 90% of the hospice care delivered in the United States is provided in the patient's home via RHC, which increasingly includes the settings of long-term care and assisted living. The levels of care are described in Table 13.6.

13.6.3 Hospice Care Financing

The MHB is one of the original capitated reimbursement programs. The CMS determines the adjusted cap amount and works through Medicare administrative contractors (MACs) to distribute the funds for hospice services. Individual hospices submit their claims to their assigned MAC to receive reimbursement for care provided. Hospice is reimbursed through a flat per diem, which varies with the level of care. With the RHC per diem rate of roughly 150 dollars, the hospice program is responsible to provide the professional care of skilled nurses, social workers, chaplains, and therapists and the involvement of a physician as a hospice medical director in an interdisciplinary team structure. The per diem also covers all the medications, therapies, and procedures related to the hospice prognosis and any durable medical equipment necessary to care for the patient. The MHB also specifically calls for the involvement of volunteers to provide support to the patient and family.

Saunder's original hospice model and the current hospice financial model are based on the trajectory of illness in an anticipated prognosis of cancer patients. Despite significant advances in oncology treatment, the estimated survival for oncology patients with an Eastern Cooperative Oncology Group (ECOG) functional status of 3–4 who are no longer receiving disease-modifying treatments is still

Table 13.6 Levels of hospice care

General inpatient (GIP)	Provides support for short-term inpatient care to meet the needs of hospice patients for pain control or acute or chronic symptom management, which cannot be safely and effectively managed in other settings
Continuous (crisis) care	Continuous (nursing) home care is provided during brief periods of crisis as necessary to maintain the terminally ill patient at home
Respite care	Provides a short-term (5-day) facility stay for the patient so as to facilitate caregiver respite
Routine home care	Hospice care in the home setting (LTC, ALF, group home, or private residence)

around 3–4 months [28]. As more patients with multiple significant comorbidities access hospice care at the end of life, the prognosis of complex illness is less predictable, and the time spent in hospice care may vary widely. In 2020, the average length of stay on hospice was 97 days, with a median length of stay of 18 days and 10% of patients enrolled for more than 287 day [29].

13.6.4 Challenges in Hospice Care

Although Medicare-certified hospice programs are regulated by the Conditions of Participation, there is variation in the care models they provide. Some have very active engagement of their physicians as specialists in palliative medicine; others have physician involvement limited to the administrative role of a medical director, and these physicians may have no specialty level training in the field. Likewise, hospices vary as to the interventions and supports they provide for patients. Some will accept patients into their programs that are receiving oral chemotherapy, inotrope infusions, radiation therapy, or recurrent blood transfusions; others will not. Some require patients to have a "do not resuscitate" status; others do not. Most importantly, patients and their families and the referring physician should ideally inquire as to the care model practiced by hospice programs and the role of the hospice physician in the plan of care.

13.6.5 The Physician Role in Hospice Care

The physician has distinct roles in hospice care. As a hospice medical director (HMD), the physician is responsible for the written certification and recertification of the eligibility of the patient to access their hospice benefit. This responsibility is always provided in conjunction with input from the interdisciplinary team, but only a physician may serve as a hospice medical director and certify or recertify eligibility for the patient to use their benefit. The hospice medical director is also responsible for the medical plan of care, along with the patient's attending physician, if they have one. The HMD typically has responsibilities in areas such as quality improvement, pharmacy oversight, and ethics as well as others. Only a physician of medicine or osteopathy may serve as a hospice medical director.

The attending physician or attending of record (AOR) is often a doctor of medicine or osteopathy and is identified by the individual, at the time he or she elects to receive hospice care, as having the most significant role in the determination and delivery of the individual's medical care. The hospice medical director may serve as the attending physician when necessary and when requested by the patient at the time of election of the hospice benefit. A nurse practitioner or a physician assistant may also serve at the AOR, although he/she may not serve as a hospice medical director nor provide certification of terminal illness.

As of 2011, every hospice patient must have a face-to-face encounter to reassess their ongoing clinical picture and whether it supports continued eligibility. This face-to-face is either provided by a hospice nurse practitioner or a hospice physician and must occur prior to their third and all subsequent benefit periods. These visits, although clinical in scope, are administrative in nature and are covered as part of the RHC per diem. The purpose of these visits is not to certify eligibility but to document the clinic status of the patient and provide that information to the interdisciplinary team and to the certifying HMD. If a medical issue is identified during a face-to-face visit, these may be separately documented and billed; however, a nurse practitioner may only bill and receive reimbursement under the HMB if he/she is the AOR.

Hospice patients frequently have complex medical conditions and benefit greatly from regular physician follow-up in the home. These visits are coded and billed in the usual and customary fashion but may require the attachment of modifiers depending on which physician sees the patient and for what medical problem. The modifiers are as follows:

GV Modifier—used by the AOR when seeing the hospice patient for issues related to their hospice diagnoses. In this case, the AOR is not employed or under contract by the hospice.

GW Modifier—Used by the AOR as well as the hospice physician when seeing the patient for issues unrelated to their hospice diagnosis.

Consulting physicians—clinicians who are not the AOR for a patient must be under contract with the hospice to bill and receive reimbursement for patient care. If the patient wishes to continue to see their cardiologist or oncologist while in hospice care and that individual is not the AOR, the physician must establish a consulting contract with the hospice before the visit. The consulting physician then must submit their bills to the hospice and the hospice bills on their behalf and reimburses them as per the contractual arrangement [30]. In home-based medical care, patients may be referred to hospice through their office-based oncologist or other specialist but practically benefit from having their home-based physician or nurse practitioner serve as the attending of record.

13.7 Ethical and Legal Aspects of Care in the Home

Given the advanced state of illness providers typically confront when caring for people in home-based primary and palliative care, advanced care planning becomes a more pressing priority and immediate in its necessity. Despite sometimes living for years with functional limitations and chronic complex illness, these patients, like the greater population, are unlikely to have communicated actionable directives as to the intensity of healthcare interventions that they would prefer. Meeting with people and their families in the home is an ideal location for these discussions as the patient is in a less vulnerable environment to explore goals of care and care preferences. In addition, the time spent in a home visit is typically longer than that in the ambulatory setting such that these conversations may have more time to evolve. Likewise the setting more naturally lends itself to patient-centered discussions of meaning and value as there may be present many physical cues to initiate or bridge to these discussions—such as pictures of family members, mementos of life achievements, or evidence of hobbies and interests. Ideally, advance care planning is a series of conversations over time that starts with authentic interest in what matters most to the patient and to their family and how their priorities are impacted and informed by their health conditions.

The culmination of these discussions of "what matters most" is to create an actionable directive that can be honored by healthcare professionals. First and foremost, every patient needs to designate a decision-maker to speak for them in the event they are unable to communicate their preferences. This individual is often a family member but does not have to be. Ideally, the person identified as the surrogate decision-maker is an individual who can support and advocate for the preferences and directives of the patient. Surrogate decision-makers who are not aligned with the patient care preferences may experience significant stress in the role or seek to redirect interventions to care goals that are inconsistent with the patient's stated or implied preferences. The home-based medical care provider has a unique opportunity to counsel patients and families to identify a surrogate decision-maker who understands and supports the patient's goals of care and furthermore to support and educate the surrogate when they must assume the responsibility.

It is imperative that the home-based medical provider is knowledgeable as to the state laws that govern the identification and documentation of who serves as the surrogate decision-maker or healthcare power of attorney. Documentation of the care preferences of individuals can take several forms and may be identified by several different labels such as Living Wills, 5Wishes, Ethical Wills, etc. These care preference documents may be very helpful when they exist but are not actionable documents—meaning that emergency medical personnel called to the home cannot utilize a healthcare directive such as a Living Will to guide or, in any way, modify emergency interventions.

Increasingly, states are adopting documents based on the Physician Orders for Life-Sustaining Treatment or POLST [31]. The POLST paradigm was initiated in Oregon by several medical ethicists in 1991 as a means to better honor the advance directives and end-of-life preferences of patients and families. POLST has been steadily adopted and adapted by other states throughout the United States by aligning with the local legal, medical, and cultural contexts and has been renamed in some settings as Physician Order for Scope of Treatment (POST), Medical Orders for Life-Sustaining Treatment (MOLST), and Medical Orders for Scope of Treatment (MOST). State law authorizes certain healthcare professionals to sign medical orders, and these individuals may also sign a POLST document.

POLST is not for everyone and is not an advance directive [32]. It does not replace the designation of the healthcare power of attorney. POLST is indicated for people with serious advanced illness and limited life expectancy who would benefit from having medical orders for treatment readily available to emergency personnel.

People whose life expectancy is such that their primary care provider would not be surprised if they died in the next year will particularly benefit from the discussion and shared decision-making that is then reflected in the creation of a POLST document. In some states, the patient or family signs the completed POLST document to indicate agreement and consent to the treatment plan.

References

1. Ritchie CS, Leff B. Population health and tailored medical care in the home: the roles of home-based primary care and home-based palliative care. J Pain Symptom Manag. 2018;55(3):1041–6.
2. American Academy of H, Palliative M, Center to Advance Palliative C, Hospice, Palliative Nurses A, Last Acts P, et al. National consensus project for quality palliative care: clinical practice guidelines for quality palliative care, executive summary. J Palliat Med. 2004;7(5):611–27.
3. Herman C. National consensus project updates palliative care guidelines. Aging Today Online. 2013. https://www.nationalcoalitionhpc.org/ncp/. Accessedd 22 May 2023.
4. Roberts B, Robertson M, Ojukwu EI, Wu DS. Home based palliative care: known benefits and future directions. Curr Geriatr Rep. 2021;10:141–7.
5. Temel JS, Greer JA, Muzikansky A, Gallagher ER, Admane S, Jackson VA, et al. Early palliative care for patients with metastatic non-small-cell lung cancer. N Engl J Med. 2010;363(8):733–42.
6. Brumley RD, Enguidanos S, Cherin DA. Effectiveness of a home-based palliative care program for end-of-life. J Palliat Med. 2003;6(5):715–24.
7. Quinn KL, Stukel TA, Campos E, Graham C, Kavalieratos D, Mak S, Steinberg L, Tanuseputro P, Tuna M, Isenberg SR. Regional collaborative home-based palliative care and health care outcomes among adults with heart failure. Can Med Assoc J. 2022;194(37):E1274–82.
8. Hamano J, Takeuchi A, Mori M, Saitou Y, Yamaguchi T, Miyata N, Shimizu M, Yamamoto R, Kimura Y, Kamiyama Y, Arai Y, Matsuo H, Shishido H, Nakano K, Nishi T, Nagaoka H, Yokomichi N, Maeda I, Yamaguchi T, Morita T, Shinjo T. Comparison of survival times of advanced cancer patients with palliative care at home and in hospital. PLoS One. 2023;18(4):e0284147.
9. Ernecoff NC, Hanson LC, Fox AL, Daaleman TP, Kistler CE. Palliative care in a community-based serious-illness care program. J Palliat Med. 2020;23(5):692–7.
10. Glare PA, Sinclair CT. Palliative medicine review: prognostication. J Palliat Med. 2008;11(1):84–103.
11. Matzo ML. Palliative care: prognostication and the chronically ill: methods you need to know as chronic disease progresses in older adults. Am J Nurs. 2004;104(9):40–9; quiz 50.
12. Wajnberg A, Ornstein K, Zhang M, Smith KL, Soriano T. Symptom burden in chronically ill homebound individuals. J Am Geriatr Soc. 2013;61(1):126–31.
13. Rozans M, Dreisbach A, Lertora JJ, Kahn MJ. Palliative uses of methylphenidate in patients with cancer: a review. J Clin Oncol. 2002;20(1):335–9.
14. Rayner L, Higginson IJ, Price A, Hotopf M. The management of depression in palliative care: european clinical guidelines. London: Department of Palliative Care, Policy & Rehabilitation. European Palliative Care Research Collaborative; 2010.
15. Taylor MJ, Freemantle N, Geddes JR, Bhagwagar Z. Early onset of selective serotonin reuptake inhibitor antidepressant action: systematic review and meta-analysis. Arch Gen Psychiatry. 2006;63(11):1217–23.
16. Chochinov HM, Hack T, Hassard T, Kristjanson LJ, McClement S, Harlos M. Dignity therapy: a novel psychotherapeutic intervention for patients near the end of life. J Clin Oncol. 2005;23(24):5520–5.

17. De Vincenzo F, Lombardo L, Iani L, Maruelli A, Durante S, Ragghianti M, Park CL, Innamorati M, Quinto RM. Spiritual Well-being, dignity-related distress and demoralisation at the end of life-effects of dignity therapy: a randomised controlled trial. BMJ Support Palliat Care. 2023;13:e1238.
18. Dignity IN CARE toolkit [Internet]. Dignity IN CARE. 2010. https://dignityincare.ca/en/dignity-enhancing-interventions.html. Accessed 22 May 2023.
19. Engel JH, Siewerdt F, Jackson R, Akobundu U, Wait C, Sahyoun N. Hardiness, depression, and emotional well-being and their association with appetite in older adults. J Am Geriatr Soc. 2011;59(3):482–7.
20. Berenstein EG, Ortiz Z. Megestrol acetate for the treatment of anorexia-cachexia syndrome. Cochrane Database Syst Rev. 2005;(2):CD004310.
21. Volicer L, Stelly M, Morris J, McLaughlin J, Volicer BJ. Effects of dronabinol on anorexia and disturbed behavior in patients with Alzheimer's disease. Int J Geriatr Psychiatry. 1997;12(9):913–9.
22. Fox CB, Treadway AK, Blaszczyk AT, Sleeper RB. Megestrol acetate and mirtazapine for the treatment of unplanned weight loss in the elderly. Pharmacotherapy. 2009;29(4):383–97.
23. Hunter CN, Abdel-Aal HH, Elsherief WA, Farag DE, Riad NM, Alsirafy SA. Mirtazapine in cancer-associated anorexia and cachexia: a double-blind placebo-controlled randomized trial. J Pain Symptom Manag. 2021;62(6):1207–15.
24. Yu S, Sun K, Xing X, Zhong Y, Yan X, Qiu W, Yan M. Fan therapy for the relief of dyspnea in adults with advanced disease and terminal illness: a meta-analysis of randomized controlled trials. J Palliat Med. 2019;22(12):1603–9.
25. Inciardi JA, Surratt HL, Cicero TJ, Beard RA. Prescription opioid abuse and diversion in an urban community: the results of an ultrarapid assessment. Pain Med. 2009;10(3):537–48.
26. Twaddle ML, Kelley S. Chapter 46. Hospice. In: Berger AM, editor. Principles and practice of palliative care and supportive oncology. 4th ed. Philadelphia, PA: Wolters Kluwer Health/Lippincott Williams & Wilkins; 2012.
27. Centers for Medicare & Medicaid Services. Medicare benefit policy manual chapter 9: coverage of hospice services under hospital insurance. https://www.cms.gov/Regulations-and-Guidance/Guidance/Manuals/Downloads/bp102c09.pdf.
28. Oken MM, Creech RH, Tormey DC, Horton J, Davis TE, McFadden ET, et al. Toxicity and response criteria of the eastern cooperative oncology group. Am J Clin Oncol. 1982;5(6):649–55.
29. NHPCO facts and figures report, 2022 edition. In: NHPCO's facts & figures: Hospice care in America. 2022. https://www.nhpco.org/wp-content/uploads/NHPCO-Facts-Figures-2022.pdf.
30. Medicare Claims Processing Manual: Processing Hospice Claims. https://www.cms.gov/Regulations-and-Guidance/Guidance/Manuals/downloads/clm104c11.pdf.
31. History [Internet]. The National POLST paradigm. https://polst.org/history/. Accessed 22 May 2023.
32. POLST: What It Is and What It Is Not [Internet]. The National POLST paradigm. https://polst.org/2013/06/20/polst-what-it-is-and-what-it-is-not/. Accessed 22 May 2023.

Chapter 14
Caregiving

Helen Kao

14.1 Who Are Caregivers?

Informal caregivers in the United States are a diverse but largely unrecognized and undervalued group. Traditionally, caregiving has been considered a family obligation. However, since the American family has changed over time, many older adults do not live with or near children or grandchildren. As family structures evolve, the United States faces an ever-growing population of older adults who need caregiver support for functional deficits.

14.2 Overview of the Caregiver Population

A recent study found that one in six Americans provides care to an adult age 50 or older. Among all adults providing some amount of unpaid care, 79% are caregivers for someone who is age 50 or older. This equates to almost 42 million informal caregivers for someone age 50 or older. Since 2015, more of these caregivers are providing care to two or more individuals (24% vs. 18% in 2015). Most caregivers (56%) of older adults are themselves age 50 or older, and over half of their care recipients are age 75 or older (53%) [1].

Caregivers of adults aged 50 or older are diverse. Most (61%) are women. Approximately 17% are Hispanic/Latinx, 14% are African American, and 5% are Asian American and Pacific Islander [1].

H. Kao (✉)
Lumina Hospice and Palliative Care, Corvallis, OR, USA
e-mail: Helen.kao@luminahospice.org

J. L. Colburn et al. (eds.), *Geriatric Home-Based Medical Care*,
https://doi.org/10.1007/978-3-031-68786-0_14

As life expectancy increases, and adults live longer with disability, caregiving has changed from a short-term familial role to one that can last for years. Compared to 2015, significantly more caregivers of older adults are providing care for 5 years or more. As care recipient age rises, the proportion of their caregivers who have provided care for 5 years or more also rises. For care recipients aged 85 or older, up to 36% of their caregivers have served them for 5 years or more [1].

Patients may need a caregiver for a multitude of reasons. The most common main problem for which caregiving is implemented include "old age" (18%), mobility issues (13%), dementia (12%), surgery or wounds (6%), cancer (6%), stroke (5%), and falling (5%) [1]. These conditions can coexist and complicate care.

The intensity and time commitment of caregiving are variable and fluctuate over time, in large part due to the variable needs of the care recipient. In 2020, the percentage of caregivers who aided with at least one activity of daily living (ADL) was 60%. Among the ADLs, caregivers assisted most frequently with getting in and out of bed and chair (41%) and least with incontinence (18%). Furthermore, caregivers increasingly help with instrumental activities of daily living (IADLs): 80% assist with transportation, 78% with shopping, 76% with housework, 64% with meal preparation, and 58% with finances [1].

While two-thirds of caregivers provide care for 20 h or less per week, one-third provide care for 21 or more hours per week. When a caregiver lives with the patient, the time dedicated to providing care almost equals a full-time job, averaging 37.4 h per week [1].

Even when a loved one lives in an assisted living facility (ALF), informal caregivers provide substantial care, up to 65 h per month. Among assisted living residents, 55% received informal care for household activities, 17% for mobility, and 8% for self-care [2].

14.3 The Economic Impact of Informal Caregiving

Informal caregivers are estimated to provide approximately 30 billion hours of care annually. This amounts to $522 billion in opportunity cost annually (in 2011/2012 dollars) [3]. This is significantly more than the estimated total ($200.1 billion) spent by Medicaid on formal long-term care services in 2020 [4]. Another study of informal caregivers of persons with dementia estimated that 3.2 million caregivers provided 4.1 billion hours of care for persons with dementia. At a non-skilled hourly median rate of $10.28, this results in a value of $41.5 billion [5].

Most informal caregivers receive no income or employment benefits for the care they provide. Additionally, these caregivers can accrue significant personal costs that impact their financial well-being and security. Approximately 20% of caregivers report a high degree of financial strain. Financial impacts are significant: 28% stopped savings, 23% took on more debt, 22% used up personal short-term savings, 19% left bills unpaid or paid them late, and 15% borrowed money from friends and family. Almost half of caregivers (45%) experience at least one of these financial impacts. Black and Hispanic caregivers experience significantly greater financial impacts compared with non-Hispanic white and Asian caregivers, across income levels [1]. Some individuals receiving unpaid care supplement their care needs with paid caregivers, at substantial added costs [6]. A 2014 survey of family caregivers for older adults found that 42% of them spent >$5000/year on caregiving expenses [7].

Approximately 61% of adult caregivers maintain other jobs in addition to their caregiving responsibilities. Among caregivers who maintained employment, 60% worked 40 or more hours per week and 25% fewer than 30 h per week [1].

Caregivers who maintain employment in addition to caregiving find value from workplace benefits. Approximately 58% had paid sick days, and 39% had paid family leave. Among caregivers who worked, 56% had flexible work hours, and 52% had unpaid family leave [1].

Many family caregivers reduce hours or stop working outside the home to provide care. Around 61% of employed caregivers have experienced a negative impact on their work as a result of caregiving. Negative impacts include changing from full- to part-time and reducing hours, taking a leave of absence, receiving formal warnings about performance or attendance, turning down promotion, giving up work or retiring early, and losing job benefits [1].

If family caregivers can no longer provide care, then they must either hire in-home support or place their loved one outside the home. Some households supplement unpaid care with private paid help, though this can come at a significant cost [8].

14.4 Caregiver Burden and Assessment

14.4.1 Overview

Caregiving is associated with physical, psychological, and financial burdens. Caregiver burden is a major public health problem affecting the well-being of both caregivers and patients.

14.4.2 Incidence and Risk Factors for Caregiver Burden

Among Medicare beneficiaries needing long-term services and supports, 43% receive unpaid care, 15% paid care, with 42% that did not receive any help. These proportions are not significantly different by income level if the individual does not have Medicaid. For those who also receive Medicaid, 30% perceive they receive paid care, and 32% do not receive any care [9]. Unpaid family members provide most of the long-term care and are at particularly high risk for burnout. Over half of caregivers experience caregiver burden [10].

Care needs, such as ADL and IADL assistance, are determined by numerous patient-related factors, including medical and psychiatric conditions. Caring for a patient with dementia is associated with a higher level of burden than caring for someone without dementia. Individuals with dementia often require supervisory care and are less likely to express gratitude to their caregivers [11]. Individuals with dementia account for 10% of noninstitutionalized adults, but their family and unpaid caregivers account for one-third of caregivers and 41% of care hours provided in the United States [12]. As an individual's cognitive function declines, the caregiver's perceived burden increases [13]. Worsening dementia is associated with an increased need for caregiving and supervision, with a mean of 113 h per month for a patient with mild dementia, increasing to a mean of 298 h per month in a patient with severe dementia [14]. Increases in neuropsychiatric symptoms and behavioral manifestations of dementia, ADL and IADL impairment, and geriatric syndromes, such as falls and sleep disorders, also increase caregiver burden [13, 15].

Caregiver burden is not only influenced by patient characteristics but also by caregiver characteristics (Table 14.1) [15]. Women partner caregivers experience more burden than men partner caregivers [17]. Cultural differences among racial and ethnic groups may influence the perspective and expectations about caregiving, as well as the amount of extended family support.

14.4.3 Impact of Caregiver Burden

Caregiver burden can have adverse effects on patients, their caregivers, and society (Table 14.2). Caregivers perceiving burden are at a higher risk for committing elder mistreatment [19].

The mental health of caregivers is often affected with high rates of depression and anxiety. In one study of caregivers for individuals with dementia, a third of the caregivers met criteria for depression [21]. Two-thirds of caregivers feel moderate or high emotional stress [1]. Caregivers have less time for other friends and family and often neglect self-care, such as healthy sleep, exercise, and diet [22]. Maladaptive

Table 14.1 Risk factors for caregiver burden

Patient characteristics	Caregiver characteristics
Dementia, especially with neuropsychiatric symptoms or behavioral disturbances [11] Increasing ADL/IADL dependence Presence of geriatric syndromes (e.g., falls, sleep disturbance) [13, 15]	Spouse of patient and/or live with care recipient [15, 16] Lower education level [16] Perceive little or no choice in caregiver role Younger age Depressive symptoms [15] Emotion-focused coping style [18]

Table 14.2 Impact of caregiver burden

Impact of caregiver burden on:		
Patients	Caregivers	Society
Individual may feel like a burden to his/her family and friends	Have high rates of depression and anxiety [21]	Informal caregivers receive no income or employment benefits
Individual may be subject to elder abuse or neglect by overwhelmed caregiver [20]	Have high rates of dissatisfaction with their lives [1]	Caregivers may use their own savings to cover caregiving expenses [7]
Individuals may spend down their savings to supplement informal caregiving with hired help [8]	Have less time for other family or friends [22]	Informal caregiving often has negative effect on one's formal job (e.g., forced caregiver to arrive late, leave early, or take time off work) [8]
Individual may move out of private home to higher level of care due to burdens on family caregivers	Neglect self-care and rate personal health as poor or declining [16]	Informal caregivers provide care with estimated value of $522 billion annually [3]

coping strategies such as self-blame or wishful thinking have been linked with more anxiety and depression [18].

Caregivers report lower levels of physical and overall health. Approximately 23% of adults who have been caregiving for over 5 years consider their personal health as fair or poor, compared to 13% of the general adult population [8]. Furthermore, 23% of caregivers believe that their health has deteriorated as a result of caregiving [1]. Older adult spouses who experienced caregiver burden had a 63% increase in mortality risk compared to controls [23]. However, subsequent studies have found that informal caregiving is associated with reduced mortality risk, which may reflect selection of healthier individuals into the caregiving role [24, 25].

While caregiving is associated with significant burdens, it can also have many benefits for the caregiver. Positive outcomes include enjoyment of role and personal fulfillment from helping a loved one. Caregivers at home are often family members or friends of the recipient, and caregiving allows them to have a continued rewarding relationship with their loved one.

14.4.4 Assessment of Caregiver Burden

Given the impact of caregiver burden, home-based medical care clinicians should assess caregiver's well-being. Multiple scales exist [26], but the most widely used is the 22-item Zarit Burden Interview (ZBI) (Table 14.3) [27]. This questionnaire was designed for research rather than clinical use in daily practice; however, we include it in this chapter to describe the scope of issues to consider when assessing caregiver burden, with higher scores reflecting higher levels of burden. A 4-item screening version (Table 14.4) and a 12-item short version of the questionnaire were

Table 14.3 Zarit Burden Interview (choose the response that best describes how you feel)

	Never	Rarely	Sometimes	Quite frequently	Nearly always
1. Do you feel that your relative asks for more help than they need?	0	1	2	3	4
2. Do you feel that because of the time you spend with your relative that you do not have enough time for yourself?	0	1	2	3	4
3. Do you feel stressed between caring for your relative and trying to meet other responsibilities for your family or work?	0	1	2	3	4
4. Do you feel embarrassed over your relative's behavior?	0	1	2	3	4
5. Do you feel angry when you are around your relative?	0	1	2	3	4
6. Do you feel that your relative currently affects your relationships with other family members or friends in a negative way?	0	1	2	3	4
7. Are you afraid what the future holds for your relative?	0	1	2	3	4
8. Do you feel your relative is dependent on you?	0	1	2	3	4
9. Do you feel strained when you are around your relative?	0	1	2	3	4
10. Do you feel your health has suffered because of your involvement with your relative?	0	1	2	3	4
11. Do you feel that you do not have as much privacy as you would like because of your relative?	0	1	2	3	4
12. Do you feel that your social life has suffered because you are caring for your relative?	0	1	2	3	4
13. Do you feel uncomfortable about having friends over because of your relative?	0	1	2	3	4
14. Do you feel that your relative seems to expect you to take care of them as if you were the only one they could depend on?	0	1	2	3	4
15. Do you feel that you do not have enough money to take care of your relative in addition to the rest of your expenses?	0	1	2	3	4
16. Do you feel that you will be unable to take care of your relative much longer?	0	1	2	3	4
17. Do you feel you have lost control of your life since your relative's illness?	0	1	2	3	4

(continued)

Table 14.3 (continued)

	Never	Rarely	Sometimes	Quite frequently	Nearly always
18. Do you wish you could leave the care of your relative to someone else?	0	1	2	3	4
19. Do you feel uncertain about what to do about your relative?	0	1	2	3	4
20. Do you feel you should be doing more for your relative?	0	1	2	3	4
21. Do you feel you could do a better job in caring for your relative?	0	1	2	3	4
22. Overall, how burdened do you feel in caring for your relative?	0	1	2	3	4

Reprinted from Zarit SH, Reever KE,Bach-Peterson J. Relatives of the impaired elderly: correlates of feelings of burden. Gerontologist. 1980;20(6):649–55. Reference [27] by permission of Oxford University Press
Interpretation of score:
0–21 little to no burden
21–40 mild to moderate burden
41–60 moderate to severe burden
61–88 severe burden

Table 14.4 Zarit Burden Interview screening version

Do you feel…	Never	Rarely	Sometimes	Quite frequently	Nearly always
That because of the time you spend with your relative that you do not have enough time for yourself?	0	1	2	3	4
Stressed between caring for your relative and trying to meet other responsibilities (work/family)?	0	1	2	3	4
Strained when you are around your relative?	0	1	2	3	4
Uncertain about what to do with your relative?	0	1	2	3	4

Reprinted from Bédard M, Molloy DW, Squire L, Dubois S, Lever JA, O'Donnell M. The Zarit Burden Interview: a new short version and screening version. Gerontologist. 2001;41(5):652–7. Reference [28] by permission of Oxford University Press
A score of 8 of higher is suggestive of high burden, though an exact cutoff has not been established

developed and validated for easier screening of caregivers of community dwelling older adults with cognitive impairment [28].

During the home visit, clinicians should ask questions to assess caregivers' mental health, coping, behavioral management, social support, and resources [28]. Examples of useful questions include the following:

- Are you feeling a lot of stress?
- Have you been feeling anxious or down?

- What do you do to relieve your stress?
- Does your relative/care recipient have behaviors that are difficult to manage or frustrating? How do you manage these?
- Does anyone help you with caregiving? Who and how often?
- Are you involved with any local support groups? If not, are you interested in learning about them?

After assessing caregiver burden, clinicians should provide education, support, and assist caregivers with identifying resources for support. These issues are addressed in the subsequent sections. The Family Caregiver Alliance National Center on Caregiving also has an online toolkit to help clinicians assess caregivers (https://caregiver.org/caregivers-count-too-toolkit). This resource provides a helpful overview of caregiving and resources, as well as a guide to conducting a caregiver assessment in Sect. 14.3.

14.4.5 Support for Caregivers

The primary support for most caregivers is their informal social networks, and clinicians should inquire about friends or family that may be assisting them. Clinicians can provide education, as well as involve other skilled resources as needed. Finally, caregivers should be informed of local and national resources, including in-person and online support groups, counseling, education and skills trainings, and respite care [29].

Most support groups and organizations focus on sharing the caregiver's experience, as well as learning strategies and skills for caregiving. An intervention including counseling sessions and conversation groups resulted in a 6-month delay in nursing home placement [23]. Skilled therapy, such as cognitive behavioral therapy, is not as widely available but has been shown to reduce depression in caregivers [30, 31]. Interventions have been developed to address coping strategies, reduce anxiety, and increase satisfaction. A focus on problem-solving and acceptance styles of coping is likely helpful for caregivers and can lead to a more positive caregiver experience [32].

Educational and supportive interventions have been shown to positively impact family and caregivers. Home visiting programs can help support caregivers and are most helpful in reducing burden among caregivers who live with patients [33]. Additional resources are discussed at the end of this chapter.

14.4.6 Abuse and Neglect

While most caregivers provide devoted, quality care, abuse and neglect of older, vulnerable adults remain prevalent. Elder abuse is intentional or neglectful acts by a caregiver or trusted individual that harm a vulnerable older adult. One in ten older adults experiences abuse or neglect by a caregiver each year, and the incidence is expected to increase [20]. Elder abuse occurs most commonly in home situations.

Risk factors for elder abuse include shared living arrangements, cognitive impairment with disruptive behaviors, social isolation, caregiver's mental or physical health problems, and financial dependence on the older adult [20]. The US Preventive Services Task Force found insufficient evidence to assess the balance of benefits and harms of screening for abuse of older or vulnerable adults. Clinicians have professional and state-based legal obligations to report and refer persons who are suspected of being victims of abuse [34]. Clinicians that perform home-based medical care are uniquely able to assess the dynamic of the caregiver and patient, as well as the safety of the home environment. Clinicians should be familiar with signs of and risk factors for elder abuse, so they can appropriately identify this underrecognized problem. Chapter 12 addresses the complexities of assessment for abuse or neglect in these vulnerable patients.

Clinicians should ensure that they interview the patient alone without the caregiver present. Suggestions on how to interview the patient alone are described in detail in Sect. 14.6 under Sect. 14.6.3. The Elder Abuse Suspicion Index, available online, is a six-item validated screen for use in primary care settings with cognitively intact patients [35]. The goal of the screen is to help identify possible cases of abuse to prompt providers to conduct more in-depth evaluation. Questions focus on neglect, emotional, financial, and physical abuse.

For patients with cognitive impairment, clinicians will need to rely on other possible red flags, such as:

- The caregiver often interrupts the patient to answer for him/her.
- The patient has:
  - Bruising in unusual locations.
  - Burns, hand slap, or bite marks.
  - Evidence of dehydration or malnutrition.
  - Poor eye contact or withdrawn behavior.
  - An unusual delay in seeking medical attention for injuries.
  - Frequently missed medications.
  - Dirty clothing and poor hygiene.

Any time elder abuse or neglect is suspected, the case must be reported to the local Adult Protective Services.

14.5 Levels of Care

Home-based medical care can be delivered in a variety of community settings: from private residences and small board and care homes to large assisted living facilities and entire "campuses" of a continuing care retirement community (CCRC) (Table 14.5). These settings provide varying levels of structural and programmed care that can enable an older adult to remain more independent while also reducing

Table 14.5 Levels of care in the home or community (not including long-term care in skilled nursing facilities)

Level of care	Care available	Costs	Comments
Private home			
Senior center/adult day program	• Centralized and supervised services/activities • Socialization • Physical and cognitive stimulation (exercise, art, music, games, etc.) • Maintenance PT/OT • Transportation • Meals • Field trips	• National average ~ $78/day • Private pay • Medicaid HCBS • Veteran's administration • Some state/local funding • Some long-term care insurance	• Range of services varies per site • Patient participation can enable family caregiver to maintain outside employment
Low-income government-funded in-home caregiving	• I/ADL support • Supervisory care for dementia • Usually does not cover 24/7 care	• Income eligibility (often Medicaid thresholds or higher +/− share of cost)	• Must reside in county where care subsidy is provided • May enable family caregiver to get paid for their services
Paid in-home caregiving (agency)	• I/ADL support • Supervisory care for dementia • Can fit together shifts to provide 24/7 coverage • Usual "minimum" shift is 4 h at a time • Agency caregivers usually restricted from performing paramedical services	• $23–40/h • Rate varies by geographic area and level of care needed • Long-term care insurance covers (and requires paid caregivers to be affiliated with an agency)	• Increasing legal protections for formal paid caregivers (maximum hours, mandated breaks, overtime, etc.) • Agencies generally conduct basic background checks
Paid in-home caregiving (independent contractor)	• Same as agency caregiver but no restrictions on paramedical services • May enable more flexible scheduling	• Rate may be cheaper than for agency caregiver • May enable flexibility of offering live-in (room and board) arrangements in exchange for services	• Increasing legal protections for caregivers limit previously commonplace arrangements • Caregiver agreement contracts recommended

Residential care facility for the elderly (RCFE)	• Daily support with I/ADLs • Home-like, community-based setting • Socialization • Similar activities to senior centers above • Inclusive of all meals • Transportation • Medication dispensation	• National average (2021) ~ $4500/month • Cost ranges greatly by location, size, level of care needs (e.g., $2500–$10,000/month) • Private pay • Some long-term care insurance covers/subsidizes • Some Medicaid HCBS waivers cover	• Many individuals who, in past decades, would have been institutionalized in nursing facilities are able to reside in RCFEs
Continuing care retirement communities (CCRCs)	• Same as above • But resident can enter at fully independent stage • Care extends to and includes on-site skilled nursing and rehabilitation • "Tiered" approach to care	• Monthly fee ($900–$10,500/month) ranges by level of contract and up-front entrance fee ($80,000–$600,000) • Private pay • Some long-term care insurance subsidizes	• Most expensive option • Enables resident to "age in place"
Respite care	• Short-term time-limited care to relieve an informal caregiver • Can be provided in the home or through temporary placement of individual in a facility	• Private pay prorated for amount of time a formal caregiver is brought into the home or an individual is placed in a facility • May be supported through some state programs or Medicaid HCBS waiver benefits • Some long-term care insurance covers	

burden on informal caregivers. Understanding the levels of care available to patients and caregivers in these settings, as well as the variable costs and availability of coverage through public programs or long-term care insurance, is useful for providers.

14.5.1 Private Home

The vast majority of older adults wish to live and die in their own home surrounded by loved ones. However, homebound older adults often require assistance to remain at home. Options for caregiving in a private home include informal/unpaid and formal/paid caregiving or a combination of both. In-home care can enable an adult to stay at home but does not necessarily address social isolation and other needs. In some states, Medicaid home- and community-based services (HCBS) waivers have allowed innovative partnerships to improve access to affordable housing and develop integrated case management and support services to enable older adults receiving Medicaid to stay independent. Some HCBS programs may also assist older adults with assistive technology or adaptive equipment installation (e.g., ramps, grab bars, safe lighting, etc.) to maximize independence and safety.

14.5.2 Senior Centers and Adult Day Programs

Community-based senior centers and adult day programs offer a wide array of centralized services and activities in a supervised and social environment. They provide physical, cognitive, and social stimulation, such as exercise classes, group recreation, art or music sessions, and book clubs. Some provide transportation to and from home and may even offer scheduled group "field trips" to museums, parks, or other local cultural settings. The average cost for a full day of services in 2021 was $78 [36]. While many individuals pay out of pocket for these programs, public funding sources that support adult day participants include Medicaid HCBS waiver programs, the Veteran's Administration, and other state and local funding [37]. Some long-term care insurance will cover or subsidize participation in these programs, and some employers may offer dependent care spending accounts. Adult day programs may enroll adults by the hour or, more commonly, in half- or full-day increments. Senior centers and adult day programs can enable informal caregivers to maintain outside employment or provide family caregivers much needed daily respite from around-the-clock caregiving.

14.5.3 Residential Care Facilities for the Elderly

Residential care facilities for the elderly (RCFE) are settings that provide daily supportive services and often socialization and activities to older or disabled adults. RCFEs vary tremendously in size, services, and cost. Smaller, more intimate and home-like board and care homes, sometimes called group homes or adult foster homes, are homes in residential neighborhoods that have been renovated to care for an average of 5–10 disabled adults. In contrast, an assisted living facility (ALF) is usually a large complex designed and built to house a higher number of residents, e.g., 100–200, in single or double-occupancy apartments. The increasingly higher level of care offered by some RCFEs has contributed to a notable shift in long-term care over the past few decades. Individuals with disabilities, who in the past would have required a nursing facility for long-term care, can now safely remain in the community at an RCFE if they have sufficient financial resources or their state covers RCFEs under Medicaid long-term care funding. RCFEs that have special dementia units or "hospice waivers" can sometimes even manage the complex and time-intensive care of a bedbound resident who requires total care, including hand-feeding. Family members can continue to play a valuable "informal" caregiving role in these settings but with the comfort of knowing that most of their loved one's needs are attended to by formal staff.

RCFEs do not fall under the same strict regulatory requirements faced by skilled nursing facilities. Older adults choose an RCFE based on the type of setting, degree of care needs, "culture" of the facility, and cost they can afford.

All RCFEs provide meals and housekeeping and may provide medication management, transfer assistance, and help with ADLs. Most RCFEs provide some type of social or cultural activities. Board and care homes with fewer resources may have visiting pet therapy, art, and birthday parties or holiday celebrations. In addition to these activities, ALFs may provide group exercise and art classes, film nights, bingo and card games, outings to shopping malls or cultural sites, and transportation to medical appointments. Some ALFs even provide on-site hair salons and nail care. Board and care homes are generally more affordable than ALFs. The average cost of an RCFE in the United States in 2021 was $4500 a month [36]. However, in some geographic regions, costs can increase up to $9000–10,000+/month, particularly if a resident has a higher level of care needs, which are often priced a la carte depending on the activity or memory care. Long-term care insurance may cover part or all of the fees depending on plan benefits and cost of the chosen facility.

14.5.4 Continuing Care Retirement Communities

Continuing care retirement communities (CCRCs) integrate the services older adults needs all in one community, as he or she transitions from independent living to assisted living to skilled nursing and hospice-level care. Often referred to as "tiered" approach to care, CCRCs are the most expensive of the long-term care options. They generally offer the same types of services and social activities as an ALF but with the additional security that an older adult can enroll while independent, transition into assisted care, and receive skilled nursing level support if needed in the same setting over time. An individual applies for and enrolls into a CCRC with an entry fee which can be anywhere from $80,000 to as much as $600,000, depending on contract level. Monthly fees then range $900–$10,500 but may increase if the resident has growing care needs [38]. As with RCFEs, long-term care insurance may cover part or all of the fees depending on plan benefits and cost of the chosen facility.

14.5.5 In-Home Caregiving

Informal or paid in-home caregivers can fulfill the needs of adults who require help with ADLs or IADLs in their own private residence or who may need to augment the services provided by an RCFE.

When paid formal caregivers are needed, patients or their families must choose a type of caregiver based on affordability and level of care needed. One option is hiring a caregiver through an agency. This is usually the most expensive hourly rate but provides several benefits to the employing adult. Agencies generally conduct background checks and manage the legal hiring and taxes. Additionally, some agencies provide basic caregiver training and health insurance to employees and take the responsibility for finding a replacement for the client if a caregiver calls in sick. Another option is hiring an independent caregiver as a private contracted employee. The responsibility lies with the "employer" (patient or their family member) to conduct any background or reference checks, to train the caregiver for specific tasks, and to abide by federal and state laws regarding payment and taxes. If the caregiver calls in sick or resigns, the employing adult is responsible for finding a replacement caregiver.

For anyone hiring an independent caregiver, even one who is a family member, it may be helpful to complete a formal caregiver agreement to define the roles and responsibilities and detail the flow of payment. Caregiver agreement templates are readily available for free online. Caregiver agreements protect the paid caregiver and enable them to build employment history, establish credit, and have access to disability insurance, workers' compensation, and public benefits. Agreements protect the employer from being taken advantage of especially when an adult is hiring a friend or relative [39]. Long-term care insurance can cover in-home paid caregivers but usually stipulate that the paid caregiver must be affiliated with an approved agency (i.e., not just a friend or independent contractor).

14.5.6 *Respite Care*

Respite care is short-term, time-limited care for an individual that can be provided in his or her own home, though more commonly is provided in a community program, an RCFE, or nursing facility. Respite services at home usually entail a formal caregiver coming to the home in place of the usual informal caregiver. Facility respite care entails moving the older adult to an RCFE or nursing facility for a short period of time. Respite care may be supported through special state programs or Medicaid, as well as through long-term care services and support programs and long-term care insurance. Most long-term care insurance policies provide respite options. Medicare generally only covers limited respite care for patients enrolled in hospice services. For private pay, some respite programs offer sliding scale payment schedules, and others prorate their monthly fee to the duration of time the individual is receiving respite services. Respite care provides a necessary break for informal caregivers to address their own personal needs, such as medical care, recovery from injury, travel to important family events, or simply to prevent burnout.

14.5.7 *How to Assess the Level of Care Needed*

Knowing when to hire caregivers or to move into a "higher level of care" and which level to move to is one of the hardest decisions older adults and their families must make. Home-based medical providers can play a vital role in evaluating and counseling patients and families when it is no longer safe to live at home. An individual's capacity to live at home can be evaluated through formal clinical assessments, as well as common-sense checklists available to the public via online Web resources.

14.5.8 *Kohlman Evaluation of Living Skills*

Kohlman Evaluation of Living Skills (KELS) is an occupational therapy evaluation that has been shown to be an effective predictor of one's ability to live safely and independently in the community. Providers can request occupational therapy for KELS as part of a Medicare-approved home healthcare plan. The evaluation is more useful than simply assessing an adult's function with ADLs and IADLs [40, 41]. KELS evaluates an adult's living skills in areas of self-care, safety, health, money management, transportation, telephone, work, and leisure. KELS can be inaccurate for individuals with visual impairment and has not been validated for all cultural backgrounds.

14.5.9 Functional Assessment

Any clinician practicing home-based medical care should be skilled in the thorough assessment of a patient's functional status. While it may not be as thorough as a formal comprehensive geriatric assessment or KELS, it can provide the clinician, the patient, and the family with key information about the general areas of support someone needs to remain functionally and safely in his or her home. The functional assessment includes ADLs—bathing, toileting, dressing, grooming, and transferring/mobility—and IADLs: food preparation, housekeeping, transportation, medication management, finances, and telephone use. Any impairment in these functional domains should warrant a discussion with the patient and family on how to assist the patient with identified deficits to enable the patient to remain at home. This could include non-personnel options such as monthly delivery of prefilled pill packs, automatic bill pay, home delivered meals, laundry service, and community transportation services. Alternatively, this could include personnel options ranging from family members taking over finances, medication management, and cooking to hired housekeepers, companions, or caregivers in the home.

14.5.10 Online Checklists

Several Web-based resources provide free online "checklists" for families to have a systematic way in which they can assess a loved one's needs. These checklists are a valuable tool to aid in decision-making regarding the safety and feasibility of an older adult remaining at home. The tools are easily accessible and educate caregivers how to identify practical and actionable issues.

Family Caregiver Alliance's website, www.caregiver.org, suggests families and caregivers consider not only ADL and IADL needs of the patient but also three other domains: healthcare, emotional care, and supervision. If an individual does not have a preceding advance healthcare directive or power of attorney for health, it is critical to establish one before she or he loses capacity. Emotional care is as important to patients' well-being as functional support. Isolation and loneliness have a significant impact on depression, wellness, and mortality. Caregivers must consider how to provide companionship, conversation, social engagement, and meaningful activities. Finally, for individuals with dementia, 24/7 supervisory care is essential if there is risk of wandering or home hazards, such as forgetting to turn off stoves or water faucets, even if the individual remains independent with his or her ADLs [42].

The Web resource, Consumer Affairs, provides a useful guide to families and caregivers who want to know when the time has come to move a loved one to a more supportive environment such as an RCFE. The guide (updated March 23, 2022) has a 17-item list of observable signs or changes that suggest the individual needs more help: https://www.consumeraffairs.com/health/time-for-assisted-living.html.

14.6 Caregiver Education

14.6.1 How to Interact with Caregivers in the Home

Home-based medical providers play a critical role in the education of patients and caregivers. There are several best practices to keep in mind in this educator role.

14.6.2 Setting the Stage

- The clinician should address the patient first.
- Distinguish between the hands-on caregiver and the legal surrogate decision-maker, who may not always know how the patient is doing day-to-day or may not be present for the visit.
- Be clear in communication when you are seeking collateral history from a caregiver and when you need to discuss decision-making with the legal surrogate.
- If the patient has cognitive impairment or is severely hearing impaired such that direct interview is difficult, set the stage by first addressing the patient and then by explaining that you will be asking the caregiver some questions as well.
- If needed, reserve time to speak to the caregiver in private away from the patient for sensitive history, e.g., the patient has paranoia, disinhibited sexual behaviors, violent aggression, depression, or other concerns, or to assess the caregiver's level of burnout.
- Always be explicit that the purpose of the visit is healthcare delivery and not a social visit.

14.6.3 Interacting with Caregivers: Key Language and Techniques

When meeting a patient who has a caregiver, even if the caregiver is the more reliable informant, always greet and acknowledge the patient. Let the patient know you will be asking the caregiver questions or ask the patient for permission to speak to the caregiver. For example:

> Hi Mr. Smith (patient), I'm here to follow up on your leg pain. I'll be asking Ms. Jones (caregiver), some questions about how you're doing as well.

You may ask the caregiver for time to meet with the patient alone, if needed. For example:

> I like to have some time to meet with my patients privately just as I would in clinic. Do you mind going to another room while I speak with Mr. Smith? I'll call you back in when we're done.

Home visits also provide an excellent opportunity to assess the caregivers' skills and knowledge with caregiving. Clinicians can provide in-person education and feedback. For example:

> Can you show me how you assist him in bed? How do you organize and give his medications? Can you assist me in rolling him to his side so I can examine his back?

Listening and observation are critical to understand the caregivers' challenges and educational needs. Clinicians should:

- Validate the challenges of the caregiver role and give encouragement and "permission" for them to ask for help.
- Encourage caregivers to take time for self-care.
- Provide anticipatory guidance regarding disease progression.

14.6.4 Addressing Barriers to Communication

- Ensure televisions and radios are turned off or muted during visits.
- Use the quietest room available with privacy, including closed door and windows with curtains that can be drawn.
- Use in-person contract interpreters, if financially possible for the practice, or telephone-interpreters for non-English-speaking patients/caregivers. This avoids miscommunications that can occur when using family or informal caregivers to interpret.
- If caregivers only work certain hours, try to arrange home visits during the time that the caregiver is present for the most reliable in-person collateral history.
- If more than one caregiver rotates through the week, recommend that all caregivers make notes in a log to share key events and changes in condition, such as appetite, sleep patterns, urination and bowel movements, and falls, with each other and with the healthcare team.

14.6.5 Care Plan and Directions

Unless a portable printer is available or all involved parties are accessing a shared electronic care plan portal, clinicians should be sure that key instructions for patients/caregivers/facility staff are clearly written down before leaving. RCFEs require written or printed and signed orders for any care plan changes. Clinicians should provide caregivers with "levels of urgency" and red flag instructions for when to call the practice for phone advice and when, if within a patient's goals of care, calling 911 and emergency care are appropriate. When caregiver education is required and if home health nursing is not involved, clinicians can consider rotating days and times of visits in order to interface with other caregivers. This allows the clinician to obtain additional collateral and provide education and support to other caregivers. Family care plan meetings are often more easily arranged in the home than in clinic and hospital settings. Home-based medical providers can make use of this valuable forum to have meetings to establish goals of care or educate multiple caregivers or family members at once.

Most informal caregivers receive no training on how to provide care. Approximately 81% of caregivers feel inadequately trained for the tasks that they perform and have never received any formal education in caregiving [43]. They are expected to provide care for a complex adult with many needs with minimal to no instruction. Caregivers often feel overwhelmed and unsure about how to assist an adult, usually a spouse or parent, with ADLs or how to manage behaviors in dementia. Some caregivers simply learn through trial and error or from informal interaction with social contacts.

14.6.6 Educational Resources for Caregivers

Home-based medical clinicians are a valuable educational resource for the caregiver and can provide guidance regarding disease-specific issues and behavioral management. They also can give insight, information, and anticipatory guidance about the patient's medical condition. During the medical encounter at home, clinicians can evaluate the caregiver-patient dynamic in the context of the home, assess home safety, provide counseling regarding behavioral management, and give suggestions based on their observations of the caregiver and patient at home.

Clinicians may involve other skilled professionals for education. Skilled home care is covered by most health insurances, including Medicare. Physical and occupational therapists assess the safety of the home environment and functional status of the patient. They may provide recommendations regarding environmental modifications, durable medical equipment needs, mobility and exercise, and caregiver education for safe transfers. In addition to addressing speech difficulties or dysphagia, many speech therapists perform cognitive rehabilitation and discuss ways to more effectively engage patients. Registered nursing may help with medication management, educating caregivers on how to assist with ADLs, and symptom monitoring. Pharmacists provide medication counseling, and some provide prefilled medi-sets or blister packs. Finally, social workers (e.g., a home health social worker if a clinical practice social worker or community social worker is not available) can refer individuals to resources, such as respite care, transportation services, support groups, adult day programs, and higher levels of care, such as RCFEs. Development of an ADL impairment due to illness or physical or cognitive decline can qualify a patient for skilled home care. Home nurses, physical therapists, and occupational therapists can educate caregivers on how to assist a patient with ADLs.

In many communities, there are growing independent or franchise services which provide free or low-cost guidance to patients and families on choosing caregiver agencies or finding an appropriate RCFE. These range from national Web resources to more personalized local services that conduct in-person patient evaluations and interviews. These services receive a placement fee from RCFEs for a successful match between a patient and facility. Clinicians may want to evaluate or meet with local franchise services to vet their commitment to patients and families and their track record for successful placements before recommending a particular local service.

Private pay services are also available, though perhaps not in all locations nationwide. Patients or families may pay for a private geriatric consultation, geriatric care manager (www.caremanager.org), or dementia behavioral specialist. Though not covered by Medicare, these consultants can help with care coordination and challenges with behavior management. Generally, the goal of these case managers is to minimize healthcare costs while optimizing function, independence, and communication.

14.6.7 Resources for the Caregiver

Access to education and support is essential for caregivers. Clinicians should provide education but can also direct caregivers to national, state, and local organizations for additional support and information. Importantly, clinicians should give caregivers "permission" to ask for help and validate the challenges of caregiving. Most caregivers receive the majority of support informally from families and social networks. Caregivers may benefit from increased social support, skills education regarding caregiving tasks, and assistance with coping. Many national organizations and state services have online websites, with resources and educational materials for caregivers, as well as links to local chapters (discussed below).

14.6.8 National Organizations

National caregiver support organizations, such as the Alzheimer's Association and Family Caregiver Alliance, are an excellent resource for caregivers. These organizations, in addition to the others listed below, have websites that provide online educational materials about caregiving, dementia, and other chronic illnesses. In addition, national organizations can connect caregivers to local chapters and resources, such as respite care.

Alzheimer's Association: http://www.alz.org
Caregiver Action Network: https://www.caregiveraction.org/
Eldercare Locator: https://eldercare.acl.gov
Family Caregiver Alliance, National Center on Caregiving: https://www.caregiver.org
AARP Caregiving Resource Center: https://www.aarp.org

14.6.9 Support Groups

National organizations such as the Alzheimer's Association and National Family Caregiver Support program have local chapters and in-person and online support groups for caregivers. Support groups are also often available through health systems, hospice agencies, community organizations, and senior centers. Groups may be run by peers or professionals and provide a venue for caregivers to discuss shared experiences, learn skills and techniques about caregiving, develop more effective coping strategies, and foster camaraderie. These groups are effective at educating and increasing social networks, and satisfaction with groups is usually high [22].

14.6.10 Counseling, Education, and Skills Training

Individual or group counseling led by a professional can be effective at addressing psychological concerns, such as anxiety or depression. Caregivers work with a practitioner to develop skills and techniques, such as through cognitive behavioral therapy, to address mental health issues and coping strategies [30]. Clinicians can provide trainings and education to increase caregiver knowledge and self-efficacy [44, 45].

As discussed previously, clinicians may refer patients to skilled home care services, including physical therapy, occupational therapy, speech therapy, registered nursing, and social work. Medicare requires a skilled need for a patient to qualify for skilled home care services. These home care professionals can help to address a variety of caregiver needs.

14.6.11 Online Articles

Written for clinicians, these articles are available publicly online and include an overview about caring for caregivers. In addition, the articles include a handout for caregivers, as well as lists of additional online resources.

- American Medical Association. Caring for the caregiver: a guide for physicians. 2018: https://www.ama-assn.org/sites/ama-assn.org/files/corp/media-browser/public/public-health/caregiver-burnout-guide.pdf
- Swartz K, Collins LG. Caregiver care. Am Fam Physician. 2019;99(11):699–706.
- Parks SM, Novielli KD. A practical guide to caring for caregivers. Am Fam Physician. 2000;62 (12):2613–22.

References

1. National Alliance for Caregiving and AARP. Caregiving in the U.S. 2020. Washington, DC. May 2020. https://doi.org/10.26419/ppi.00103.001.
2. Coe NB, Werner RM. Informal caregivers provide considerable front-line support in residential care facilities and nursing homes. Health Aff (Millwood). 2022;41(1):105. https://doi.org/10.1377/hlthaff.2021.01239.
3. Chari AV, Engberg J, Ray KN, Mehorta A. The opportunity costs of informal elder-care in the United States: new estimates from the American time use survey. Health Serv Res. 2014;50(3):871–82.
4. Mudrazija S, Johnson RW. Economic impacts of programs to support caregivers: Final Report. Washington, DC: Urban Institute; 2020.
5. Rabarison KM, Bouldin ED, Bish CL, McGuire LC, Taylor CA, Greenlund KJ. The economic value of informal caregiving for persons with dementia: results from 38 states, the District of Columbia, and Puerto Rico, 2015 and 2016 BRFSS. America. J Public Health. 2018;108:1370–7.
6. Fabius CD, Wolff JL, Willink A, Skehan ME, Mulcahy J, Kasper J. Community-based long-term services and supports: are the needs of older adults and their caregivers being met. The Commonwealth Fund Issue Brief, October 27, 2021.
7. Senior Care Cost Index 2014, based on family caregiver usage and attitudes survey [internet]. 2014. https://www.caring.com/static/senior_care_cost_index_2014.pdf. Accessed 1 Sept 2022.
8. Anderson LA, Edwards VJ, Pearson WS, Talley RC, McGuire LC, Andresen EM. Adult caregivers in the United States: characteristics and differences in well-being by caregiver age and caregiving status. Prev Chronic Dis. 2013;10:E135.
9. Willink A, Davis K, Mulcahy J, Wollf JL. Use of paid and unpaid personal help by medicare beneficiaries needing long-term services and supports. The Commonwealth Fund Issue Brief, November 2017.
10. Riffin C, VanNess PH, Wolff JL, Fried T. Multifactorial examination of caregiver burden in a national sample of family and unpaid caregivers. J Am Geriatr Soc. 2019;67(2):277–83.
11. Ory MG, Hoffman RR, Yee JL, Tennstedt S, Schulz R. Prevalence and impact of caregiving: a detailed comparison between dementia and non-dementia caregivers. Gerontologist. 1999;39(2):177–85.
12. Kasper JD, Freedman VA, Spillman BC, Wolff JL. The disproportionate impact of dementia on family and unpaid caregiving to older adults. Health Aff. 2015;34(10):1642–9.
13. Kamiya M, Sakurai T, Ogama N, Maki Y, Toba K. Factors associated with increased caregivers' burden in several cognitive stages of Alzheimer's disease. Geriatr Gerontol Int. 2014;14(Suppl 2):45–55.
14. Haro JM, Kahle-Wrobleski K, Bruno G, Belger M, Dell'Agnello G, Dodel R, et al. Analysis of burden in caregivers of people with Alzheimer's disease using self-report and supervision hours. J Nutr Health Aging. 2014;18(7):677–84.
15. Shankar KN, Hirschman KB, Hanlon AL, Naylor MD. Burden in caregivers of cognitively impaired elderly adults at time of hospitalization: a cross-sectional analysis. J Am Geriatr Soc. 2014;62(2):276–84.
16. Collins LG, Swartz K. Caregiver care. Am Fam Physician. 2011;83(11):1309–17.
17. Swinkels J, van Tilburg T, Verbakel E, Broese van Groenou M. Explaining the gender gap in the burden of partner caregivers. J Gerontol. 2017;74(2):309–17.
18. Snyder CM, Fauth E, Wanzek J, Piercy KW, Norton MC, Corcoran C, et al. Dementia caregivers' coping strategies and their relationship to health and well-being: the Cache County study. Aging Ment Health. 2014;19:390–9.

19. Orfila F, Coma-Sole M, Cabanas M, Cegri-Lombardo F, Moleras-Serra A, Pujol-Ribera E. Family caregiver mistreatment of the elderly: prevalence of risk and associated factors. BMC Public Health. 2018;18:167.
20. Lachs MS, Pillemer KA. Elder abuse. N Engl J Med. 2015;373:1947–56.
21. Covinsky KE, Newcomer R, Fox P, Wood J, Sands L, Dane K, et al. Patient and caregiver characteristics associated with depression in caregivers of patients with dementia. J Gen Intern Med. 2003;18(12):1006–14.
22. Connell CMC, Janevic MR, Gallant MP. The costs of caring: impact of dementia on family caregivers. J Geriatr Psychiatry Neurol. 2001;14(4):179–87.
23. Schulz R. Beach SR caregiving as a risk factor for mortality: the caregiver health effects study. JAMA. 1999;282(23):2215–9.
24. O'Reilly D, Rosato M, Maguire A, Wright D. Caregiving reduces mortality risk for most caregivers: a census-based record linkage study. Int J Epidemiol. 2015;44(6):1959–69.
25. Mikkola TM, Kautiainen H, Manty M, von Bonsdorff MB, Kroger T, Eriksson JG. Age-dependency in morality of family caregivers: a nationwide register-based study. Aging Clin Exp Res. 2021;33:1971–80.
26. Robertson ML, Phung A, Bhatnagar S, Li L, Schuchman M, Wolff J, Ritchie C, Leff B, Sheehan OC. Assessing the wellbeing of family caregivers of multimorbid and homebound older adults-a scoping literature review. J Am Geriatr Soc. 2023;71(1):268–75.
27. Zarit SH, Reever KE, Bach-Peterson J. Relatives of the impaired elderly: correlates of feelings of burden. Gerontologist. 1980;20(6):649–55.
28. Bedard M, Molloy DW, Squire L, Dubois S, Lever JA, O'Donnell M. The Zarit burden interview: a new short version and screening version. Gerontologist. 2001;41(5):652–7.
29. Bourgeois MS, Schulz R, Burgio L. Interventions for caregivers of patients with Alzheimer's disease: a review and analysis of content, process, and outcomes. Int J Aging Hum Dev. 1996;43(1):35–92.
30. Chang BL. Cognitive-behavioral intervention for homebound caregivers of persons with dementia. Nurs Res. 1999;48(3):173–82.
31. Wiegelman H, Speller S, Verhaert LM, Schirra-Weirich L, Wolf-Ostermann K. Psychosocial interventions to support the mental health of informal caregivers of persons living with dementia—a systematic literature review. BMC Geriatr. 2021;21:94.
32. Kneebone II, Martin PR. Coping and caregivers of people with dementia. Br J Health Psychol. 2003;8(Pt 1):1–17.
33. Melis RJ, van Eijken ML, van Achterberg T, et al. The effect on caregiver burden of a problem-based home visiting programme for frail older people. Age Ageing. 2009;38(5):542–7.
34. Hoover RM, Polson M. Detecting elder abuse and neglect: assessment and intervention. Am Fam Physician. 2014;89(6):453–60.
35. Yaffe MJ, Wolfson C, Lithwick M, Weiss D. Development and validation of a tool to improve physician identification of elder abuse: the elder abuse suspicion index (EASI). J Elder Abuse Negl. 2008;20(3):276–300.
36. https://www.genworth.com/aging-and-you/finances/cost-of-care/cost-of-care-trends-and-insights.html. Accessed 28 Jul 2022.
37. The MetLife Mature Market Institute, National Adult Day Services Association (NADSA), The Ohio State University College of Social Work. The MetLife national study of adult day services: providing support to individuals and their family caregivers. New York: MetLife Mature Market Institute; 2010.
38. https://www.care.com/c/continuing-care-retirement-community-cost. Accessed 4 Sept 2022.
39. https://www.caregiver.org/resource/personal-care-agreements/. Accessed 4 Sept 2022.
40. Naik AD, Burnett J, Pickens-Pace S, Dyer CB. Impairment in instrumental activities of daily living and the geriatric syndrome of self-neglect. Gerontologist. 2008;48(3):388–93.

41. Burnett J, Dyer CB, Naik AD. Convergent validation of the Kohlman evaluation of living skills as a screening tool of older adults' ability to live safely and independently in the community. Arch Phys Med Rehabil. 2009;90(11):1948–52.
42. https://www.caregiver.org/caregiver-resources/all-resources/. Accessed 26 Aug 2022.
43. The National Center on Caregiving at Family Caregiver Alliance. Caregiving: state of the art, future trends. Chicago: The American Society on Aging; 2007.
44. Coen RF, O'Boyle CA, Coakley D, Lawlor BA. Dementia carer education and patient behavior disturbances. Int J Geriatr Psychiatry. 1999;14(4):302–6.
45. Burns R, Nichols LO, Martindale-Adams J, Graney MJ, Lummus. Primary care interventions for dementia caregivers: 2-year outcomes from the REACH study. Gerontologist. 2003;43(4):547–55.

Index

J. L. Colburn et al. (eds.), *Geriatric Home-Based Medical Care*,
https://doi.org/10.1007/978-3-031-68786-0

MIX
Papier aus verantwortungsvollen Quellen
Paper from responsible sources
FSC® C105338

If you have any concerns about our products,
you can contact us on
ProductSafety@springernature.com

In case Publisher is established outside the EU,
the EU authorized representative is:
Springer Nature Customer Service Center GmbH
Europaplatz 3, 69115 Heidelberg, Germany

Printed by Libri Plureos GmbH
in Hamburg, Germany